Treating Functional Abdominal Pain in Children

Treating Functional Abdominal Pain in Children

A Clinical Guide Using Feeling and Body Investigators (FBI)

Nancy L. Zucker
Duke University Medical Center, Durham

Katharine L. Loeb
The Chicago Center for Evidence-Based Treatment, Chicago

Martha E. Gagliano
Duke University Medical Center, Durham

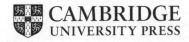

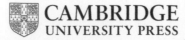

Shaftesbury Road, Cambridge CB2 8EA, United Kingdom

One Liberty Plaza, 20th Floor, New York, NY 10006, USA

477 Williamstown Road, Port Melbourne, VIC 3207, Australia

314–321, 3rd Floor, Plot 3, Splendor Forum, Jasola District Centre,
New Delhi – 110025, India

103 Penang Road, #05–06/07, Visioncrest Commercial, Singapore 238467

Cambridge University Press is part of Cambridge University Press & Assessment,
a department of the University of Cambridge.

We share the University's mission to contribute to society through the pursuit of
education, learning and research at the highest international levels of excellence.

www.cambridge.org
Information on this title: www.cambridge.org/9781009073745

DOI: 10.1017/9781009072595

First published 2024

Printed in the United Kingdom by CPI Group Ltd, Croydon CR0 4YY

A catalogue record for this publication is available from the British Library.

Library of Congress Cataloging-in-Publication Data
Names: Zucker, Nancy L., author. | Loeb, Katharine L., author. | Gagliano, Martha E.,
author.
Title: Treating functional abdominal pain in children : a clinical guide using feeling
and body investigators (FBI) / Nancy L. Zucker, Katharine L. Loeb, Martha E.
Gagliano.
Description: Cambridge, United Kingdom ; New York, NY : Cambridge University
Press, 2023. | Includes bibliographical references and index.
Identifiers: LCCN 2023017928 | ISBN 9781009073745 (paperback) | ISBN
9781009072595 (ebook)
Subjects: MESH: Abdominal Pain – diagnosis | Abdominal Pain – therapy | Child |
Clinical Protocols | Abdominal Pain – psychology | Psychology, Child
Classification: LCC RJ446 | NLM WI 147 | DDC 616/.0472083–dc23/eng/20230605
LC record available at https://lccn.loc.gov/2023017928

ISBN 978-1-009-07374-5 Paperback

To the children with sensory superpowers and their parents whose insightful and creative observations of their bodies inspired me to design this intervention. To my dear husband for his continued support, patience, and guidance. Our shared moments of calm and joy made writing possible.

NLZ

To all my patients with chronic abdominal pain, in the hope that kids in the future can be helped by this work.

MEG

For my own sensory superhero at home.

KLL

Contents

Acknowledgement   viii

Part I.   The Background Science Behind Feeling and Body Investigators

1. Becoming a Feeling and Body Investigator – Pain Division   1

2. Visceral Sensitivity as a Superpower   9

3. Responsive Parenting and Creating Safety   22

4. Discriminating Safe from Threatening Body Sensations: The Science of Interoceptive Exposures   32

5. The Medical Evaluation of Abdominal Pain in Children – One General Pediatrician's Approach   37

Part II.   A Session-by-Session Guide to Feeling and Body Investigators

6. Session 1: Initiation into Feeling and Body Investigators   43

7. Session 2: The Eats   54

8. Session 3: The Explosions   66

9. Session 4: The Zoomies and the Shakies, Part 1   78

10. Session 5: The Blahs   89

11. Session 6: The Ouchies   97

12. Session 7: The Drowsies   106

13. Session 8: The Zoomies and the Shakies, Part 2   116

14. Session 9: The Soothies   123

15. Session 10: The Celebration … and the Next Leg of Our Journey   129

Part III.   Sample Workbook Pages, Handouts, and Additional Resources for Feeling and Body Investigations

Appendix 1   135

Appendix 2   147

Appendix 3   168

Index   185

The additional resources can be found at www .cambridge.org/fbi-clinical-guide

Acknowledgements

What A Wonderful World

Words and Music by George David Weiss and Bob Thiele
Copyright © 1967 Range Road Music Inc., Quartet Music and Abilene Music
Copyright Renewed
All Rights for Range Road Music Inc. Administered by Round Hill Carlin, LLC
All Rights for Quartet Music Administered by BMG Rights Management (US) LLC
All Rights for Abilene Music Administered by Concord Sounds c/o Concord Music Publishing
All Rights Reserved Used by Permission
Reprinted by Permission of Hal Leonard LLC

Be Still

Words and Music by Brandon Flowers, Dave Keuning, Mark Stoermer, Ronnie Vannucci and Daniel Lanois
Copyright © 2012 SOMEBODY TOLD ME GMR and DANIEL LANOIS SONGS
All Rights for SOMEBODY TOLD ME GMR Administered by UNIVERSAL MUSIC WORKS
All Rights for DANIEL LANOIS SONGS Administered by PENNY FARTHING MUSIC c/o CONCORD MUSIC PUBLISHING
All Rights Reserved Used by Permission
Reprinted by Permission of Hal Leonard LLC

Closer To Fine

Words and Music by Emily Saliers and Amy Ray
Copyright © 1989 GODHAP MUSIC
All Rights Controlled and Administered by SONGS OF UNIVERSAL, INC.
All Rights Reserved Used by Permission
Reprinted by Permission of Hal Leonard LLC

Time In A Bottle

Words and Music by Jim Croce
Copyright © 1971 Time In A Bottle Publishing and Croce Publishing
Copyright Renewed
All Rights Administered by BMG Rights Management (US) LLC
All Rights Reserved Used by Permission
Reprinted by Permission of Hal Leonard LLC

Happy

from DESPICABLE ME 2
Words and Music by Pharrell Williams
Copyright © 2013 EMI April Music Inc., More Water From Nazareth and Universal Pictures Global Music
All Rights on behalf of EMI April Music Inc. and More Water From Nazareth Administered by Sony Music Publishing (US) LLC, 424 Church Street, Suite 1200, Nashville, TN 37219
All Rights on behalf of Universal Pictures Global Music Controlled and Administered by Universal Music Works
International Copyright Secured All Rights Reserved
Reprinted by Permission of Hal Leonard LLC

Sister Golden Hair

Words and Music by GERRY BECKLEY
Copyright © 1975 (Renewed) WC MUSIC CORP.
All Rights Reserved Used by Permission of ALFRED MUSIC

Cheeseburger In Paradise

Words and Music by JIMMY BUFFETT
Copyright © 1975 (Renewed) WC MUSIC CORP.
All Rights Reserved Used by Permission of ALFRED MUSIC

Becoming a Feeling and Body Investigator – Pain Division

Becoming a Feeling and Body Investigator

Welcome! This program will help you support and treat children who experience frequent and impairing abdominal pain. You will help these children trust their bodies and feel safe in them, a mission we accomplish by training everyone (yourself included) to be Feeling and Body Investigators – FBI agents – Pain Division. Through this training, we create an emotional context of exploration and inquisitiveness toward body sensations and provide concrete strategies so that the experience of pain is not scary, but rather a clue, an object of curiosity, and a mystery to be investigated. We treat our strategies as cryptographic tools that help children decipher and respond to the various messages their bodies are communicating, whether these messages are the cramps of hunger pain, the butterflies of anxiety, or the pressure of gas pain.

It may surprise you to think that focusing *more* on physical sensations can actually reduce the frequency and intensity of pain experiences and improve children's emotional awareness and regulation. The key to improvement lies in the *quality* of that attentional focus: it should be one of playful inquiry rather than of anxious hypervigilance. We teach children a new way to interpret their bodies' physical signals. And perhaps equally important, we foster this same mindset in the parents of these children – both in how they relate to their own bodies and in how they respond to the experiences of their children.

Who can put the FBI program into practice? We have written for a broad audience. Any health professional who works with children in pain, whether in a primary care, school, or therapy setting, can implement this treatment. It should be accessible enough for a trainee but also interesting enough for seasoned clinicians.

By the time you have learned this program, the way in which your practice engages with patients about body symptoms generally and pain specifically will have become a lot more fun as well as more effective. You may even find that your own relationship to your body will have improved. You are officially on the path to becoming a certified Feeling and Body Investigator – Pain Division. Congratulations! We are an elite group of special forces.

How It All Started

The FBI intervention actually arose from my work with an entirely different patient population – children, adolescents, and adults with eating disorders. Amidst numerous other complexities, individuals with eating disorders did not trust the messages their bodies were sending. For example, instead of recognizing a growling stomach as a sign of hunger, they might interpret this discomfort as the body trying to trick them into eating. They saw the emotions and drives of the body as threatening. They treated the body not as an essential life-partner, but as an enemy – something that needed to be subdued, ignored, or punished. This kind of thinking led to life-threatening disorders such as anorexia nervosa; but also, at a more basic psychological level, these individuals did not know themselves – what they wanted, needed, or cared about. Thinking about their experiences led me to wonder how children learn to develop a sense of trust in their body's wisdom and how to teach this trust when it was not present.

I began to ask myself a lot of very interesting questions. How do children learn to develop a sense of trust and awe at their bodies' power and wisdom? What type of life experiences could interfere with the emergence of this sense of trust? Could you teach children to trust their bodies when they already had some life experiences that challenged this sense of trust? When do you start? If you do intervene early, can you actually prevent the emergence of psychiatric disorders rooted in distrust of the body? Among many answers to these questions, one theme appeared repeatedly: children with early medical conditions, particularly those resulting in pain, may come to distrust their bodies.

My colleagues and I began to look for a target population of children for whom an intervention might make a difference. Our goal was lofty. If we could (a) take children who were vulnerable to developing feelings of distrust toward their bodies (or perhaps already had) and then (b) help them experience, instead, that their bodies were invincible, and then (c) show them that this invincibility actually arose from the very thing that they thought made them weak – their pain or other prior vulnerability – *that* could be something very powerful! We wanted to design an intervention that would help vulnerable children (or really any children) to learn to trust deeply in their bodies, to feel safe, and to feel equipped to handle all of life's challenges.

The FBI program was thus born. Through funding by the National Institutes of Health in the United States, we conducted a clinical trial targeting five- to nine-year-old children with chronic abdominal pain.

Why This Age Group?

Young children are just learning to make sense of their bodies. A developing child must learn how to decipher the various messages that the body sends, to respond to those messages, and to observe the effects of those responses. In turn, these experiences generate data that help to shape future responses. For example, a child senses a pang in their gut, learns to decipher that sensation as hunger, and grabs a small snack.

The presence of chronic or recurrent pain can disrupt this emerging adaptive self-awareness. Children with chronic pain may fail to link uncomfortable body feelings to common, benign sensations, such as hunger or gas. They may begin to avoid or fear a variety of normal body signals. They may even come to fear their bodies.

Our job as FBI agents is to change this trajectory, to alter this framework so that body sensations are viewed with wonder rather than trepidation. As you will see, we take a holistic approach to this awareness: we teach children to recognize all aspects of their experience – not just to develop an awareness of pain and the ability to delineate between types of pain. Children learn to recognize their emotions, to savor sensations like relaxed muscles or a cheery moment, to improve their awareness of basic motivational drives such as hunger, thirst, and fullness, to know what sleepiness feels like and not to become alarmed when Mind-Racing Mikella pays them a visit in bed.

In addition to intervening during a key developmental period, we targeted this age group for another very important reason. We wanted to equip children with tools in body trust so that they were ready for the onslaught of puberty. Think about all the intense, unpredictable, and complicated sensations that erupt as puberty begins. Cramps. Bloating. Surges of anger. Profound waves of sadness. Rejection. Maddening crushes. As puberty starts to unfold, unpredictable hormone fluctuations produce novel body sensations and new levels of emotional intensity (which can also be experienced as intense body sensations). These surges in body intensity may occur at inconvenient and unwanted times – or may be unwanted by their very nature and intensity. Not surprisingly, someone who enters puberty with a deep distrust of their body is going to be very vulnerable. This may set the context for eating disorders, and other psychiatric disorders rooted in fear of the body, to emerge during puberty and early adolescence, their typical age of onset.

Therefore, arming vulnerable children with a profound sense of trust in their bodies seemed like an optimal idea – not only to protect children from experiencing intense sensations as threatening, but also to provide them with a sense of self-awareness that would prepare them for the onslaught of puberty. Imagine what you could accomplish if, at the age of five, you deeply trusted in the power and wisdom of your body and had achieved a sense of profound self-awareness. There would be no stopping you!

Yet, children who are five to nine years old are tough customers. They are not going to stick with a treatment that is not fun, does not make sense, and does not help. We viewed this tough-minded set of consumers as our greatest challenge: if we could satisfy this group, we knew we were onto a winning formula for an intervention strategy. Thus, starting young gives us several critical advantages and keeps us on our toes. We will next touch briefly on our current understanding of recurrent abdominal pain and relate this to the core components of FBI – Pain Division.

Why Children with Abdominal Pain?

Approximately one in ten children or adolescents experience recurrent abdominal pain episodes, episodes of pain that are severe enough to interfere with their daily functioning.[1] For some, this pain is chronic. For example, children who experienced recurrent abdominal pain at the ages of two, eight, or ten years old were more than twice as likely to have pain at the age of 17.[2]

Children with pain often avoid activities. For example, 80.5% of children with recurrent abdominal pain missed school during the past quarter relative to 44.6% of children without pain. Chronic absenteeism (missing > 15 days of school) was six times greater in children (6 to 17 years old) with various forms of pain, including abdominal pain, relative to children with no pain,[3] a consistent finding across studies.[4] Notably, only 7.2% of children with recurrent abdominal pain participated in six to ten hours of sports per week, relative to 92.8% of children without pain![5] Child pain is also associated with family-level suffering: parents report reduced healthcare quality of life that they attribute to the emotional consequences and time demands of having a child with recurrent pain.[5,6]

Early pain is also a vulnerability marker for psychopathology. In children who presented to their primary care physician with recurrent abdominal pain, the odds of receiving a current or lifetime anxiety disorder diagnosis were approximately five times greater, and for a lifetime depression diagnosis two times greater when compared to children without a pain presentation.[7] Several population-based studies have reported similar findings: the presence of pain in children increases the likelihood for both a concurrent and prospective depression or anxiety diagnosis, in addition to increasing risk for chronic pain.[8]

As these findings highlight, it is challenging to parent a child with recurrent pain. Take, for instance, the remarkable discrepancy in sports participation between children with or without pain and consider this particular choice point for parents: deciding whether to enroll your child with recurrent pain in organized team sports. On the one hand, you know the social and emotional benefits of participating in organized sports and have been told by doctors about the benefits of exercise to facilitate pain management.[9–11] On the other hand, given that pain is unpredictable, you do not want your child to get down on themselves or feel that they have let their team down because they are not able to play one day. As a parent, you do not want to risk reneging on your commitments to the team, and you worry that further pressure will actually precipitate more pain episodes. We can all appreciate how difficult navigating these choices can be for parents.

Thus, recurrent abdominal pain is costly to both the individuals experiencing pain and their families. It contributes to the restriction of a child's activities during key developmental periods when they are learning and practicing skills to improve academic and social competence.[12] It contributes to diminishing feelings of mastery and increases guilt and worry in parents. These studies point to two necessary components for an intervention for recurrent abdominal pain: (1) Start with young children, and (2) Include tools not only to help manage pain, but also to manage intense emotions.

These findings also point to another essential ingredient of an intervention for recurrent abdominal pain: we need to give parents tools so that they feel confident and comfortable with the decisions they make about pain management and related questions, like when to encourage their child to participate in activities such as organized sports.

A Word About Words

In the latest nosology for diagnosing gastrointestinal disorders of gut–brain interaction (also referred to as Functional Gastrointestinal Disorders) published by the Rome Foundation,[13] the diagnosis of Functional Abdominal Pain – Not Otherwise Specified is defined by the criteria listed in Table 1.1.

It is notable that the use of the term functional has a rather complicated history and was used to refer to gastrointestinal disorders that were related to problems in function, rather than structure. However, an unfortunate connotation of this definition is that the etiology of functional pain disorders is behavioral or psychological rather than biological (i.e., individuals' descriptions of pain have a "function" – to avoid an unwanted activity, to get attention, etc.), a formulation that is increasingly outdated given researchers' and clinicians' increasingly refined understanding of the complex, influential, and constant reciprocal interactions of the gut–brain axis.[14]

As our conceptualization of these disorders has gotten more nuanced (see the next section), the term functional is still employed, more for historical reasons, and disorders of gut–brain interaction is a term that is thought to better reflect the complex etiology and maintenance of these disorders.

Table 1.1 Functional Abdominal Pain, Not Otherwise Specified[13]

A child has episodes of abdominal pain at least four times a month. These episodes have a variety of possible triggering or exaggerating events and do not occur solely during eating or other physiological events such as menstruation. While children can be diagnosed with multiple functional gastrointestinal disorders, there is not sufficient criteria for other disorders such as irritable bowel syndrome, functional dyspepsia, or abdominal migraine, or, if present, episodes of pain would be beyond what is expected for those disorders. After a reasonable (i.e., not overwhelming the child and family with unnecessary diagnostic tests, see Chapter 5 in this book), the abdominal pain cannot be fully explained by another medical condition.

Notes: Functional Abdominal Pain – Not Otherwise Specified (NOS) falls into the class of Functional Abdominal Pain Disorders within the *Rome IV Pediatric Functional Gastrointestinal Disorders, Disorders of Gut-Brain Interaction*, classification guidelines, first edition, 2016 with guest editors Carlo Di Lorenzo and Samuel Nurko and the Rome IV Pediatric Committee. Dr. Douglas Drossman (senior editor), Lin Chang, John Kellow, William D. Chey, Jan Tack, and William E. Whitehead are the editors of the series. For the clinical trial of FBI – Pain Division, we screened children directly from primary care. They had to meet the Rome III criteria for Functional Abdominal Pain in terms of pain frequency or intensity (e.g., weekly pain or a particularly impairing pain episode over the past month), but we were liberal in the presence of other abdominal, pain-related functional gastrointestinal disorder (AP-FGID). We reasoned that the strategies employed in FBI – Pain Division would be applicable across the spectrum of abdominal pain predominant functional GI disorders. The name Functional Abdominal Pain, Not Otherwise Specified is new to the Rome IV classification and is meant to help with greater specificity of diagnosis for research purposes. For the purpose of this guide, we use the term Recurrent Abdominal Pain to reflect this broad inclusion of pain-related functional gastrointestinal disorders.

To bypass this complexity in nosology, we will use the term recurrent abdominal pain (RAP) throughout the remainder of this book to refer to children who have recurrent episodes of abdominal pain that impair functioning. That said, the strategy of this intervention, with its focus on body awareness and body curiosity, would arguably be appropriate to aid in the management of the class of pain-predominant pediatric functional gastrointestinal disorders classified in the ROME IV classification system.[15]

Approach To This Book

This book is divided into three sections. Part I reviews the scientific background that supports our intervention strategy. This material will help you understand the fundamental principles that guide the intervention so that you can be flexible in its application – not bound to a rigid script or set of techniques performed in prescribed ways. Part II presents the intervention, walking you through each session and its components, translating the scientific principles into suggestions of implementation strategies. If you are eager to get started, you could skip to Part II and begin the treatment. Then, when you are curious about why it is working, you can go back and read Part I to enhance the meaning of your observations as an FBI provider. Just as there is no one right way to implement this intervention (the implementation itself is also in the spirit of investigation), such may be your attitude toward this book: there is no one right way to read it. Finally, Part III provides you with handouts, workbook pages, resources for additional trainings, web-based family communities your patients may join, and therapist communities you may access to augment your treatment delivery.

Throughout, when referring to singular individuals, we will include the use of the pronouns they/them to be as inclusive as possible.

We hope you enjoy reading this book as much as you will enjoy conducting the FBI – Pain Division intervention.

Conceptualizing Disorders of the Gut–Brain Axis

There has been a transformative reconceptualization in the way in which a particular class of gastrointestinal disorders, functional gastrointestinal disorders, are understood. Disorders such as functional abdominal pain – not otherwise specified are understood to arise in vulnerable individuals. What makes an individual vulnerable differs, but vulnerability can arise from a complex interplay of early life experiences that sensitize the gut–brain axis to pain, from genetic contributions, and/or from environmental stressors including those experienced as traumatic. For example, Thapar et al.[16] describes a model of sensitizing medical events, sensitizing psychosocial events, and genetic predispositions that increase the vulnerability of

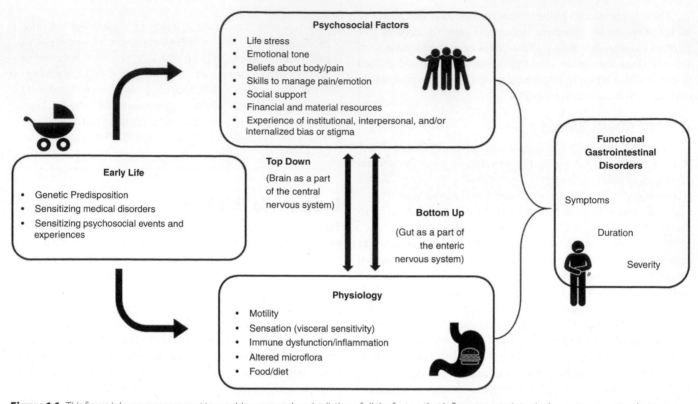

Figure 1.1 This figure is by no means meant to provide a comprehensive listing of all the factors that influence gastrointestinal symptom onset and maintenance. Rather, the central messages of this figure are that various categories of influences (e.g., psychosocial, physiological,) are reciprocal in influence – each impacting the other, while early developmental factors may increase vulnerability to the potentiation of these processes. This conceptualization actually offers hope regarding clinical intervention: addressing any part of the model may impact multiple facets. However, this model also presents challenges: how do we choose one intervention powerful enough to influence other factors? Furthermore, we must recognize that some aspects of the model may be more modifiable than others (e.g., beliefs about pain).

the microbiota gut–brain axis (see Thapar et al.[16] for a review). Upon this vulnerable backdrop unfolds complex interactions between bottom-up influences related to gut physiology and top-down influences from the central nervous system that both influence and are influenced by input from the gut (Figure 1.1). In other words, interacting influences from the central nervous system (e.g., vigilance and attention directed toward detecting symptoms, fear about body sensations, perceived stress); sensory systems (e.g., individual differences in the intensity of sensory signaling, capacities to notice changing visceral sensations and the experienced intensity of those sensations – a construct known as visceral hypersensitivity); the gut environment (e.g., the communities of gut bacterial flora composition that influence host health); and the body's defensive responses against disease or perceived somatic threats (e.g., immune responses, inflammation) all interact to influence the symptoms and severity of functional GI disorders – i.e., disorders of gut–brain interaction. One theme that emerges from this conceptualization of disorders of the gut–brain axis is that no process occurs in isolation, but, of course, is part of a dynamic system.

The first impression one may gather from looking at Figure 1.1 is that disorders of gut–brain interaction are complicated. On the one hand, one can appreciate that this model is a beautiful reflection of an individual's unique journey across development, one that is embedded within a social and emotional context that impacts physiology which, in turn, influences that

context. Yet, as intervention developers, at first glance such models can be a tad overwhelming. Where does one begin to influence change? How does one take into account all of these interlocking and mutually reinforcing factors? Where do we start?

This is where FBI – Pain Division comes in. Here we briefly outline our intervention and show how it interfaces with key nodes of this model to effect change. An important assumption in our approach is that you do not have to target all elements of a system simultaneously; you just have to pick some key nodes, nodes in the system that are powerful enough to have clinically meaningful downstream effects. In Figure 1.2 we highlight how elements of FBI address what we view as key nodes in the system.

An alternative, and complementary, manner to approach the biopsychosocial model is the attempt to alter the entire backdrop on which this model is unfolding. Figure 1.3 illustrates how FBI – Pain Division also attempts this approach. By creating a context of humor and a mindset that a child's body is wicked smart and capable of adapting and learning from the most painful and distressing of circumstances, we hope to influence not only events as they unfold in the current moment, but also how one's history is viewed and how one's future is regarded. Rather than walk you through each of these components right now, we will gradually work you through them as we go through these chapters.

We integrate the entire social support network into treatment and give everyone tools to map their body sensations onto meanings and actions so that we create a contact of safety of an individual within themselves and between each other. **Chapter 3.**

We provide further resources such as our online community and suggestions for practices so that the mindsets and tools mastered in this intervention can be further sustained and strengthened. **Chapter 15.**

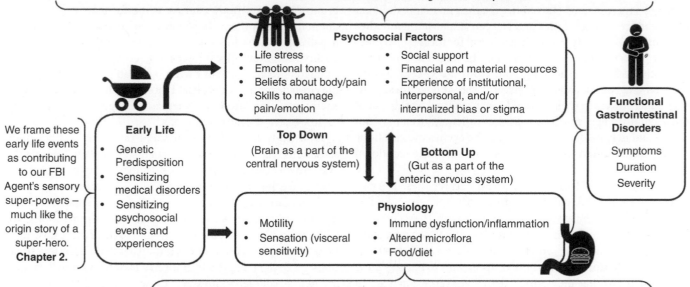

Psychosocial Factors
- Life stress
- Emotional tone
- Beliefs about body/pain
- Skills to manage pain/emotion
- Social support
- Financial and material resources
- Experience of institutional, interpersonal, and/or internalized bias or stigma

We frame these early life events as contributing to our FBI Agent's sensory super-powers – much like the origin story of a super-hero. **Chapter 2.**

Early Life
- Genetic Predisposition
- Sensitizing medical disorders
- Sensitizing psychosocial events and experiences

Top Down
(Brain as a part of the central nervous system)

Bottom Up
(Gut as a part of the enteric nervous system)

Functional Gastrointestinal Disorders

Symptoms
Duration
Severity

Physiology
- Motility
- Sensation (visceral sensitivity)
- Immune dysfunction/inflammation
- Altered microflora
- Food/diet

Body sensations are linked to playful characters that we investigate to further establish the wisdom of the body. Thus the initial attention allocated to body sensations is one of playful familiarity and curiosity. **Chapter 4.**

Figure 1.2 We present a very broad-strokes, conceptual overview of how to think about FBI – Pain Division in relation to disorders of gut–brain interactions.

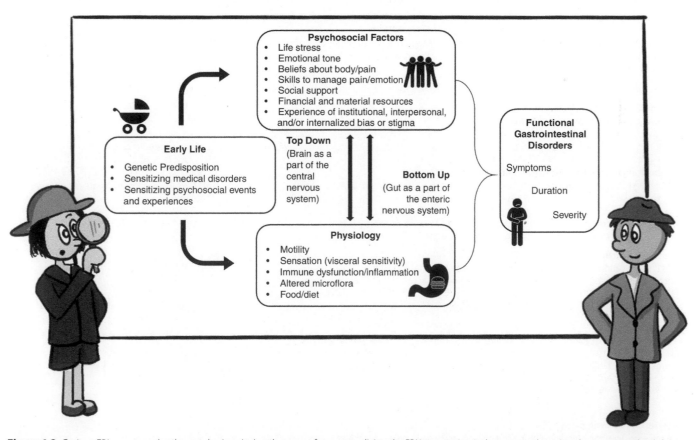

Figure 1.3 Curious FBI agents probe the gut–brain axis. Another way of conceptualizing the FBI intervention is that we are changing the context or backdrop on which disorders of gut–brain interaction operate: all these complex pathways unfold against backdrop of discerning, investigative wonderment.

The Logic and Core Components of FBI – Pain Division

We believe that children with recurrent abdominal pain have "sensory superpowers." They notice changes in their bodies that other children do not notice and feel sensations in their bodies with unusual intensity. The technical term for these "superpowers" is "visceral hypersensitivity," i.e., having low thresholds for noticing and experiencing pain from the viscera and for experiencing other changing visceral sensations. These sensory superpowers may also extend to the external world, in that these children may notice things that other children may not notice and may be deeply affected by the events and emotions of the world around them; these children are little emotional sponges.

Through the FBI program we re-interpret these sensory superpowers as a gift: children with sensitive superpowers live life out loud! They have vivid lived experiences. Their deep and intense feelings make them – quite literally – sensitive children who can make the world a better place in which to live. FBI – Pain Division teaches these children how to harness these superpowers so that they enrich their lives rather than get in the way.

Table 1.2 summarizes the core components of the FBI – Pain Division intervention.

Each weekly session consists of several consistent elements – Body Sensations, Body Investigations, Body Map, Body Brainstorms, and Body Clues – while focusing on the introduction of a new theme (e.g., eating and drinking, high-energy negative emotions, low-energy negative emotions, high-energy positive emotions, digesting food, sleeping, relaxing) and silly characters related to that theme (see Table 1.2). For example, the Groovies and Shakies, Part 1, are sensations related to high-energy negative emotions, whereas the Blahs are the category for low-energy negative emotions.

The **Body Sensations** characters represent distinct body sensations (e.g., Gassy Gus, Patricia the Poop Pain, Georgia the Gut Growler). Each playful cartoon illustrated in the workbook (Part 3) teaches the meaning of a bodily sensation.

Body Investigations are conducted every session to learn new things about how the body handles certain situations. We will learn much more about the art and logic of these investigations in Chapter 4, but for now, know that these body investigations are designed to teach children a lesson about their bodies and help strengthen a mindset in these children that their bodies are strong, capable, and wicked smart.

Table 1.2 Common components across sessions

1. Learning new body sensation characters that correspond to the theme of the session (starting in Session 1).
2. Performing Body Investigations to learn more about the wisdom and power of the body (starting in Session 1).
3. Summarizing what we have learned on a Body Map (starting in Session 1).
4. Using our Body Brainstorms Worksheet to generalize what we learn to sensations outside of the session (starting in Session 1).
5. Using our Body Clues Worksheet to figure out what our bodies were trying to tell us, to plan what we might try next time, or to investigate a moment (starting in Sessions 2 and 3).

While Session 1 is the Introduction that introduces a variety of sensations, each of the remaining sessions has a unique theme as summarized below.

Rituals That Begin the Sessions

1. **Henry Heartbeat Warm-Up Activity**
   We meet Henry Heartbeat and practice raising and lowering our heartbeat. Each session begins with a Henry Heartbeat investigation so we can keep emphasizing how wicked smart the heart is and get our minds and bodies ready for the session (it also helps for five- to nine-year-olds to run around a bit to gear up for a session).
2. **Checking In with Our Energy and Fueling Up.**
   Starting in Session 2, we meet body sensation characters related to hunger, thirst, fullness, and food deliciousness. We learn to check in with our energy as we eat with our energy meter. Checking in with our energy and eating a snack becomes one of the rituals that starts off every session, starting with Session 3.
3. **Homework Review.** We pull out our Body Maps and write down all the wisdom we have learned about the body this week from our Body Clues Worksheet and from any Body Investigations we did at home.

Session 1: The Introduction
This is the initiation ceremony. Families are introduced to the rationale for FBI, design their Body Map, and meet their first group of body sensation characters. Henry Heartbeat, Betty Butterfly, and Samantha Sweat are a few of the characters introduced this session. Children are given their first investigative assignment and off we go!

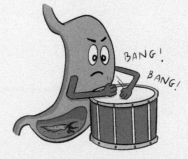

Session 2: The Eats
Hunger. Fullness. The deliciousness of savoring a tasty morsel. Thirst. These are the sensations we learn here and we practice tuning into what hunger and fullness feel like with our energy meter. Georgia the Gut Growler, Harold the Hunger Pain, Solomon Satisfied, Sabrina Stuffed, Umm-ma Uma, and Thirsty Theo are the body sensations we explore. We learn the first two steps of our Body Clues Worksheet.

Session 3: The Explosions
Passing gas. Vomiting. Gagging. Having to poop. All the clever ways your body gets rid of things – sometimes in a huge hurry and with a lot of noise and fanfare – is the focus of Session 3. Gassy Gus, Victor Vomit, and Gordon Gotta Go are some examples of friends we meet in this session. We learn the last few steps of our Body Clues Worksheets so we are ready for some pretty sophisticated investigations.

Table 1.2 (cont.)

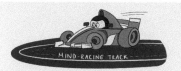

Session 4. The Zoomie and Shakies, Part 1. High arousal, negative emotions are the focus of this session. The feeling that your mind is racing (Mind-Racing Mikella), your heart is pounding (Henry Heartbeat), you have the jitters (Julie Jitters), or butterflies in your stomach (Betty the Butterfly) are the friends we meet this session. Parents are taught how to design body investigations in high-intensity moments and we try to bring on the butterflies!

Session 5. The Blahs. Blah Bertha, Nauseous Ned, Empty Eliza, and Ricky the Rock are some of the low-arousal sensations that we learn that may accompany feelings of sadness, guilt, or emptiness. We see what happens to these feelings when we get cozy and get support or try fixing a problem. Lots of snuggling in this session. We work with parents on the challenges of parenting a child with sensory superpowers this session.

Session 6. The Ouchies. Pain. We have finally gotten here! Investigations focus on seeing all the amazing things our bodies can do – even when uncomfortable. Ella the Emotional Pain, Sore Muscle Stan, and Harriet the Headache join all the pain characters we have met already (e.g., Patricia the Poop Pain, Harold the Hunger Pain). Parents are given more tools to design investigations in these uncomfortable moments to investigate what is going on.

Session 7. The Drowsies. Sleepy Stan, Tired Tina, Cozy Celeste, Cool Cyrus, Comfortable Cayla, Stuck Stephanie, Dark Debra – so many sensations associated with getting sleepy and feeling cozy in bed. We design body investigations exploring different sleep routines so we can learn the most fun and efficient ways to get tucked in and enjoy the peace of the dark.

Session 8. The Zoomies and Shakies, Part 2. Our last two sessions focus on joyous and peaceful sensations. The Zoomies and Shakies, Part 2 are high arousal sensations that often accompany positive emotions: Ernie the Energy Ball, Laughing Pain Lulu, Bursting Bella, Giggling Gena, Crying Cassie, and Dancing Darrin. In this session, we practically explode with joy. It feels wonderful to learn to focus our attention on all the moments of joy that we get to experience.

Session 9. The Soothies. We end our treatment with the sensations associated with calm, peaceful, and relaxing feelings that allow us to feel really awake and alive in the moment. We investigate different ways to bring on these sensations and see what we notice. Cheery Cathy; Day-Dreamy David; Slow Thinking Stewart; Ahhhh Annie; Focused Frankie; and Alert Arnold are the friends we meet this session.

Session 10. The Celebration. We play games reviewing all the characters we have learned. We perform an official graduation ceremony now that we are fully FBI Agents – Pain Division, complete with a certificate of graduation. We explore ways to stay in touch with the FBI community via our online groups for therapists and other groups for children and parents. We are ready to live life out loud!

Each week the forensic team (child, parent, and therapist) summarize all that they have learned on a **Body Map** unique to that child, much as a detective would organize clues on a crime map.

Body Brainstorms help children generalize what was learned in a treatment session to the world around them. Body Brainstorms guide them to think about other situations in which they have experienced the same body sensations that were the focus of the session.

Finally, as the intervention progresses, children and parents are trained in our **Body Clues** worksheet. This worksheet helps children link sensations to meanings and then to take whatever action is needed to meet the need communicated by that sensation. For those of you who are well-versed in cognitive behavioral approaches for pain management, a key differentiator of FBI – Pain Division is the focus here on sensations rather than on thoughts to guide monitoring and to increase self-awareness. All these activities are facilitated by therapists and parents who also embody the spirit of inquisitive and playful investigators, a topic we spend time delving into in Chapter 3 and throughout the intervention.

The first three sessions of the workbook and the corresponding worksheets with these sessions are found in Part III of this handbook in black and white. The entire color workbook and color worksheets are available via download from links found throughout the book, because we thought this was the easiest way to deliver the materials. In the clinical trial, we gave parents the workbook pages session by session – mainly because

the children got so excited to learn the new characters in a big "reveal" each week.

Before we leave this chapter, let's revisit the dilemma of a parent who is deciding whether to enroll their child with recurrent abdominal pain in an organized sports program. Since we last visited this family, they have been trained as official FBI Agents – Pain Division. Armed with the spirit of adventure, the parent decides that they will enroll their child in baseball. When an episode of pain occurs on the day of a practice or game, parent and child will design a series of investigations that they are going to explore. Here are a few examples:

If I think I'm feeling Gassy Gus, can I swing the bat hard enough or run fast enough that it makes me fart?

What happens to the pain when I run? Does it stay in the same place? Move around? If it does move around, can I do a couple experiments where I try to see where I can move it exactly where I want it?

If I do fart when I run, does that make me run faster? Like the gas from the fart is propelling me onward?

When they get home, they will add what they have learned to their Body Map. As it turns out, the child decided they needed a new character to capture the bouncing nature of the pain as they ran. And thus, Bouncy Bart Butt was born.

And that is an example of one part of the science and "elegance" of FBI – Pain Division.

Let's start our first mission.

References

1. Korterink, J.J., Diederen, K., Benninga, M.A., et al. (2015). Epidemiology of pediatric functional abdominal pain disorders: a meta-analysis. *PloS One 10*, e0126982. https://doi.org/10.1371/journal.pone.0126982

2. Stein, K., Pearson, R.M., Stein, A., et al. (2017). The predictive value of childhood recurrent abdominal pain for adult emotional disorders, and the influence of negative cognitive style. Findings from a cohort study. *PloS One 12*, e0185643. https://doi.org/10.1371/journal.pone.0185643

3. Groenewald, C.B., Giles, M., Palermo, T.M. (2019). School absence associated with childhood pain in the United States. *Clin J Pain 35*, 525–531. https://doi.org/10.1097/ajp.0000000000000701

4. Mehta, V., D'Amico, S., Luo, M., et al. (2020). Food habits, stressors, and use of complementary medicine therapies among pediatric patients who attend an integrative medicine pediatric pain clinic. *J Altern Complement Med 26*, 691–700. https://doi.org/10.1089/acm.2019.0253

5. Devanarayana, N.M., de Silva, D.G., de Silva, H.J. (2008). Recurrent abdominal pain syndrome in a cohort of Sri Lankan children and adolescents. *J Trop Pediatr 54*, 178–183. https://doi.org/10.1093/tropej/fmm114

6. Calvano, C., Warschburger, P. (2018). Quality of life among parents seeking treatment for their child's functional abdominal pain. *Qual Life Res 27*, 2557–2570. https://doi.org/10.1007/s11136-018-1916-2

7. Shelby, G.D., Shirkey, K.C., Sherman, A.L., et al. (2013). Functional abdominal pain in childhood and long-term vulnerability to anxiety disorders. *Pediatrics 132*, 475–482. https://doi.org/10.1542/peds.2012-2191

8. Ayonrinde, O.T., Ayonrinde, O.A., Adams, L.A., et al. (2020). The relationship between abdominal pain and emotional wellbeing in children and adolescents in the Raine Study. *Sci Rep 10*, 1646–1611. https://doi.org/10.1038/s41598-020-58543-0

9. Vierola, A., Suominen, A.L., Lindi, V., et al. (2016). Associations of sedentary behavior, physical activity, cardiorespiratory fitness, and body fat content with pain conditions in children: The Physical Activity and Nutrition in Children Study. *J Pain 17*, 845–853. https://doi.org/10.1016/j.jpain.2016.03.011

10. Sollerhed, C., Andersson, I., Ejlertsson, G. (2013). Recurrent pain and discomfort in relation to fitness and physical activity among young school children. *Eur J Sport Sci 13*, 591–598. https://doi.org/10.1080/17461391.2013.767946

11. Kichline, T., Cushing, C.C., Ortega, A., et al. (2019). Associations between physical activity and chronic pain severity in youth with chronic abdominal pain. *Clin J Pain 35*, 618–624. https://doi.org/10.1097/ajp.0000000000000716

12. Meijer, S.A., Sinnema, G., Bijstra, J.O., et al. (2000). Social functioning in children with a chronic illness. *J Child Psychol Psychiatry 41*, 309–317. https://doi.org/10.1111/1469-7610.00615

13. Drossman, D.A. (senior ed.), Di Lorenzo, C., Nurko, S., (guest eds.), with editors Chang, L., Chey, W.D., Kellow, J., Tack, J. Whitehead, W.E., & the Rome IV Committee. (2016). Rome IV Pediatric Functional Gastrointestinal Disorders: Disorders of Gut-Brain Interaction. Rome Foundation, Raleigh, North Carolina.

14. Drossman, D.A. (2005). Functional GI disorders: what's in a name? *Gastroenterology 128*, 1771–1772. https://doi.org/10.1053/j.gastro.2005.04.020

15. Hyams, J.S., Di Lorenzo, C., Saps, M., et al. (2016). Functional disorders: children and adolescents. *Gastroenterology 150*, 1456–1468. https://doi.org/10.1053/j.gastro.2016.02.015

16. Thapar, N., Benninga, M.A., Crowell, M.D., et al. (2020). Paediatric functional abdominal pain disorders. *Nat Rev Dis Primers 6*, 89. https://doi.org/10.1038/s41572-020-00222-5

Visceral Sensitivity as a Superpower

Overview

In this chapter we aim to rewrite the narrative of a child with recurrent pain. We make the case that visceral sensitivity is a superpower rather than a vulnerability. Examples of these superpowers include spell-binding powers of perception, awe-inspiring self-awareness, and breath-taking self-trust.

Yet, despite the potential for visceral sensitivity to act as an asset, this may not have been the experience of many patients and their families. We will reflect on the implications of over-simplifying the etiology of pain as purely psychological, rather than appreciating the complex effects of the reciprocal, interacting pathways of the gut–brain axis. This misunderstanding may lead patients to believe that their symptoms of pain are being relegated to psychological causes and thus not "real." To help remedy this invalidation on behalf of our small clients, we leave you with some ideas to challenge the naysayers.

Visceral Sensitivity as a Sensory Superpower

As we alluded to in Chapter 1, children with pain are sensitive children. It is worth spending a minute thinking about the use of the term "sensitive" in our lay vernacular and how our historical use of that term may negatively influence the optimal growth and development of children with pain. Such negative influences end here.

When someone is described as a "sensitive person," what comes to mind for you? Here are some consistent responses that arose when we posed this question to parents and professionals:

- Feels everything too intensely
- Cannot handle things
- Needs to be protected
- Fragile
- Is an emotional sponge – soaks up the emotions around them

As you can see from these answers, being "sensitive" carries a negative connotation. Yet, the sensitivity that these children experience is actually a valid physiologic state. Visceral sensitivity, a feature we introduced you to in Chapter 1 and remind you of here, is defined as a heightened awareness of sensations in the gut and other visceral organs. It is a feature that has been shown to be elevated in individuals with disorders of gut–brain interaction.

So yes, children with recurrent abdominal pain (RAP) are objectively sensitive. And, as one may expect, this increased sensitivity has been associated with and is predictive of more intense experiences, including pain.[1] When this objective sensitivity is combined with beliefs that sensitive children are fragile, we can inadvertently create an environment where we treat sensitive children as weak and limit their experiences in an effort to protect them. Our intention is to harness this sensitivity as an asset.

An alternative narrative of these capacities is that children with recurrent pain are sensory supercomputers – children who have a more nuanced and vivid perception and experience of the worlds in and around them. Thus, while a cost of visceral sensitivity may be more intense experiences of pain when pain occurs, this is offset by a life of vividness, meaningfulness, and beauty created by other intense feelings and sensations – a life, perhaps, that the majority of people will never have the benefit of experiencing.

To appreciate why one core tenet of FBI – Pain Division is to treat this sensitivity as an asset – a Sensory Superpower! – let's take a minute to think about the opposite: a world of muted sensibilities. Perhaps the best illustration of this is in the 1998 film *Pleasantville*. This movie features a town in which life was incredibly predictable and days were routine. To achieve such simplicity of life, passions and emotions were suppressed, as depicted visually by the early part of the story being cast in black and white – an absence of color. As the individuals in the town started connecting with and expressing their emotions, the individuals and things they were passionate about became increasingly colorized. The people woke up and became alive.

Similarly, sensory superpowers and the emotions these sensations create can make the world beautiful. We believe that individuals with sensory superpowers have been gifted the potential for "living a life out loud"; however, it's easy to understand that these children also are at risk of avoiding experiences that may bring about such intense sensations. This is a double-edged sword. Because these children feel everything intensely – positive as well as negative things – they may try to manage this intensity by making everything predictable and rigid. Individuals with sensory superpowers may fall into the Pleasantville trap, living a ritualized and routine life that avoids all risks. This can even manifest as a fear of letting oneself love or care about something "too deeply" for fear that it may be lost.

Thus, these individuals are at risk of living a very safe but very uninspired and potentially dysthymic kind of life.

"Prolonged bodily pain, if not amounting to an agony, generally leads to the same state of mind [low spirits]. If we expect to suffer, we are anxious; if we have no hope of relief, we despair."

Charles Darwin (1872), *The Expressions of the Emotions in Man and Animals*

What if we could help children who are sensitive, such as those who experience frequent pain, to not only be unafraid of pain but to also be unafraid of all the other experiences that body and sensory sensations constitute – such as emotional experience. What a life that would be!

Thus, a fundamental tenet of FBI – Pain Division is that we can harness this sensitivity as an asset and by doing so, we capture all the beauty of being a sensitive individual and triumph over the fragility. That is where we are headed.

To provide some evidence backing up why this is truly the case – that sensitivity can be an asset – we will spend this chapter focusing on certain features of gut–brain communication. Specifically, we focus on emotions: their function, the interpretations we make about their value, and what emotions feel like in our bodies – such that they are a particularly precise and useful resource for those with sensory superpowers. In fact, these individuals' sensitivity to their bodies, and correspondingly, their ability to tell what emotion they are feeling, to experience their emotions strongly, and to act on them adaptively, paves the way for their most essential sensory superpowers: awe-inspiring self-awareness and self-trust.

Second, we focus on gut-feelings and decision-making and provocatively suggest intuitive decision-making as a sensory superpower. We end with a brief reflection on the profound journey these children are traveling. By tuning into their bodies and learning to know and trust themselves, they are learning to self-parent, the foundation for feeling safe and ready to explore the world. In Chapter 3, we further explore this concept of self-parenting by considering the role of parents in the FBI intervention. In Chapter 4, we consider how the Body Investigations that we perform can help us manage the intense memories that can form when you have sensory superpowers.

The Wisdom of Emotions

"… [My lab has been] concerned with the bodily changes which occur in conjunction with pain, hunger, and the major emotions. A group of remarkable alterations in the body economy have been discovered, all of which can reasonably be regarded as responses that are nicely adapted to the individual's welfare and preservation."

"The conditions favorable to proper digestion are wholly abolished when unpleasant feelings such as vexation and worry and anxiety, or great emotions such as anger and fear, are allowed to prevail."

Walter Cannon (1925), *Bodily Changes in Pain, Hunger, Fear, and Rage*

Emotions are full-body responses that rapidly communicate what is happening or needed in a given situation, both to ourselves and others. Emotions are "salience signalers": emotions communicate that there is something important or valuable that requires our attention. However, emotions go well beyond appraising the meaning of a situation.[2] That appraisal activates responses that help get our needs met. In other words, emotions communicate needs, and the corresponding neurological, physiological, cognitive, and other components of an emotional experience help to mobilize the response that satisfies those needs. Because satisfying needs typically involves performing an action, it makes sense that part of an emotional experience involves bodily changes that help us act.

Emotions are thus essential solutions that we discover within ourselves to complex problems in our environment. This conceptualization of emotion is often referred to as the functionalist perspective of emotions.[3] We assume that emotions have a function, a purpose in communicating to ourselves and others what is important. According to this logic, different emotions communicate different functions,[4] and thus different emotions will also tend to elicit different feelings in our bodies that help us communicate and organize our responses to diverse problems – or, if you are an FBI agent, to mysteries.

Let's consider some examples to demonstrate how wise the body is when experiencing emotions. Consider fear. The quote above is from Walter Cannon. This famous physiologist studied the physiological manifestations, particularly alterations in the gastrointestinal tract, that constitute and accompany various states of stress and emotional experience, as well as the neurological and related origins of these experiences.[5] He, as well as others, have documented that digestion is impeded in states of "great emotion" such as anger and fear. Why might this be?

What might fear communicate? Danger. So, what might be the function of fear? To protect us from danger. Fear is an emotion that is experienced when danger and associated threat are imminent and thus require the rapid mobilization of defensive responses. Such responses may include fighting, fleeing, or freezing, extremely adaptive and reliable behavioral responses that defend against danger.

What does fear feel like? Heart pounding. Sweating profusely. Shaking. "Butterflies" in the stomach. (These feelings will take the form of FBI characters, namely Henry Heartbeat, Samantha Sweat, Julie Jitters, and Betty Butterfly, respectively.) All these sensations have a function – they index different physiological changes that are occurring to help mobilize the protective responses to fear. So, what would this have to do with digestion? Digestion is a process that helps us build up energy stores and replenish. In fear, we are using our energy to fight, flee, or freeze.[6] In a state of danger, blood flow, and with it oxygen and nutrients, increases to muscles that facilitate the body's capacity to escape danger while decreasing to the gut. Thus, some body components of fear, such as gut butterflies, may actually reflect the changes the body is undergoing to help activate these protective responses.[7] Butterflies, nausea, or other gut indicators of fear may actually index how shrewd your body is in mobilizing resources to help you cope with potential danger.

Consider another example of a strong emotion: rage. What does rage communicate? Perhaps that someone has violated your rights and you need to defend yourself. What is the function of rage? Protection. What does rage feel like? Heat. Muscles clenching. Chest tightening. Energy bubbling up like you are about to explode. All in the service of helping you take action to defend and protect your rights.

If we put these pieces of information together, we can begin to see how children with visceral hypersensitivity can have sensory superpowers like awe-inspiring self-awareness and breathtaking self-trust. If emotions convey important information about what we like and need, and if we feel emotions in our bodies, and if children with visceral hypersensitivity are extraordinarily good at sensing what their bodies are feeling, then there is only one logical conclusion: the body is wicked smart and children with sensory superpowers are uniquely capable of sensing and understanding their body's wisdom. We now expand on each of these superpowers.

Superpower Number 1: Spell-Binding Powers of Perception
Individuals with Sensory Superpowers Notice Things That Others Do Not Notice

In more technical terms, interoceptive accuracy is the ability of a person to accurately sense changes in their viscera (e.g., being able to accurately count the number of times their heart beats without resorting to taking their pulse).[8] Individuals who are more accurate in sensing what their bodies are telling them have been shown to have more intense emotional experiences and to be better at regulating these emotions.[9,10]

This is one of the capacities that gives children with sensory superpowers their edge: their ability to notice. As emphasized earlier, different emotions can be experienced as different feelings in the body.[11] The weight of a sad mood can feel like your body is filled from head to toe with sand. It can be hard to even move (you'll meet Bertha Blah a little later in the book). If you are anxious about an impending work deadline, you may feel agitated, like you have excess energy (Julie Jitters). Our body sensations provide clues about our emotional state. The body is the source of all this vital information.

> FBI agents are experts at detecting these body clues and figuring out what is going on. Learning to discriminate body sensations and linking them to different emotions is an essential skill mastered by elite FBI agents.

The mindset one brings into noticing a sensation is important to determine what happens next when a body sensation captures attention. Will this sensation be greeted with the curiosity of an FBI agent or with fear? Figure 2.1 outlines two different pathways that can occur when a child with sensory superpowers first notices a sensation. The path on the left is the classic fear avoidance model of pain – the path of self-fear and avoidance (a bit more on this later and in Chapter 4). The pathway on the right

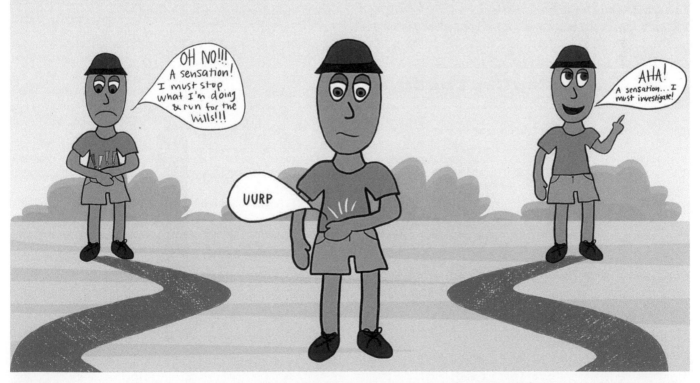

Figure 2.1 Diverse mindsets in response to a body sensation. The left pathway represents a step on the fear–avoidance of pain cycle: children fear sensations and become increasingly avoidant of activities that have the potential to provoke a range of sensations, including those that are harmless. The right pathway is the gateway to greatness: a mindset of curiosity toward the body that can build self-knowledge and self-trust.

is the path to greatness: it is the path of curiously investigating a body sensation on the road to self-knowledge and self-trust.

Because children with sensory superpowers are so good at noticing what is happening in the worlds within and outside them, they can achieve Superpower Number 2 – awe-inspiring self-awareness and self-trust. However, to acquire this superpower we must first harness the child's awesome powers of perception and then help them reframe their mindset into one of engaged curiosity. This mindset forms the lynchpin of FBI training.

So, you ask, how can we get children to be CURIOUS about PAIN? Before we answer that question, let's talk a little about how pain affects us and how we respond to it.

Pain is an intense and potentially threatening experience. Because pain can be a threat, the acute experience of pain and the threat of future pain can be accompanied by emotional experiences designed to protect us from threat. Thus, fear and pain often travel together: individuals can experience fear when they sense a body sensation that they think is predictive of future pain.

One challenge for individuals with spell-binding powers of perception is learning to discriminate harmless from harmful sensations. This can become tricky when one has experienced repeated episodes of intense pain. Pain leaves intense memories. In fact, they may also have vivid memories of the context and circumstances that surrounded that intense pain experience. Things that are close replicas of those prior experiences may remind us of our prior pain and may become feared.

However, the system is more sophisticated than that. Our fear reaction may generalize to body sensations, features, and contexts that are similar to our original experience, much as a pebble creates widening rings when dropped into a pond. In some sense, this generalization can be seen as a very wise and efficient thing for the body to do: it is a good idea to be able to form categories of things that are painful or potentially painful rather than having to experience each thing individually (e.g., extremely sharp pointy objects may be painful if you bump into them vs. a nail is painful, a screw is painful, a sharp corner is painful, etc.). The challenge and art for an elite FBI agent, however, is learning how to increase the accuracy of prediction: learning to discriminate what bodily signals or experiences are likely to lead to pain and which ones do not.

For example, imagine that you eat a new type of shellfish and immediately have an anaphylactic reaction that necessitates an emergency room visit, following which you have several days of intense gastrointestinal pain. Now, you ate a specific type of shellfish in a specific context – let's say it was a fancy new seafood restaurant. The next week you go to a different restaurant, but there it is – that same shellfish on the menu. Given the intense reaction that you had before, it is logical to conclude that your allergic reaction will follow you into this new context. You do not have to keep re-learning anew, in every restaurant that serves that shellfish, that you are deathly allergic to this type of shellfish. Thus far, this seems like a really efficient, adaptive system.

But how far might your system go to protect itself? It is reasonable to be cautious around other types of shellfish and to investigate their effects (e.g., through medical testing in an immunologist's office with Epi-pens at the ready) to better understand the boundaries of the allergy. But what if you stopped eating in restaurants altogether? And then what if you also began avoiding carbohydrates because there were dinner rolls on the table when you had the anaphylactic reaction? Those responses would represent a form of maladaptive conditioning (Figure 2.2); that is, the fear gradient has generalized to stimuli to which avoidance is not adaptive.

Maladaptive Conditioning

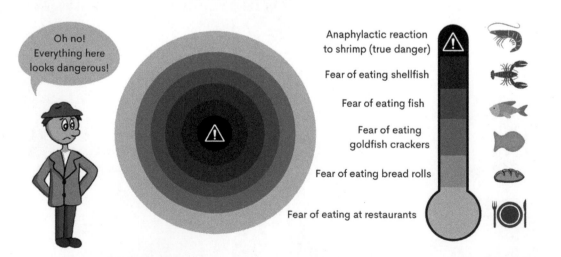

Figure 2.2 Maladaptive fear conditioning from pain. When someone has had an intense and potentially harmful pain experience, it is adaptive for one's alert system (often their fear-learning system) to be activated to avoid future pain. However, if this system is too imprecise and over-general, then broad avoidance can ensue, avoidance that can be threatening to one's mental and physical health as one restricts potentially joyous and enjoyable activities. In this example, while it would be adaptive to be cautious around shellfish until one has learned the boundaries of one's allergy (and fish to be extra certain), generalizing the fear to goldfish crackers and beyond would just increase avoidance (and risk for unhappiness) without increasing safety.

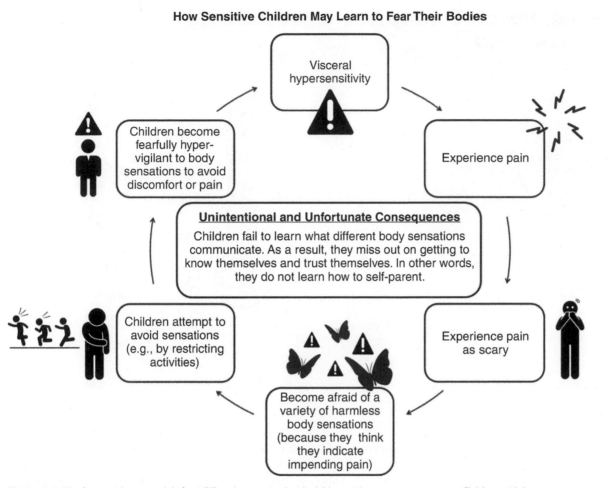

How Sensitive Children May Learn to Fear Their Bodies

Figure 2.3 The fear avoidance model of pain[12,13] as characterized with children with sensory superpowers. Children with "sensory superpowers" have the power of noticing changes in visceral sensations. The combination of pain experiences with the fear-learning architecture may set the stage for a fear of pain to generalize to innocuous body sensations and promote avoidance. Avoidance, in turn, may exacerbate pain via restricted activities, among other mechanisms.

Continuing with the allergy example, imagine the different sensations you might feel as hives develop. Your skin feels hot. You begin to itch. Yes, you could be having an allergic reaction. Realistically, though, there are lots of reasons skin can feel hot and itchy, only one of which is a dangerous allergic reaction. If you started to avoid all the situations that generated hot or itchy sensations, life would become boring fast. This cycle is illustrated in Figure 2.3. In a maladaptive fear gradient, any sensation with the least potential for pain becomes something to be feared and avoided. Maladaptive generalization sets a vicious cycle spinning, perhaps uncontrollably.

Given this potential for maladaptive conditioning, children with a history of pain often have an automatic "knee jerk" fear reaction when they notice an unknown or unclear sensation in their bodies. This is similar to individuals with anxiety disorders, such as those with panic disorder. Individuals with panic disorder may fear body sensations like an increasing heartbeat because they think this sensation may predict a threatening event like a heart attack. Research in individuals with panic disorder has demonstrated that these individuals exhibit an exaggerated startle response – an intensified fear "knee jerk" reaction to initial encounters with stimuli – even when those stimuli are safe.[14] Likewise, in children with a history of pain, it is not hard to imagine the learning history that could lead to a "knee-jerk" fear response when noticing an unknown sensation in the body. If children learn to fear all body sensations, then over time, they will avoid all activities that generate these sensations. They become less and less able to discern what their body is communicating and to act on that effectively because rather than listening to their bodies they are trying to avoid feeling. They may fail to develop self-knowledge and self-trust. They have entered another vicious cycle.

Now we know what we need to do. We need to teach children to treat body sensations as wise messengers. We need to help them be curious rather than fearful about body sensations. We need to train our FBI agents to detect and discriminate among a variety of body sensations, knowing which sensations signal safety and which signal threat. Figure 2.4 shows the new mindset of our elite special forces – calculated and thoughtful explorations in a world of inviting experiences.

Shaping Perception

One way to think about the FBI – Pain Division intervention is to see it as a means of altering the mindset or appraisal that children have toward *all* sensations. A key strategy we employ is altering the initial reaction a child has to a body sensation.

Shrewd, Precise Adaptive Conditioning
(the FBI-Agent Way)

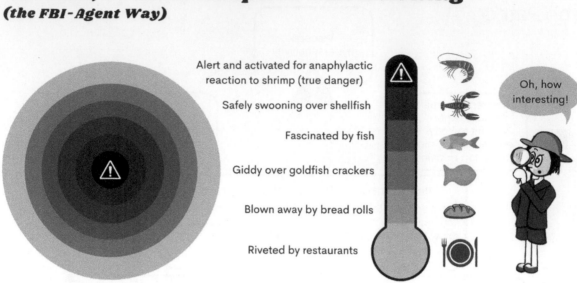

Figure 2.4 The shrewd, precise adaptive conditioning of an FBI agent. Fueled by fascination yet appropriately cautious, our elite forces ensure that approach rather than avoidance is their guiding tenet.

"It is indeed possible for your brain to know what is good or bad before it knows exactly what it is."

Joseph LeDoux, *The Emotional Brain*, p. 69

Consider an interesting study.[15] Students who experience test anxiety often worry that their anxiety will impede their test performance. This, of course, creates a loop in which anxiety about anxiety makes one even more anxious. In this study, researchers informed the students that the physiological changes that they experience prior to an exam were actually helpful: their bodies and minds were getting "pumped up" to dominate this exam. Indeed, this may be much like the strategy of an athletic coach in the locker room before game time, channeling pre-game anxiety into pure performance adrenaline. Sure enough, in this study, the students that received this reappraisal of their arousal as performance-enhancing performed better on the exam than students with test anxiety who did not receive this intervention.

This study leads us to one of the key components of the FBI intervention: the children learn and practice their new mindset BEFORE the sensations appear. Children learn to identify a vast array of body sensations and to label these sensations with playful (and adorable) characters. Just as the coach re-framed anxiety as adrenaline, we de-toxify scary sensations by associating them with playful characters. Figure 2.5 illustrates a few of the silly characters we associate with body sensations; it's easy to see why children would love these guys! Identifying these sensations as silly characters makes children more willing to experience these sensations instead of avoiding them. We want to prepare children for unexpected body sensations so that they do not simply have those "knee-jerk" negative reactions and descend into the fear/pain cycle. For example, as children become skilled FBI agents, they can explore and learn to discriminate many different pain sensations (e.g., hunger pain, emotional pain, laughing pain, poop pain, gas pain), all in the service of making pain

less scary. Curiosity and humor can break the problematic cycle, changing fear and avoidance to curiosity and investigation.

We also attempt to increase awareness and attention toward pleasant and peaceful sensations. Thus, not only do we try to make potentially scary sensations less threatening, but we also try to amplify the attention paid to the sensations associated with positive emotions, such as the feelings of being joyous, giggly, calm, and cheery. The last three sessions of the program are devoted to such beautiful sensations such as Bursting Bella, a sensation that comes around when you are having a moment that is so filled with love, joy, or happiness that your body is filled from head to toe with a warm energy that feels like it may explode from your chest, or Dancing Darrin who has a rhythm in their heart and a beat in their feet – they just feel like dancing.

> Thus, you may be wondering why many chapters in this book begin with a song lyric. Our journey has started. We are all becoming more alert and awake for sensations that signal feeling joyous, alive, and deeply moved – such as those that come from powerful music.

Our Body Clues Worksheet helps children to identify and organize the different body sensations they perceive. In Part II of this book, you will learn a great deal about the Body Clues Worksheets. These worksheets help children notice the various sensations they may be feeling. Step 1 of the Body Clues Worksheet relates to our first superpower: awesome powers of perception. This step guides children and adults to label what we notice in our bodies. Step 1 depicts all of the body sensation characters that the children have learned thus far (Figure 2.6).

When exploring what is going on in a given moment, parents, children, and therapists "interrogate" each other about

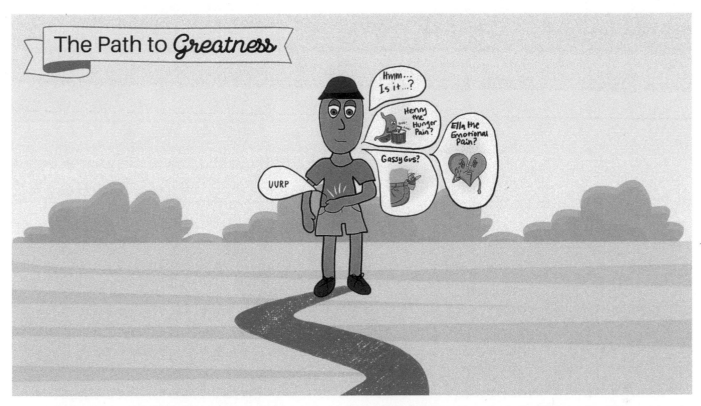

Figure 2.5 The path to greatness of an FBI investigator. Noticing a sensation, the trained elite investigator explores the depth of their sensation dictionary, integrates it with the context of the moment, and arrives at a hypothesis as to what they may be feeling. Armed with that information, they are ready to formulate a plan.

STEP 1: LISTEN TO YOUR BODY.

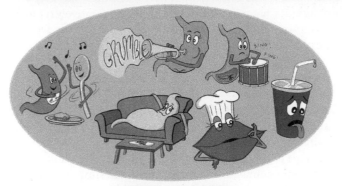

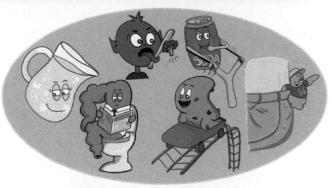

THE EATS

THE EXPLOSIONS

Figure 2.6 In Step 1, FBI agents consider each body sensation that they have learned so far. These pictures show the characters that are learned in two of the sessions: "The Eats" and "The Explosions". Each category (e.g., the Eats) gets filled up with characters as the children learn these body sensations. They consider whether they are feeling that sensation at the current moment or during the moment that is the focus of the Body Clues Worksheet. If so, they circle that character. The intensity of the sensation is matched by the degree of completion of the circle (quarter circle, half circle, full circle, double circle, etc.).

what they may be feeling. They name each character and ask the child (or person being interviewed) to indicate whether they were feeling a given body sensation. If so, the character will be circled. However, the degree of completion of the circle indexes how intense the sensation is. By going through each of the characters, we can help children to more fully realize all the different sensations they may feel when there are experiencing a certain type of emotion or type of pain (Figure 2.6). To help parents remember the characters (the children generally remember them), each week includes a summary character sheet that lists all the characters learned so far (Figure 2.7).

Superpower Number 2: Awe-Inspiring Self-Awareness

Children then learn to map those body sensations to different meanings. Awareness of our emotions helps us to learn more about ourselves (e.g., what we like or dislike; what excites or scares us) and acts as a guide to help us get our needs met. Thus,

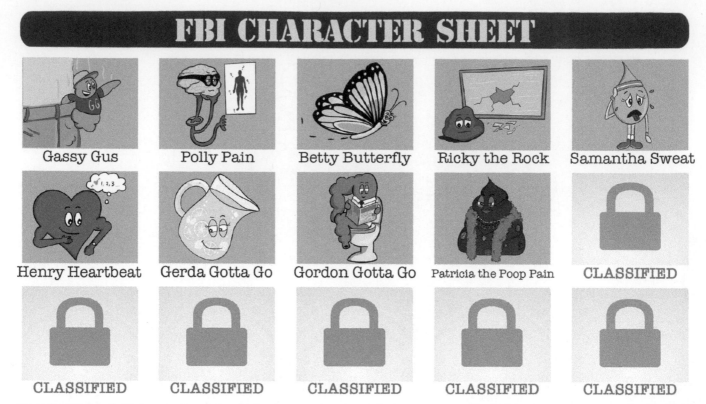

FBI CHARACTER SHEET

Gassy Gus

Polly Pain

Betty Butterfly

Ricky the Rock

Samantha Sweat

Henry Heartbeat

Gerda Gotta Go

Gordon Gotta Go

Patricia the Poop Pain

CLASSIFIED

CLASSIFIED

CLASSIFIED

CLASSIFIED

CLASSIFIED

CLASSIFIED

Figure 2.7 The weekly FBI character sheet. Each week, families get a "cheat sheet" of the characters learned so far. These characters then populate Step 1 of the Body Clues Worksheet. As the weeks go by, more and more characters are "de-classified," a testament to all the child has learned about their bodies.

being able to decode and respond to what are bodies are telling us can help us to know ourselves, trust ourselves, and feel safe in our own bodies. It stands to reason then that children with sensory superpowers would be the best at this because they are so good at noticing what their bodies are telling them. In other words, visceral hypersensitivity is a sensory superpower because children who are sensitive and open to experience learn to figure out the messages their bodies are sending them. As a result, they get to know themselves. By learning to respond to those messages, they come to trust themselves. The end result of tuning into and responding to your body? You feel safe in your own body and are ready to explore the world. Steps 2 and 3 of our Body Clues Worksheet help with this emerging self-awareness.

In Step 2 of the Body Clues Worksheet (Figure 2.8), the therapist or parent asks the child to describe what they were doing when they were feeling that sensation. In other words, the child contextualizes these sensations. Different sensations can tell us different things depending on what we are doing. A keen FBI agent knows this and learns to investigate a sensation fully. Henry Heartbeat can come about when we are about to take a test, open up a surprise present, sing in a concert – innumerable situations. A wise FBI agent knows how to put these clues together and figure out what is going on.

In Step 3, the therapist and parent help the child put these pieces of information together. By combining what they were feeling and what they were doing, they collaboratively try to figure out what their body was telling them. Were they feeling a type of emotion, a type of pain, a motivational drive like hunger or the need for sleep (Figure 2.9)?

With repeated, playful practice in mapping sensations to contexts and meanings, children become increasingly more confident in decoding what their body is trying to tell them and in discriminating the subtleties of different sensations. Specifically, we aim to minimize their false alarms (Figure 2.2), to discern the meanings of different types of pain, to label innocuous sensations as innocuous, and to learn all the interesting and informative messages their bodies send.

Building Self-Trust

FBI agents are experts at self-reflection. Consider the aftermath of an episode of fear or rage you experienced. If you were to take the time to reflect about what had just happened, what caused you to become so enraged or terrified, you would actually learn a great deal about yourself. You might increasingly make a connection between stimuli within yourself or your environment that contributed to the creation of these powerful emotions.

STEP 2: CONDUCT AN INVESTIGATION.
What were you doing? What was going on?

Figure 2.8 Step 2 of a Body Clues Worksheet. After figuring out the sensations that they are feeling (Step 1), individuals contextualize the sensations (Step 2).

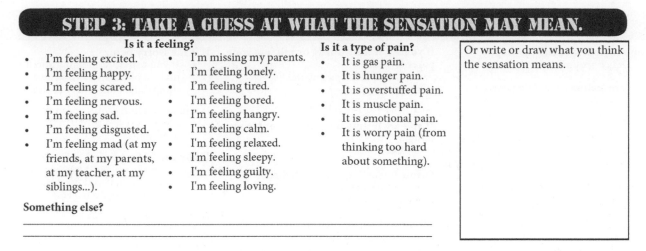

STEP 3: TAKE A GUESS AT WHAT THE SENSATION MAY MEAN.

Is it a feeling?

- I'm feeling excited.
- I'm feeling happy.
- I'm feeling scared.
- I'm feeling nervous.
- I'm feeling sad.
- I'm feeling disgusted.
- I'm feeling mad (at my friends, at my parents, at my teacher, at my siblings...).

- I'm missing my parents.
- I'm feeling lonely.
- I'm feeling tired.
- I'm feeling bored.
- I'm feeling hangry.
- I'm feeling calm.
- I'm feeling relaxed.
- I'm feeling sleepy.
- I'm feeling guilty.
- I'm feeling loving.

Is it a type of pain?

- It is gas pain.
- It is hunger pain.
- It is overstuffed pain.
- It is muscle pain.
- It is emotional pain.
- It is worry pain (from thinking too hard about something).

Or write or draw what you think the sensation means.

Something else?

_____

_____

Figure 2.9 Step 3 of the Body Clues Worksheet. FBI agents use information from Step 1 (what sensations they notice in their bodies) and Step 2 (what they were doing) to figure out what their bodies are trying to tell them.

Depending on how you responded, your satisfaction with that response, and the subsequent outcome, you might also use that episode to become better prepared for the future. For example, if your rage manifested in a hurtful rant that did not yield the desired outcome, you might mentally rehearse a different strategy that you could try next time you notice your anger starting to evolve into rage. Rehearsing a more adaptive response will make it more readily available to you in moments of intense feeling. But more than that, such reflections help us to know ourselves really, really well.

Steps 4 and 5 of the Body Clues Worksheets help FBI agents figure out what they might need in a given situation depending on what their body is communicating (Figure 2.10). We go over these steps in more detail in Chapter 3, but we will take a peek at them now so you can visualize the entire Body Clues Worksheet. Step 4 gives suggestions of things we might try when we notice certain messages in our body. However, ultimately, figuring out what our bodies are trying to tell us demands an investigation: trying something out and seeing what happens. Reliably sensing and responding to internal needs builds trust – self-trust.

Superpower Number 3: Faster-Than-Lightening Intuitive Decisions

Thus far, we have discussed how a child's sensitivity to sensations in their body can aid in their self-awareness by helping them to identify different emotions and motivational states and use that information to engage in behaviors to get their needs met. In addition to their superpowers of perception, it may also be the case that children with disorders of gut–brain interaction also have amplified visceral input that may further augment that perception.

Research examining the impact of stress on the gut has revealed that individuals with disorders of gut–brain interaction may experience more stressful life events and/or changes in their physiological responses to stress relative to individuals without these disorders.[16] Further, early adverse life events are associated with alterations in stress responsiveness that may increase vulnerability for the development of disorders of gut–brain interaction.[17]

There are numerous feedback loops that influence gut–brain communication. Think of gut–brain communication as a superhighway. This superhighway has various on-ramps that can amplify, mute, or alter the nature and intensity of somatic signals, including those that communicate pain. For example, neuroimmune and neuroendocrine systems impact this communication network via electrophysical and biochemical influences.[18] The composition of the gut microbiome, microorganisms that live symbiotically in the gut, may be both influenced by environmental factors such as stress, but also may influence top-down stress responses.[19] These influences may impact gut sensory experiences and gut motor responses – a powerful reciprocal system. In his review on gut–brain communication, Dr. Emeran Mayer, Director of the Oppenheimer Center for Neurobiology of Stress at the University of California, Los Angeles, describes how in gut–brain responses to stress, prolonged autonomic nervous system signaling to the gut can actually change target cells of the gut. These changes may influence the relative influence or salience of gut-to-brain signaling. It is like signals from your gut are driving a Ferrari sports car on a super-highway to your brain and other somatic signals are driving beat-up, sluggish used cars on muddy country roads. These changes may be associated with altered emotional states such as anxiety and depression.[20] Such examples show how profoundly these on-ramps can affect traffic on the gut–brain super-highway.

If we continue with our superhighway metaphor, consider the impact of the weather – particularly bad weather like heavy rain and high winds – on this traffic system. FBI aims to change the weather, functioning like the shift when the rain stops and the sun begins penetrating the clouds. That change in climate eases the ride, even when traffic is congested on the on- or off-ramps. To this point, perhaps we can influence the whole gut–brain system by creating a context of safety for the child: a curious context surrounding body sensations combined with responsive self-parenting that can alter a child's stress reaction.

STEP 4: DESIGN AN INVESTIGATION AND SEE WHAT HAPPENS.

If you are feeling excited or happy
- Dance around!

If you are feeling scared or nervous
- Talk to someone.
- Take some slow, deep breaths and close your eyes.
- Count your butterflies as you face your fears.
- Do something that makes you laugh.

If you are feeling mad or disgusted
- Yell really loudly.
- Do slow deep breathing and walk around.
- Make a firms but polite request about what you need.

If you are feeling sad or have emotional pain
- Get a hug from someone or hold someone's hand.
- Draw a picture or write about it.
- Snuggle with something.
- Make up a song about it.

If you are feeling loving
- Share that feeling with someone or something.

If you are feeling lonely or missing your parents
- Call or talk to someone.
- Write a letter.
- Play with an animal.

If you are feeling hunger pain or feeling hangry
- Eat.

If you are feeling overstuffed pain
- Lay on the couch.
- Go on a slow walk.

If you are feeling gas pain
- Go to the bathroom, or pass gas.

If you are feeling calm or relaxed
- Keep doing what you are doing! Make sure to write about it in your journal so you remember what things help you feel relaxed.

If you are feeling muscle pain
- Get someone to rub your muscles or your ears.
- Lay on a heating pad.
- Take a nice hot bath.

If it is a worry pain
- If you can do something about it, make a plan. If you can't do anything, boss your worry around!

If you are feeling guilty about something
- See if there is a problem that you need to fix.

If you are feeling bored
- Make a list of 50 things you can do (ask for help if you need it). You can use this list again later.

If you are feeling sleepy
- Rest

Something else?
_____
_____

Write or draw what you tried, how it went, or what you are planning to try!

STEP 5: PLAN YOUR NEXT INVESTIGATION.

Is there anything exciting coming up that we can investigate? Let's make a plan!

Write down the plan for your investigation.

Figure 2.10 Steps 4 and 5 of the Body Clues Worksheet. Once you have figured out what your body is feeling, you can respond to those messages and see what happens – you are performing Body Investigation! Over time, as you become more attuned to what your body is communicating and more adept at responding to those messages, you get to know yourself better and better.

In other words, by helping children respond to their bodies differently, we can also help them respond to the experience of stress-induced sensations differently. When children can manage stress more adaptively, they possess the power to change the weather (see Figure 1.3 in Chapter 1).

> In Hans Selyve's classic definition, stress is a condition in which one's demands exceed the body's available resources to deal with those demands. In training FBI agents, we intend to help children increase their available resources and maximize their ability to utilize those resources effectively. Children are then ready and able to meet any challenge.

This brings us to another superpower to consider in children who are viscerally hypersensitive and may have altered gut physiology, particularly in response to stress. This superpower relates to the impact of gut sensations on decision-making – what is often referred to as intuitive decisions.

Most if not all of us may have had a rapid and charged gut intuition about a situation that was hard to shake. To appreciate the impact of this, put yourself in the following situation. Your friend sets you up on a date with someone they know from work. Your friend describes this person's attractive appearance and their impressive professional credentials and successes. So far, so good. Then, you meet them in person and immediately get this creepy feeling in your gut (in more technical terms: you have an intense visceral reaction to them). You have trouble shaking this gut feeling throughout dinner together. Will you go out with them again?

The influence of emotions on the process of rational decision-making is complicated and important. Whether that feeling of uneasiness in your gut becomes one data point in making a decision or _the_ data point in determining the decision is likely an individual difference. People differ in how much they "trust their gut."

Our trust in the messages our gut signals may be a reflection of the influence of the enteric nervous system. The wisdom of the enteric nervous system (ENS) is another super-power tool that those who are viscerally hypersensitive can use. The ENS is comprised of sensory and motor nerve complexes and has been referred to as a second brain, monitoring the state of the gut, much like the central nervous system (CNS) is monitoring the state of the environment. The ENS can directly influence the CNS: gut stimuli are sensed in the ENS, which communicates them to the CNS, thereby forming or shaping emotional experience and cognition. One example of this bottom-up influence is when your stomach rumbles, you perceive this rumbling, you recognize the sensation from prior experience and discriminate it as a hunger signal, and you grab a snack.

From an evolutionary perspective, the enteric nervous system is older than the central nervous system.[20] From a developmental perspective, neurons from the vagal crest of the CNS migrate to the gut and differentiate to become the neuronal complexes of the ENS. It is as if you and your sister, to whom you are very attached, both got super-speed wireless internet service so that you could talk frequently at rapid speed all the time. So, we all have this old wise "brain" in our gut. Children with visceral hypersensitivity potentially have more sensitized capacities to notice the messages of this brain; these messages may influence their decision-making. Research establishing these links is just emerging, notwithstanding, it is an exciting area for future research that is fun to think about.

> We are fortunate to have our friend and colleague, Emeran Mayer, author of the *Mind–Gut Connection* and the *Gut–Immune Connection*, advise us over the years about the wisdom of gut–brain communication.

Visceral hypersensitivity presents an opportunity and a challenge. Let's imagine another situation. It is before school. The child with sensory superpowers perceives an uneasy feeling in their gut and has a strong gut intuition that they should avoid school. While we will spend all of the next chapter talking about parenting and the challenge of parenting a child with pain, for now focus on how FBI – Pain Division addresses situations in which a decision needs to be made as to whether to approach or avoid something. It is time for a Body Investigation!

First, we pull out our Body Clues Worksheet and complete Step 1: we label these gut sensations. Is it Ricky the Rock? That pit of dread you feel in your stomach when you are not looking forward to something? Yes, it is. How strong is Ricky the Rock? Quarter circle? Half-circle? We determine it is pretty strong: a half circle. We then figure out that in addition to Ricky the Rock, the child is also experiencing Betty the Butterfly and Polly the Pain – a ¾ circle and ¼ circle, respectively. On to Step 2! We know that the situation is the child getting ready for school. Time for Step 3! We determine that the child is feeling a little nervous and a little sad. Step 4: we make a plan. We decide we are going to perform an investigation and go to school with our FBI journals and check in to see what happens to Ricky the Rock, Betty the Butterfly, and Polly the Pain at 10 AM and after recess at 11 AM. We can then figure out the effect of recess on

butterflies and rocks. One important emphasis of this investigation (and all investigations that we design) is that we are not trying to prove something or achieve a given outcome. We are not trying to reduce Betty the Butterfly or abolish Ricky the Rock. There is no failing an investigation. We are just curious about what happens. So, in this example, the parent is validating the child's experience in their gut as real and important and is helping them to figure out what their bodies are telling them and then designing an investigation to learn a bit more about what their body is trying to communicate. Hopefully, this is a much more rewarding interaction between parent and child than just informing them that they have to go to school, a topic we spend Chapter 3 exploring.

So, how this does this process of investigation apply to the creepy feeling you experienced on a date with a new person? In some situations, you go with your gut. Learning when to do so is part of learning to know yourself.

The Sensory Superpower Narrative and the Medical Community

We were nervous in the writing of this chapter. Our work is with children, children who are at risk of developing chronic pain conditions and comorbid psychopathology, such as depressive and anxiety disorders. Our goal was to reframe visceral hypersensitivity – something considered a liability – as an asset in these children. However, in giving children and their families behavioral and psychological tools to channel the sensitivity into an asset, we by no means wish to dismiss real gastrointestinal symptoms as "psychological." Rather, as discussed previously, there is good evidence for the physiologic interplay between the gut and the brain. Our intention is to take charge of what we can influence within the gut–brain axis and see how far that influence goes in improving the management of gastrointestinal symptoms such as abdominal pain.

Why is it so important to validate the symptoms that these children have? The individuals that you see may have been negatively impacted by well-intentioned but potentially over-simplified conceptualizations of gastrointestinal pain. Individuals may come to you with a history of interactions that they experienced as invalidating and dismissive, perhaps from the healthcare community or their own family. While children may be impervious to these messages, their parents are certainly not. Parents of children with pain may have had to manage their own family histories of pain. They may have had experiences in which they felt their physical symptoms were not treated seriously by the medical community and instead, were regarded as "psychological" in their etiology and maintenance.

We have spent this chapter discussing processes of self-attunement – the feelings of safety and trust that one can gain as one feels increasingly competent in deciphering and responding to their own experience. In the next chapter we will talk about the interpersonal processes that facilitate self-attunement. Suffice to say, feeling that one's symptoms are not being seen, heard, and understood by the medical community can elicit profound feelings of invalidation and self-mistrust.

We want this treatment to be helpful for all members of the family. In the first session, we spend a great deal of time with the parents. For a parent who has had their own history of pain, engaging in this treatment with their child can be quite emotional. If we are successful in the first session in setting up this treatment, we will have created hope that these sensitive children have the capacity to live beautiful lives. If the parent themselves did not have this experience, there may be feelings of grief that arise in this initial session, but also hope that perhaps this intervention can provide some healing for themselves as well.

In his discussion about physician–patient relationships, Dr. Douglas A. Drossman, the head of the Rome Foundation and an influential scholar in the study of gastrointestinal disorders, writes about the importance of incorporating a patient's narrative as one describes the nature of their disorder and to fully flush out and understand their beliefs about barriers and expectations for change.[21] The essence of his advice is to make sure patients feel seen. Dr. Frank Keefe, director of the Pain Prevention Research Program at Duke University, with his colleague Dr. Lisa Perry, examines how pain can be a traumatic event that can be viewed as central to one's identity.[22] In one study, they gave patients a measure called the Centrality of Events scale to examine differences in how individuals viewed their lives as organized and impacted by their prior and current pain experiences. Their results indicated that stronger endorsement of the centrality of pain in their life narrative was associated with impairment and diminished quality of life over and above pain intensity. If, in the first session, we have not fully heard the family's journey to this point, and their fears about this treatment are not recognized, we have already lost.

Therefore, we feel it crucial that we acknowledge the reality of children's gastrointestinal symptoms, provide some explanation of the known science behind the gut–brain interaction, and then offer – with joy and excitement! – new tools for taking charge and living life out loud. Taking this extra time will save you so much time in the long run. It also feels really good. We will need to come up with a character for that, that moment of exhilaration when you feel you have really authentically connected with another human being.

Self-Reflections

Perhaps take a few minutes to pause and reflect on what showed up for you as you worked your way through this chapter. Are there parts that you are skeptical about? Are you considering using this as an opportunity to work on your own self-attunement? It may be very impactful for you to write down some of these impressions. These moments of pausing and tuning in are essential practice for an FBI agent and we hope we get you to join the force.

This exercise in self-reflection highlights an important theme of the FBI intervention. All of us can get better at knowing, trusting, and caring for ourselves. We hope that as a clinician delivering this intervention, you are simultaneously a participant in the intervention, using it as a springboard to tune in a bit more to what your needs are.

References

1. Simren, M., Tornblom, H., Palsson, O.S., et al. (2017). Visceral hypersensitivity is associated with GI symptom severity in functional GI disorders: consistent findings from five different patient cohorts. *Gut 67* (2), 255–262 https://doi.org/10.1136/gutjnl-2016-312361

2. LeDoux, J. (1996). Blood, sweat, and tears. In *The Emotional Brain: The Mysterious Underpinnings of Emotional Life*. New York, NY: Simon & Schuster, pp. 42–72.

3. Tooby, J., Cosmides, L. (1990). The past explains the present – emotional adaptations and the structure of ancestral environments. *Ethol Sociobiol 11*, 375–424. https://doi.org/10.1016/0162-3095(90)90017-z

4. Hutcherson, C.A., Gross, J.J. (2011). The moral emotions: a social-functionalist account of anger, disgust, and contempt. *J Pers Soc Psychol 100*, 719–737. https://doi.org/10.1037/a0022408

5. Cannon, W.B. (1925). *Bodily Changes in Pain, Hunger, Fear, and Rage: An Account of Recent Researches into the Function of Emotional Excitement*. New York, NY: D. Appleton and Company.

6. Hicks, J.W., Bennett, A.F. (2004). Eat and run: prioritization of oxygen delivery during elevated metabolic states. *Respir Physiol Neurobiol 144*, 215–224. https://doi.org/10.1016/j.resp.2004.05.011

7. Camilleri, M., Lasch, K., Zhou, W. (2012). Irritable bowel syndrome: methods, mechanisms, and pathophysiology. The confluence of increased permeability, inflammation, and pain in irritable bowel syndrome. *Am J Physiol Gastrointest Liver Physiol 303*, G775–785. https://doi.org/10.1152/ajpgi.00155.2012

8. Khalsa, S.S., Adolphs, R., Cameron, O.G., et al. (2018). Interoception and mental health: a roadmap. *Biol Psychiatry Cogn Neurosci Neuroimaging 3*, 501–513. https://doi.org/10.1016/j.bpsc.2017.12.004

9. Herbert, B.M., Pollatos, O., Schandry, R. (2007). Interoceptive sensitivity and emotion processing: an EEG study. *Int J Psychophysiol 65*, 214–227. https://doi.org/10.1016/j.ijpsycho.2007.04.007

10. Schuette, S.A., Zucker, N.L., Smoski, M.J. (2021). Do interoceptive accuracy and interoceptive sensibility predict emotion regulation? *Psychol Res 85*, 1894–1908. https://doi.org/10.1007/s00426-020-01369-2

11. Kragel, P.A., LaBar, K.S. (2014). Advancing emotion theory with multivariate pattern classification. *Emot Rev 6*, 160–174. https://doi.org/10.1177/1754073913512519

12. Leeuw, M., Goossens, M.E., Linton, S.J., et al. (2007). The fear-avoidance model of musculoskeletal pain: current state of scientific evidence. *J Behav Med 30*, 77–94. https://doi.org/10.1007/s10865-006-9085-0

13. Crombez, G., Eccleston, C., Van Damme, S., et al. (2012). Fear-avoidance model of chronic pain: the next generation. *Clin J Pain 28*, 475–483. https://doi.org/10.1097/AJP.0b013e3182385392

14. Lissek, S., Rabin, S.J., McDowell, D.J., et al. (2009). Impaired discriminative fear-conditioning resulting from elevated fear responding to learned safety cues among individuals with panic disorder. *Behav Res Ther 47*, 111–118. https://doi.org/10.1016/j.brat.2008.10.017

15. Brady, S.T., Hard, B.M., Gross, J.J. (2018). Reappraising test anxiety increases academic performance of first-year college students. *J Educ Psychol 110*, 395–406. https://doi.org/10.1037/edu0000219

16. Parker, C.H., Naliboff, B.D., Shih, W., et al. (2019). Negative events during adulthood are associated with symptom severity and altered stress response in patients with irritable bowel syndrome. *Clin Gastroenterol Hepatol 17*, 2245–2252. https://doi.org/10.1016/j.cgh.2018.12.029

17. Videlock, E.J., Adeyemo, M., Licudine, A., et al. (2009). Childhood trauma is associated with hypothalamic-pituitary-adrenal axis responsiveness in irritable bowel syndrome. *Gastroenterology 137*, 1954–1962. https://doi.org/10.1053/j.gastro.2009.08.058

18. Tait, C., Sayuk, G.S. (2021). The brain-gut-microbiotal axis: a framework for understanding functional GI illness and their therapeutic interventions. *Eur J Int Med 84*, 1–9. https://doi.org/10.1016/j.ejim.2020.12.023

19. Foster, J.A., Rinaman, L., Cryan, J.F. (2017). Stress & the gut-brain axis: regulation by the microbiome. *Neurobiol Stress 7*, 124–136. https://doi.org/10.1016/j.ynstr.2017.03.001

20. Mayer, E.A. (2011). Gut feelings: the emerging biology of gut-brain communication. *Nat Rev Neurosci 12*, 453–466. https://doi.org/10.1038/nrn3071

21. Drossman, D.A. (2016). Functional gastrointestinal disorders and the Rome IV Process. In C. Di Lorenzo and S. Nurko (eds.). *Rome IV Pediatric Functional Gastrointestinal Disorders*. Raleigh, North Carolina: Rome Foundation, pp. 1–27.

22. Perri, L.M., Keefe, F.J. (2008). Applying centrality of event to persistent pain: a preliminary view. *J Pain 9*, 265–271. https://doi.org/10.1016/j.jpain.2007.10.019

Responsive Parenting and Creating Safety

The Importance of Safety

Over the years, we have witnessed the profound emotional and physical consequences that children experience when they sense that they are not safe. This chapter is about safety: what it is, how parents can facilitate that experience for their children, the difficulties in doing so when you have a child with sensory superpowers, and the strategies for enhancing a parent's own sense of safety within themselves. To begin, let's look at some classic historical influences on the creation of safety in children.

What is safety? What does feeling safe feel like? At its most fundamental level, safety is freedom from harm or danger. To experience safety, one must feel that their basic needs are reliably provided for (food, water, shelter, regular medical care, as examples). One must experience living in a non-abusive environment. These are fundamental and crucial elements of safety. However, safety is also subtler than that.

At its essence, safety is experiencing that you are seen, that your needs are witnessed, acknowledged, and understood, and that your needs are reliably responded to.[1] A crucial test of safety is observing what happens when those needs are threatened in some way. For example, it is one thing to feel safe when you are sitting at home watching a movie with your parents. But what about if you are really sad or anxious about something? What about if you really screwed something up and you have to tell your parents? The test of safety is whom you go to when that happens and whether you feel comforted (safe) after you do.

To more fully understand this concept of safety, it is helpful to go back to early classic developmental psychology studies of parent and child attachment. The developmental psychologist Mary Ainsworth devised a paradigm to test whether a child experienced safety in the presence of a caregiver,[2] what has also been described as a secure attachment.[1] Ainsworth designed a paradigm named the Strange Situation Test as a way to learn more about the relationship between a child and their primary caregiver. A child would be playing with their (mother). Then the child would be exposed to a stressor: a stranger would enter and attempt to engage with the child and the mother would leave (a situation that would be upsetting for most children). The key test as to whether the child experienced a secure attachment, a renewed sense of safety, was what happened when the mother returned to the situation. Did the distressed child seek out the mother for support and was the child comforted upon being reunited with their mother? If so, one interpretation of this pattern is that the child viewed the mother as a source of

comfort and support and did, in fact, feel comforted by her presence when they were distressed. Such theories continue to evolve and be refined as we learn more about the complexities of parent–child interaction and the various child and parent factors that can influence such interactions. Nonetheless, it is a useful framework to think about the back-and-forth dance between a parent and child – one that we can use as we help train these young investigators to become their own "self-parents" to ensure their experiences of security.

Time for Reflection

Think back to a time when you were very distressed or deeply sad about something during your childhood. What did you do with that sadness? Did you reach out for support from someone? If you did, why did you choose that person and what happened after you reached out? If you did not, can you think of experiences that may have taught you that it may not be advantageous to reach out? While you may not be able to remember a vivid event from such a long time ago, you may have a general impression of your pattern as a child, adolescent, and adult. Do you feel comforted by someone else in moments of distress? If you do not even think to share your distress with someone, that can be a powerful signal of your prior learning history regarding seeking and experiencing comfort.

So, what does it take for a child to feel safe? Is this any different for a child with sensory superpowers? We next explore the complexities of creating an experience of safety for any child, and the particular challenges of creating safety when the child is incredibly sensitive to their own experiences and to the world around them. We want to take you through the developmental journey of the emergence of safety so you can better understand where and how FBI – Pain Division attempts to create safety in young children.

Responsive Parenting and the Experience of Safety

What is important to emphasize outright is that there are a multitude of reciprocal, interacting factors that contribute to the experience of safety for a given child. We are not about to enter into a section on parent blaming or child blaming. The creation of safety is far too complicated for simplistic formulations

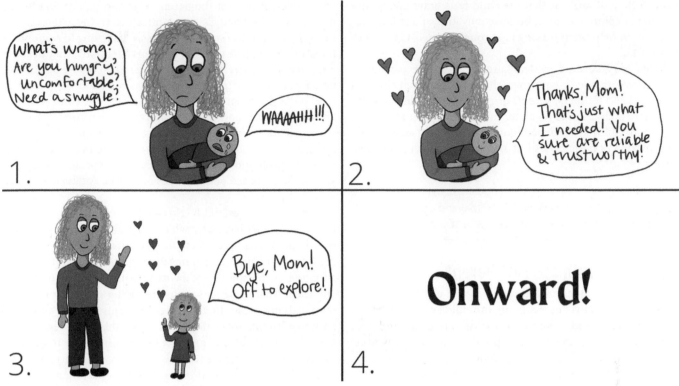

Figure 3.1 An over-simplified depiction of one of the million challenges of parenting – trying to play detective and decode the signals of distress communicated by a child (A). If all goes well, the child trusts that their needs are reliably responded to and feels safe (B). In the context of safety, they are ready to explore (C & D).

such as unilateral causation by one person. As we mentioned in Chapter 1 when we discussed the biopsychosocial model of pain, the creation of safety for a child is embedded within that same complex framework of biological, psychological, and social influences. A parent is always just doing their best to create safety against a multitude of competing forces. Let's imagine for a minute that the situation is simpler. Here, we illustrate an idyllic process of responsive parenting.

In Figure 3.1, the child communicates distress. Initially this is experienced by the parent as undifferentiated distress. How is the parent supposed to know what the child is communicating? Parents are not mind readers. Furthermore, children vary greatly in the degree to which they communicate distress. Children with more ambiguous facial or non-verbal/verbal communication may not signal distress in ways that are easily perceptible to others. The parent may miss these cues. Children with intense, easily discernible facial and/or non-verbal/verbal communication may signal such high levels of distress that it can be hard for a parent to maintain composure as they respond. But in our optimal situation, the child communicates distress and the parent acts like an elite FBI agent, performing a series of trial-and-error investigations to decipher what message is being communicated by the child's distress.

Panel A illustrates this guessing game. Is the child hungry? If so, providing nourishment may stop the crying. If that does not work, perhaps the child needs a diaper change? Maybe the child just needs a snuggle? Or to sleep? Maybe the child needs intellectual stimulation? A philosophical debate? All

the parent can do is attempt something, and see what happens. That said, they are indeed acting as well-trained investigators because they need to pay attention and notice cues and patterns. Through a process of trial and error over time, this undifferentiated distress evolves into more discernible communication signals. The parent gets better at telling a hunger cry from a sleepy cry. As a result, the child's needs are deciphered more expediently and reciprocally, the communication of those needs is made more precisely. In other words, the system (parent and child interacting) becomes increasingly efficient and responsive.

Let's place ourselves into the body and experience of the infant for a moment. The child communicates something and the environment responds. Whammo! The child is given feedback that they exist in the world. They are seen. They are heard. They are important enough to respond to. The child repeatedly expresses needs and time after time, the environment, and specifically, caregivers, are reliably there and respond to those needs. One result of this is that the child regards the world as safe and that certain individuals as particularly trustworthy – you can go to them when you need something and you will feel better. These are swell people indeed (Panel B).

Once the child starts to identify key adults as a source for reliably alleviating distress, it stands to reason that the child would learn to seek out this person in times of distress. Enter Ainsworth's Strange Situations Paradigm – the securely attached child is expected to seek out the mother to re-establish their sense of safety. Furthermore, an important consequence of this feeling of safety is that the child feels brave and secure enough to explore – in part, because they know there is someone there to help them if things get rough (Panels C and D of Figure 3.1).

What may become evident after reading (or personally experiencing this with your own child) is that when children are infants and toddlers, parents are doing a great deal of work helping their children to regulate. Parents are essential for such regulation: children are dependent on their parents not just for the provision of basic needs but also to help the child manage distress.

> The end result of this back-and-forth trial and error between parent and child is that the child feels seen, heard, and safe.

Children Learning to Self-Parent

As the child gets older, including the age of children targeted in the FBI – Pain Division program, the child becomes increasingly capable of and responsible for decoding the messages their body is telling them and responding to those messages. Essentially, the child learns to parent themselves – to "self-parent." They learn to do the same things for themselves that their parent was doing for them (Figure 3.2). Rather than having their parent engage in trial-and-error investigations to figure out what the child needs, the child learns to perform these investigations on themselves. A child will go through the same

trial and error process the parent went through: trying to figure out what their body is communicating, trying to discern the meaning of various forms of distress, etc., trying to respond to those needs and to learn what happens afterward. They become a self-parent (Figure 3.2). And just like a responsive parent can help facilitate the experience of safety in a child, so becoming an expert self-parent makes a child feel safe: the child comes to know themselves and trust themselves. One truism is that the child will always have themselves, so establishing a responsive self-parenting relationship with yourself when you are a young child has profound implications. It can set the child up to feel safe in the presence of challenges and to be willing to explore new challenges.

How do we establish this self-parenting in children? Fortunately, this is exactly what FBI trains parents and children to do. We embrace the wisdom of all sensations, including those that constitute pain or negative emotional experiences. By adopting the perspective of a wise investigator, we can observe and learn what these sensations are telling us and work to get our needs met rather than feeling like we just need to end them abruptly. Parents are facilitators: helping their children investigate these mysteries and figure out something to try to get their needs met. Thus, a parent's role has evolved from playing an essential role in their child's regulation to playing a coaching role to encourage the child to learn about and regulate themselves. What does a parent's behavior look like in this new role? To understand this, let's review what is intended when a parent validates their child's experience.

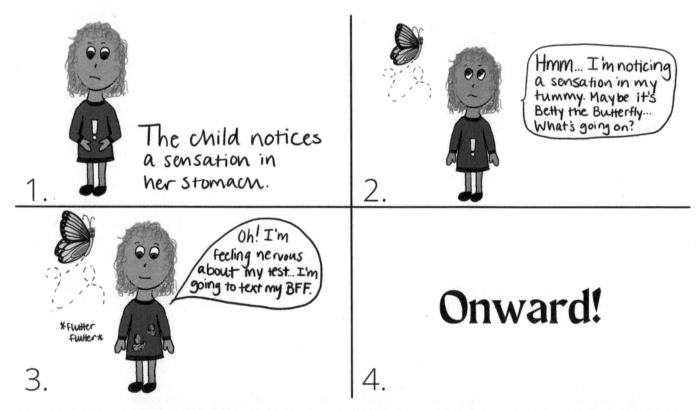

Figure 3.2 A child learning to self-parent. As children get older, they increasingly take on the responsibility for becoming their own responsive parent: noticing sensations in their body (A), figuring out what those sensations might be (B), and decoding the messages of those sensations (C).

Validation

The concept of validation is a bit tricky and nuanced to understand. Despite what your teenager may tell you, you are not being invalidating if you do not give them what they want. Thus, when a parent disagrees with a child, they are not necessarily being invalidating. However, validation is about ensuring that a/your child/patient knows they exist. It goes a step beyond perspective taking because it also requires that one understands the wisdom of a person's emotional experiences in a given context. It is not empathy either: you are not out to share the feelings of the person you are validating: just to accept the inherent logic of why it makes sense that a person, given their life experiences and capacities, may have the experience that they are having at a given moment and in a certain situation. To develop a validating stance toward someone else involves engaging in an intellectual and emotional embodiment of their experiences in that moment and the journey that brought them to that moment.

> Given all the rejection and hurt that you experienced from people close to you, I imagine it must be truly hard to share personal things with me. I would guess that is really terrifying. Is that your experience?

How might a person who had those experiences feel when they heard that from a healthcare provider?

There are several important elements in that simple communication. The provider paid attention: they know what you have been through. They are really trying to understand your experience and imagine what it would feel like to have encountered what you have been through. However, the provider is not you and thus can only guess what you (the patient) might be feeling. Thus, the quote above very deliberately poses assumptions about a person's experience as a guess and asks the expert, the person themselves, for confirmation.

> The essence of validation is that an individual feels and knows that their existence matters. It requires that the wisdom of their experience, given what that person has been through and what they understand the world to be, is acknowledged and accepted.

FBI – Pain Division makes the process of validating a child's experience very straightforward, by applying a set of concrete tools.

Table 3.1 provides a brief overview of the activities in FBI – Pain Division that provide parents and clinicians with opportunities to validate a child's experience and help teach them to self-parent. While all of these activities will be described in great detail in Part II of this book, we mention them here so you can better understand how FBI works. We also name some invalidation traps: ways that well-intentioned parents and clinicians can inadvertently invalidate a child's experience.

Table 3.1 Unintentional validation traps

FBI activity	Ways in which a child feels validated	Unintentional invalidation traps
Body Investigation	Each session, parent, child, and therapist engage in investigations to learn more about the body. The child describes their experience of their body. For example, they may describe how many heartbeats they sense or how much energy they feel as they are eating a snack. In these activities, the child is treated as the expert of their own experience. In fact, their observations are so important that we record them on their own personalized Body Map.	Correcting a child's experience of their own body. Children may sometimes provide answers that are biologically implausible if not downright impossible. It does not matter. The point is to get the child to curiously tune into what their body is doing. They will get more accurate with practice. However, we can help them to make sure they are tuning into a given sensation. For example, we help them find their pulse and work through the stages of what hunger and fullness feel like.
Body Clues Worksheet	This worksheet walks the parent and child through the process of self-parenting. In a given moment, the child indicates what sensations they are feeling (e.g., Ella the Emotional Pain? Georgia the Gut Growler?) The exercise of completing one of these worksheets basically walks parents and clinicians through the process of validating a child's experience. By having the child describe what sensations they are feeling; listening to them as they figure out what their bodies are trying to tell them (e.g., am I feeling sad); and brain-storming with them what to try to get their needs met, the parent is teaching their child how to self-parent while guaranteeing that the child feels like they have all the answers when it comes to their own experience.	If the parent, feeling bad about not having completed worksheets during the week, fills them out quickly "on behalf" of their child, this is actually the ultimate invalidation. The parent is unintentionally communicating that the parent does not even need to see or hear the child – they just "know" their experience. Now that you know what to look for, as a clinician you may be curious to observe what happens to a child's affect when they experience invalidation. You have not met them yet – but Tommy Thunderbolt is a powerful invalidation detector. Tommy Thunderbolt is the feeling of tightness and heat – sensations that may accompany feelings of anger – or even rage. Having someone tell us we are not feeling how we are feeling or should not be feeling how we are feeling is a pretty reliable way to bring Tommy Thunderbolt out in full force. The therapist not inquiring about Body Clues Worksheets and not reviewing these sheets is also invalidating. These sheets are intended to be one vehicle for a child to express their experience for greater understanding by themselves and others. Therapists communicate that this is important by asking to review these sheets.
Body Journal	For each session, we suggest optional prizes. In Session 1, one of these prizes is a journal. We give various ideas throughout the treatment of things the child can record in their journal. Anything the child records in their journal is, of course, a record of their own experience.	Similarly, a parent or therapist failing to ask the child about their journal and having them explain what they did could be perceived as invalidating. When a child feels that their experiences are not an object of interest by their parents or therapist, Bertha Blah may come to visit – the heavy, low-energy feeling that often accompanies feelings of sadness.

The importance of a child feeling seen, heard, and understood (aka validated) is so important that we try to create rituals: checking in daily to review the child's most intense moments.

Parenting in the Context of Sensory Superpowers (Responsive Parenting in FBI – Pain Division)

One of the most important activities that is learned during the FBI intervention is the Body Clues Worksheet, introduced in Chapter 2. Among other functions, this worksheet is designed to help children and parents learn to self-parent. In addition, as the intervention progresses, the Body Clues Worksheet goes one step further. As children feel safer, they have the courage to explore. In the FBI intervention, this may take the form of designing investigations that encourage the child to try something new or to approach something that they think is challenging. Figure 3.3 summarizes the different uses of the Body Clues Worksheet throughout the intervention.

As discussed in the previous chapter, in the first two sessions of the FBI intervention, the Body Clues Worksheet is used to help children to become more aware of the different sensations they are experiencing and increasingly skilled at naming these sensations. Moreover, the worksheet provides a way for children to index the intensity of a given sensation, to signal that even the fine nuances of an experience are important. Children then indicate what they were doing when they felt the sensations. This step is designed to help parent and child figure out what their bodies may be trying to tell them. Body sensations can be complicated. They can mean different things in different situations.

Starting in Session 3, parent and child are asked to figure out what their body sensations may be communicating. Are they feeling a certain type of emotion? A certain type of pain? Because body sensations convey messages about what we need, the fourth step guides parents and children to try a strategy and see what happens: to design an impromptu body investigation! Thus, the Body Clues Worksheet is essentially a "how-to" guide for children and parents to learn how to self-parent.

As treatment progresses, families get increasingly skilled at designing in-the-moment body investigations to explore unexpected or increasingly intense moments. The child may notice some sensations and the family may be trying to make a decision about what to do next. Planning an investigation and recording it (then or later) and seeing what happens will provide valuable self-parenting experiences. For example, the child may be taking on a daring mission, such as going to school when experiencing a lot of Gassy Gus and related gastrointestinal pain. In instances like this, parent and child can design an investigation (such as doing jumping jacks for 60 seconds before leaving for school to see what happens to Gassy Gus) and then they observe what happens.

Parents are instructed to use these worksheets at different moments to help facilitate self-parenting. First, they can pull out a worksheet right after an intense moment to figure out what just happened and what investigation they may like to try next time. Parents can use it as part of a daily ritual to review what happened during the day so they can ensure that they are not missing out on important things that their child may have experienced. Parents can use it to plan an upcoming investigation, helping the child approach a challenging situation by making it into an investigation (Figure 3.3). Parents can use it to role model their own self-parenting. Thus far, the conditions that we have described for engaging in responsive parenting/self-parenting interventions have been calm moments: after an intense experience, as a review of the day, or in anticipation of an upcoming challenge. Investigations may also be extremely useful in the midst of an intense moment. As this circumstance requires more nuance and skill to navigate it, we unpack the steps involved.

When to Use a Body Clues Worksheet

After an intense moment has passed, as a way to figure out what just happened and some things to try next time.

At the end of the day, as a way to review the moments in which the child had the most feelings.

As a guide to planning an in-the-moment investigation and seeing what happens.

As a way for a parent or sibling to role-model their own self-parenting.

As a way to plan investigations to explore in the future.

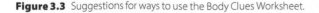

Figure 3.3 Suggestions for ways to use the Body Clues Worksheet.

The Challenge of Staying Calm in a Storm

By definition, children with sensory superpowers live life out loud. As we have already learned, they experience intense, vivid sensations – a gift that enables them to have a richer and vibrant lived experience, but one that also contributes to some tough moments.

Thus far we have talked about the establishment of safety in the child via the parent's responsiveness – the trial-and-error process that ensues while tuning in to the child's needs. Of course, there are many challenging influences on responsive parenting. Children vary in the degree to which they are able to communicate what they need. Some children are just more expressive than others. Children differ in their capacities to self-regulate – something that we help them with in FBI, but still, easier for some than others. Children differ in their snuggle propensity. While this is not a technical term, what we mean is that some children just love to nuzzle up. If they could, they would be attached to you as an appendage. For other children, it seems like they feel trapped if you try to snuggle. For these children, we have to perform some investigations on strategies that will allow them to feel safe and comfortable. Parents as investigators are constantly on the lookout for clues on how to respond in a given situation.

However, there is also another important ingredient to the establishment of safety. That ingredient is the parents own ability to self-parent and self-regulate (Figure 3.4). If one imagines the experience of a young child, one can see why this is important. We mentioned earlier that safety is tested when there is a threat. In the face of something distressing to the child, the parent not only helps the child to decipher what they need and brainstorm ways to respond, but they also communicate that they, the parent, are tough enough to handle the situation. This requires a gentle combination of active engagement while the parent's feet are firmly planted on the ground, figuratively speaking.

The energy and arousal a parent brings into the system is an interesting factor to explore and investigate. For example, in a high-arousal situation, the parent may get distressed too. This is human. The parent can still facilitate safety by communicating that even though they (parent and child) are both upset, scared, sad, etc., that they are tough enough and smart enough to figure out what to do and try it. A less obvious example occurs when parents are bringing a lot of positive energy into a system. In a high-arousal situation in which the child is distressed, parents can sometimes inadvertently increase the energy in the system by being overly positive. Trying high-energy, positive strategies to attempt to cheer up a distressed child may feel supportive for some children but may inadvertently backfire for other children. For these latter children, it just adds gas to a flame. What may be more useful are strategies that decrease arousal and lower the energy in the system. However, what works in terms of the parent's own regulation strategies and the interaction of those regulation strategies with their child calls for cleverly designed FBI investigations (Figure 3.4).

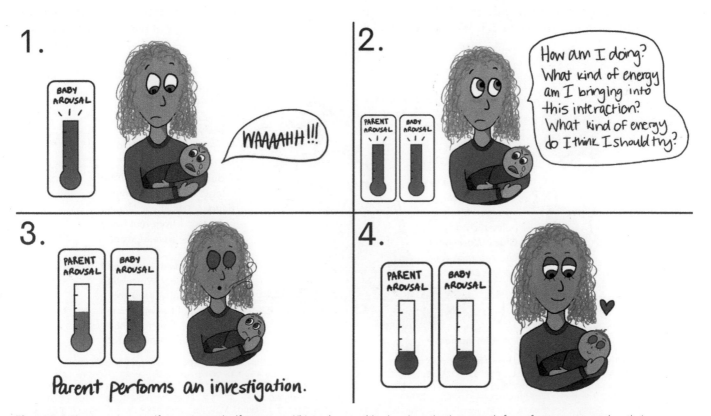

Figure 3.4 The parent's own self-parenting and self-awareness. Ultimately, everything is an investigation: a gentle frame for a parent to explore their own experiences and how those experiences interact with those of their child.

To explain what we mean, I (NZ) am going tell you a story about the lecture that my undergraduate class on psychopathology was lucky enough to hear.

Dr. Rebecca Shelby is a clinical psychologist and trained sex therapist at Duke University. She was speaking to my class on various forms of sexual dysfunction. In this particular instance, she was talking about the relational influences on sexual dysfunction. Specifically, she was describing how, when a couple is experiencing challenges with sexual intimacy, one's instinct is to increase the gas: buy sexy outfits and elaborate gadgets. What is needed, instead, is applying the brake, lowering the level of arousal in an overcharged system.

Throughout the FBI intervention, there are key moments when we have conversations with parents alone. This is for many important reasons, including ensuring that the parent feels validated and establishing the parent's own sense of safety. In Session 4, we talk privately with parents about the challenges of managing intense emotional moments and how investigations may be useful in those moments. Session 4 is called the Zoomies and the Shakies, Part 1. It is a session focused on high arousal and negatively valenced sensations that often accompany intense negative emotions like rage, anger, fear, and anxiety. For the parents, we use a metaphor of a wave, the sensory wave, as a way to index the intensity of an individual's sensory (including emotional or pain) experiences and guide parents in the use of responsive parenting strategies. A diagram of the wave and how it relates to responsive parenting is shown in Figure 3.5. We repeat a similar

figure in Session 4 in the context of directly instructing the therapist about how to teach the wave to parents.

The top of the wave is a phrase we use to refer to extremely high intensity sensations that cross the "logic line." As we discussed in Chapter 2, emotions communicate needs that we have and are accompanied by certain urges to act that can help us to get those needs met. In truly high-intensity, threatening situations, there's no time to think. Your system is set up to help you react instinctively to a perceived threat. For example, if you are in a burning building, you just need to escape. You don't have time to consider and measure the relative merits and distance of different exit strategies.

Thus, logical problem-solving strategies are generally incompatible with the "top of the wave." Because you can't think clearly when emotions are so intense, strategies that require you to be rational just will not work as well. Instead, lowering one's arousal at the top of the wave usually requires a physical or sensory strategy. Expert FBI agents learn a plethora of physical and sensory-based strategies to lower arousal and parents will have all these at their disposal to help their children manage high-intensity moments. Parents can also use these strategies to manage their own level of arousal, the regulation of which is an additional responsibility they face. They must be responsive to both themselves and their child.

To appreciate why this is so important, let's again imagine the experiences of a young child. You (as a child) are having an intense moment. Your parent is trying to work with you to figure out what is going on and what to do. However, you also sense that your parent is distressed and is having a hard time helping you figure out what to do because they are so upset. What does this feel like from the perspective of the child? Is it reasonable

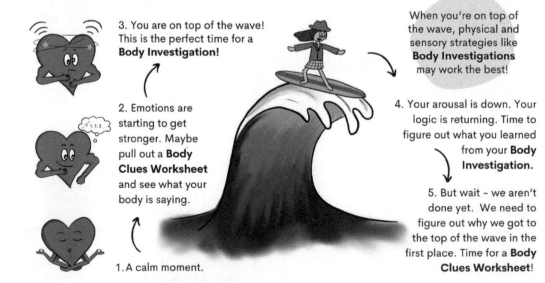

3. You are on top of the wave! This is the perfect time for a **Body Investigation!**

When you're on top of the wave, physical and sensory strategies like **Body Investigations** may work the best!

2. Emotions are starting to get stronger. Maybe pull out a **Body Clues Worksheet** and see what your body is saying.

4. Your arousal is down. Your logic is returning. Time to figure out what you learned from your **Body Investigation.**

5. But wait - we aren't done yet. We need to figure out why we got to the top of the wave in the first place. Time for a **Body Clues Worksheet!**

1. A calm moment.

Figure 3.5 The Sensation Wave and how it relates to responsive parenting. (1) We learn to pay attention to calm, peaceful sensations as well as intense warning signals. When these calm sensations arise, it may be nice to just revel in them. (2) Well-trained FBI agents notice when sensations in their body are changing. If they need help figuring out what might be happening, this is a great time to pull out a Body Clues Worksheet. (3) It is an intense moment. It might be time for the parent to join with the child and design an investigation they can try (or at least explore) together. Doing this as a team is important here: we want to preserve a person's dignity when they are having strong feelings. Makings things a "we can try" rather than "you should really try" can help with this. (4) Once the investigation has been conducted and the intense moment has passed, we have to figure out what we just learned. Finally, if you are an advanced FBI agent, you might want to fill out a Body Clues Worksheet to figure out what put you at the top of the wave in the first place.

to expect parents to be able to stay calm all the time if their children have frequent, long, intense experiences?

Well, FBI provides several solutions for intense moments. The whole basis of FBI is to make various body sensations, and what these sensations constitute, such as emotional experiences or pain, less scary. Thus, a high-intensity moment is one in which we are visited by some well-known characters. A high-intensity moment just calls out for an investigation to see what happens. The fact that a parent is also having a high intensity moment can actually be quite dignifying for the child in that it normalizes intense moments and casts them not as a sign of weakness, but merely as experiences to investigate. In fact, we encourage parents to behave in the following manner even when they are not quite having a high-intensity moment for that reason – so that the child feels joined and not judged.

Thus, in a situation in which the child is having a high-intensity moment and the parent also finds themselves having a high-intensity moment, they can say something like, "Whoa! I'm having a bunch of Betty the Butterflies right now too! Let's figure this out together! Let's try going for a walk outside and see what happens to all of our butterflies."

And that, is safety.

Table 3.2 lists some examples of things parents can do when they are experiencing their own high-intensity moments along with their child. These examples demonstrate how parents are validating their child's experience and then guiding them in the performance of an investigation to learn more about themselves.

Table 3.2 Examples of using investigations in high-intensity parent/child moments

"Ok, so we are feeling Ella the Emotional Pain. Let's go for a walk (one of their many Henry Heartbeat activities) and then we can fill out a Body Clues Worksheet and figure out what we should do next."

"I've got some Julie Jitters. Do you? Maybe we both need some Cozy Celeste – let's just snuggle for a bit."

"Oh wow!! Tommy Thunderbolt is SOOO strong! Let's both go whip a tennis ball against the wall and see what happens next."

Safety and Exploration

When children have had potentially scary experiences, such as recurrent pain, it stands to reason that a parent may have to work harder to create a sense of power and safety than for a child without that history. Thus far, we have been focused on the responsivity aspect of parenting and how this builds trust and safety. However, there are also other ways that parents help create safety: establishing routines and expectations. These help children know what to expect.

In line with our emphasis on helping children to feel seen, heard, and understood, an important consideration in setting those expectations is whether they are reasonable. Parents must therefore aim for a delicate balance of warmth (aka responsivity) and firmness (or establishing expectations). Researchers have studied different parenting styles and have attempted to classify how parents behave based on the relative influence or balance of these dimensions. Of course, this is over-simplified,

but it is useful to give parents a framework to think about how they approach parenting their child with sensory superpowers.

Figure 3.6 provides a framework to think about dimensions of warmth and firmness. While many studies support the importance of a balance between warmth and firmness, it has also been shown that parenting styles are much more complicated than that. First, the optimal balance of warmth and firmness may differ based upon the context you are parenting in and the capacities and experiences of the child you are parenting. If you are not only a clinician but also a parent of multiple children, this is probably not news to you. Responsive parents parent their children differently, each to their own needs; further, they parent an individual child differently at different times depending on the situation, needs of the child, and a multitude of other factors.

This leads us to the challenge of parenting a child with sensory superpowers and figuring out the optimal balance between warmth and firmness. Or, more plainly, when do you insist that a child with pain go to school? Join a sports team? When a child has been through a lot already, isn't the instinct to protect them rather than pushing them to do more hard things? Of course. The challenge is determining what path is truly protective. Holding children back may not make them feel safe at all, but weak and fearful that the world is unsafe. Yet putting them into situations they are not prepared for also may not build mastery. How can a parent negotiate and decide when to nudge and when to hold back? Isn't there a way to create a context in which gently nudging children to approach things can also feel safe?

Hopefully by now the logic of FBI – Pain Division is starting to make more sense. It is our intention that the investigations that children and parents design together enable the child to approach a new situation, to the degree that they are ready for, and in a manner that is impossible to fail. Critically, no matter what happens during these homemade Body Investigations, both parent and child will learn something about their bodies and know themselves a bit better than before the investigation was attempted. No matter what happens, the investigation can be tweaked so that next time we learn a bit more. Did we investigate different ways to secretly pass gas at school at recess? How many butterflies come out if we go to baseball practice for an hour?

Our intention is that the framework of investigations gives parents a way of balancing warmth and firmness that feels safe for them as well. It is devastating to feel like you may have done something that caused your child pain and triumphant to feel that you are helping to make them stronger, tougher, and wiser. What a wonderful thing if this could all be fun.

Parents' Own Journey of Pain

Parents are asked to do many things as part of the FBI – Pain Division intervention. While our intention is that these tools will eventually make their job as parents much easier and substantially more rewarding, parents are still working hard in this intervention and so we need to take care of them. As any child provider knows, you are never just treating the child, you are

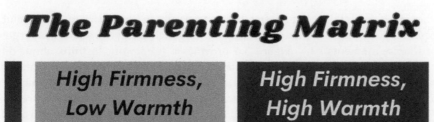

The Parenting Matrix

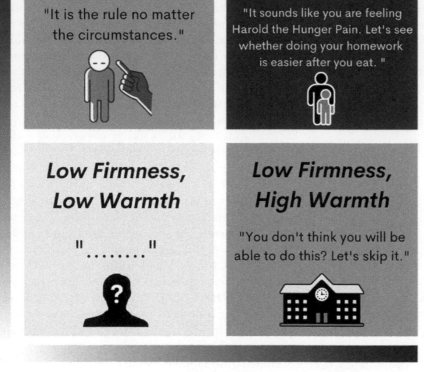

Firmness

High Firmness, Low Warmth	High Firmness, High Warmth
"It is the rule no matter the circumstances."	"It sounds like you are feeling Harold the Hunger Pain. Let's see whether doing your homework is easier after you eat. "
Low Firmness, Low Warmth	Low Firmness, High Warmth
" . . . . "	"You don't think you will be able to do this? Let's skip it."

Warmth

Figure 3.6 Parents balance different levels of warmth and firmness in how they parent. The question is not whether there is an optimal style, but rather for an elite special forces parent to investigate the optimal balance for a given mission.

helping the system in which the child exists. This includes making sure the parents themselves are okay and if not, ensuring that they have therapeutic resources of their own.

In FBI – Pain Division, we try to take some ownership of how the parent is doing by including improvement in their own compassionate self-parenting as part of our treatment goals. Parents may come to us with their own histories of pain. Their own experiences of invalidation. Perhaps they experienced a sustained and profound absence of their own feelings of safety. Imagine for a moment that you are a parent with this type of history. In the initial session, where we explain the logic of the FBI intervention and concepts such as creating safety and self-parenting, how would this make you feel? Imagine you have not experienced this yourself. What comes up for you? Perhaps fear that you will not be able to create this experience for your children. Perhaps profound sadness that you did not get what you needed when you were a child. It is critical that a parent's journey to this moment in their child's treatment for pain also be witnessed. It is imperative that we foster hope in the parent that not only can they create safety for their children, but also that going through this journey with their child provides a second chance for them – a chance for them to get the self-parenting that they so deserved.

And yet, it is not the same.

Thus, it is important that we give parents a chance to voice the injustice – that they missed out on what they needed as a sensitive child themselves. This has shown up a lot for us when implementing the FBI intervention. We think it is crucial to spend this time. As we note in Session 1, this may be a long conversation and it is a valuable investment.

Part of this conversation may involve mourning the loss of what parents deserved when they were children but did not receive. Therapists provide a gentle balance between instilling hope that parents can improve their own sense of safety, but also validating and witnessing the sense of loss that they might be experiencing as they reflect upon what they needed themselves as children but did not get.

Children with sensory superpowers are particularly adept at sensing when their parents are not okay. Thus, helping children to establish a sense of safety is also about establishing a sense of safety in the parents themselves. We have implemented the FBI intervention, as written, directly to adults. In fact, we have delivered the FBI intervention to adults who have experienced complex trauma. We framed it as "starting over" – helping parents to get what they needed when they were five years old but did not receive. So it may be with parents who have children with pain and who have been through their own history of pain. Parents may be working through their own self-exploration as they learn to help their child. Regardless, we strongly emphasize parent participation throughout the FBI intervention. Parents are essential role models for self-parenting. Our intention is that while getting to know themselves, they can be more responsive parents for their children.

Summary and Self-Reflection

We have covered a lot in this chapter. We provided a model of responsive parenting and discussed how developmentally, the intention is for responsive parenting to be increasingly subsumed by the child, so that they become their own self-parents. We discussed how the framework of FBI is designed to facilitate this and walked through the use of FBI tools in moments in which responsive parenting can be particularly challenging – such in moments of high arousal. Finally, we discussed the parents own self-parenting as a reasonable additional target in FBI, one that may help both parent and child. While it may sound like there is a lot going on in FBI, you may be surprised when you read how straightforward the intervention is. We learn new body characters. We do body investigations to explore what these sensations feel like and communicate in certain circumstances. We summarize what we learn. Ultimately, FBI is just about helping individuals to tune into and trust their bodies.

References

1. Ainsworth, M.D.S., Bowlby, J. (1991). An ethological approach to personality development. *Am Psychol 46*(4), 333–341. https://doi.org/10.1037/0003-066x.46.4.333
2. Ainsworth, M.D.S., Blehar, M.C., Waters, E., et al. (2015). *Patterns of Attachment: A Psychological Study of the Strange Situation*: London: Psychology Press, Routledge Classic Editions.

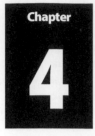

Discriminating Safe from Threatening Body Sensations: The Science of Interoceptive Exposures

The Potent Experience and Memory of Pain

Pain is an intense and potentially threatening experience. Threatening experiences can create vivid memories. These memories, and the learning that has occurred from these prior experiences, can both protect us and sometimes over-protect us. Fortunately for elite FBI agents, discerning the boundaries of safety requires investigations – right up our alley! In this chapter we further discuss fear learning and memory. We then dive a bit deeper into how different components of FBI – Pain Division are designed to maximize the helpful learning fear can teach us, while minimizing the harms of fear overgeneralization.

Misinterpreting the Stick for the Snake

One of the many tasks for trained FBI agents is establishing a curious reaction to body sensations that may be of uncertain origin. Have you ever had the experience in which your attention was grabbed by what seemed like a sudden movement? In the corner? Of your house! You did not know exactly what you saw, but something happened that alerted you to some change in lighting or movement, startling you and making you jump. Your immediate interpretation was that an uninvited mouse was keeping you company. When discussing threat perception, researchers such as Joseph LeDoux describe both a fast and slow pathway designed to process potentially threatening or salient/important stimuli by different parts of your brain.[1] The fast road (or subcortical route) is proposed to process crude features (think shadows and contours – not detailed features) – hence, in this example, a vague sense that something moved.[2] This system alerts you that something potentially important or dangerous may be unfolding before you can correctly identify just quite what is going on. Thus, in our example, we got startled by a movement that turned out to be harmless – it was your child's remote-controlled electric toy car. It makes sense that we would have a system for alerting and orienting to potential threat so responsive actions are mobilized as quickly as possible, even before we might be aware of exactly what is happening.

One can imagine that a child with sensory superpowers would be alerting to all types of features that they notice in the environment, including their bodies, due to their keen powers of perception. Having these keen powers of perception is the superpower we described in Chapter 2. Problems can arise, however, when individuals have difficulty discriminating safe stimuli from dangerous stimuli. This is what often happens in individuals with anxiety disorders. Consider the following study.

Panic disorder is an anxiety disorder in which individuals have a fear of having (and sometimes do have) intense fear reactions (panic attacks). These individuals often worry that the intense fear reaction is actually a medical emergency, such as a heart attack, rather than panic. In an (understandable) attempt to avoid a future panic attack, individuals with panic disorder are often on the alert for various body sensations that they think are warning signals for a future attack (such as their heart beating faster). They also start avoiding activities (e.g., like exercise) that provoke the sensations that they think may bring on a potential heart attack (aka, panic). Sound familiar? There are direct parallels between our fear avoidance model of pain (Chapters 1 and 2) and panic disorder. On to the research study.

In this particular study, individuals with panic disorder engaged in a fear-learning task in which they were trained to associate certain signals with danger and certain signals with safety. Individuals with panic disorder had difficulty with this discrimination training: they exhibited an exaggerated startle response to the safety cues as well as the danger cues, a pattern that was different than individuals without panic disorder who were able to learn to differentiate between these stimuli. In other words, individuals with panic disorder exhibit heightened startle responses to signals that should indicate that everything is OK and instead, they view safety signals as potentially threatening.[3] (This is akin to our earlier example of avoiding the basket of rolls following an allergic reaction to shellfish.) So that rapid, unconscious reaction to stimuli that we cannot yet identify is one of fear – as indexed by an exaggerated startle response.

Let's return to our children with sensory superpowers. We can think of one's body as one example of an environment. Children with pain have been shown to have a similar pattern of over-reaction to safety signals, in this case, safe body sensations: that is the essence of the fear avoidance model of pain that we have been discussing. The goal of Chapter 2 was to explain how FBI reframes this sensitivity into a superpower. By creating a playful context of curiosity, we intend to change the initial startle response to a body sensation and set the stage for all the activities that we do in FBI – Pain Division.

Thus, one interesting thing that we are attempting to do in FBI – Pain Division is to see if we can retrain that initial unconscious evaluation of a stimulus: rather than being viewed as threatening, it is viewed as interesting. More specifically, in the case of children with sensory superpowers, body sensations are perceived as potentially threatening. Given a child's history of pain, it would make sense that a child's system could go into a defense mode of responding when the child thought they were experiencing a body sensation they consciously or unconsciously perceived to be associated with or predictive of pain – even if the majority of time these conclusions were incorrect. The child's system has become risk averse, continually bracing itself for the possibility of pain. Better safe than sorry.

In Chapter 2, we discussed the superpower "Spellbinding Powers of Perception." We discussed how one of the strategies of FBI is to teach children a vast and diverse array of body sensations and to associate each distinct sensation with playful characters. Not only does this include a variety of types of pain, e.g., Harold the Hunger Pain, but also sensations that accompany positive emotions and relaxing body experiences. The intention is to make scary sensations more playful and pleasant sensations more salient. In fact, the last three sessions are all about positive and relaxing sensations – ending the treatment with joyous investigations about joyous sensations.

Our intention is that with practice – the regular rehearsal of reviewing each character on the Body Clues Worksheet – children learn to view body sensations as interesting clues, thereby subverting the initial preconscious alarm system.

An Expert FBI Agent's Complex Vocabulary of Pain

Agents from FBI – Pain Division will come to know more about different types of pain than the overwhelming majority of mere mortals. LuLu the Laughing Pain, Patricia the Poop Pain, Harold the Hunger Pain, Ella the Emotional Pain, Harriet Headache, Sore Muscle Stan, Polly Pain, Gassy Gus – not to mention the characters the children come up with – all represent different aspects of pain experience. In fact, by the time the child has graduated as an elite FBI agent, they will have learned more than 50 different sensations! Each sensation is a funny character, and each character can communicate different meanings that need to be investigated, presenting multiple opportunities to forge new memory pathways for each sensation signal.

Think of this analogy. Imagine that every time you ate peanut butter, you had it with strawberry jelly. Year after year, sandwich after sandwich. Then, you attended a culinary academy where you learned innumerable combinations with peanut butter: peanut butter with honey; with bacon and Sriracha sauce; with marshmallow fluff – and so on – so many combinations and some of them oh so silly. Whereas before peanut butter evoked one memory: strawberry jelly, now your brain has so many options to reminiscence about – and the fact that some of them are silly makes the old boring peanut butter and strawberry jelly pairing less automatically recollected. Thus, with over 50 sensations, all of them interesting, all of them having different meanings depending on the context, the goal is an automatic reaction of curiosity no matter which sensation the child notices first.

To understand why this may be the case, consider this interesting study led by our friend and colleague Dr. Kevin LaBar at Duke University, an expert in fear learning and memory. Dr. LaBar studies, among other things, strategies that could help people learn that something that once was fearful is now safe.

To explore this, Dr. LaBar and colleagues designed an interesting experiment using virtual reality environments.[4] Individuals learned that encountering certain people in these virtual reality environments would sometimes be followed by an electrical shock (at a safe level, of course). That was the fear-learning phase. Then, in the extinction phase, participants experienced that same virtual person in many different virtual reality scenes, but that person was never followed by a shock. What Dr. LaBar and his colleagues found was that the fear memories were less likely to be remembered when a person learned that there were no longer any shocks across multiple settings – experiencing multiple situations with no shock was the key to extinguishing fear. So back to FBI – Pain Division. With over 50 sensations and hundreds of different body investigations that we perform in all kinds of contexts, we are strengthening memories that the body is interesting and wicked smart, and weakening or eliminating fear associations.

> "A key strategy for enhancing fear extinction is to contextualize the threatening experience to a specific time and place and to generalize safety learning across various environmental settings."
>
> *Dr. Kevin LaBar, Duke University*

An Expert FBI Agent's Investigations of Body Sensations

What we have described so far in FBI – Pain Division can be considered a playful form of psychoeducation, an important part of many psychological interventions. However, there is an even more powerful tool at our disposal – a technique referred to as interoceptive exposures. Interoceptive exposures are strategies that have been developed to treat various forms of anxiety-related psychopathology such as panic disorder or social phobia, but more recently, these strategies have also been employed in the context of pain disorders.[5] What happens in therapeutic interoceptive exposure exercises is that the therapist guides the patient to try to intentionally provoke a sensation that is feared, such as an uncomfortable feeling in their gut, and then to observe what happens. Via this experience of a feared sensation in a new context – the safety of a therapy session – and with a new outcome – nothing dangerous occurred – a new memory has been created in which a gut sensation that had been feared is now experienced as non-threatening (a new association: peanut-butter with bacon and Sriracha).

Typically, therapies of this nature are designed for older adolescents and adults, age groups that have the cognitive maturation to be able to articulate their feared beliefs and make predictions about the likelihood of future harm from an event. In interoceptive exposure exercises, there is a deliberate creation of what is referred to as an expectancy violation. The therapist works with a patient to determine what they think will happen in a given situation. Then, they conduct an interoceptive exposure activity that is designed to violate those expectancies.

For example, imagine that I believe that every time I get winded, I will faint. As a result, I avoid all kinds of exercise including taking the stairs. I even walk very slowly so as not to breathe heavily. My expectation is that if I raise my heart rate and my exertion to a level at which I am breathing heavily, that soon I'll be down on the ground. This is an ideal setting for potentially potent interoceptive exposures. In the safety of a therapy session with a trusted therapist, I would engage in activities that provoke this feared sensation, heavy breathing, and then observe what happens. After repeated trials in which I keep breathing heavily and no fainting occurs, my brain now has a dilemma. When the sensation of windedness occurs, rather than one possible outcome, fainting, there is another possible outcome – nothing happens. In fact, if the *nothing happened* outcome occurred a thousand times and the fainting outcome only happened once or even only in my imagination, then the association of heavy breathing with nothing happening would be a lot more salient and easily accessible in my memory.

And there is even more learning occurring than simply disassociating heavy breathing and fainting. Exposure therapists cannot (and therefore should not) promise that the feared outcome will *never* occur. After all, I might have indeed fainted once in the context of heavy breathing! Avoidance serves several functions. Not only does it maintain distance between the anxious person and the feared outcome, but it also seemingly protects individuals from the discomfort of uncertainty. If I stay far away from heavy breathing, I can feel confident that I will not faint. Moreover, I never have to test whether I can cope with feeling faint. Therefore, exposure work also teaches the brain that one can tolerate uncertainty (about both the feared outcome occurring and whether I will be OK if it does) and the discomfort that comes along with it. It can even teach that if the worst happens, and I feel faint or do faint, that I can survive, cope, and bounce back. For all these reasons, exposure techniques are considered one of the most powerful therapeutic tools ever developed in psychology!

The technical name for the form of learning that occurs during exposure treatment is called inhibitory learning.[6,7,8] Inhibitory learning layers new associations (that bad things do not always happen when a feared stimulus is experienced, and that tolerance of uncertainty and coping are possible) on top of old associations (that the stimulus portends bad things), decreasing the "volume" and power of the feared associations over time. A prominent figure in this line of research is Dr. Michelle Craske, an authority in understanding the mechanisms whereby treatments for anxiety disorders exert their effects and an expert consultant for us in developing the FBI intervention.[9]

> The science of interoceptive exposures has been led by the work of Dr. Michelle Craske, a Professor of Psychology, Psychiatry, and Behavioral Sciences and the Miller Endowed Chair at the University of California, Los Angeles. Dr. Craske is an expert consultant for the FBI – Pain Division intervention and is one of our heroes.

Thus, the essence of interoceptive exposures is creating neutral, positive, and even triumphant memories that compete with fear-based memories. These new memories, if practiced repeatedly, eventually become more accessible to recall and helpful in facilitating extinction – the process of learning to discriminate that a given stimulus is no longer or is not dangerous.

Creating New Memories: Seeking Out Adventures

There are several strategies that we use in FBI that are designed to create and strengthen the accessibility of playful associations with body sensations. The body investigations that we conduct in FBI are our child-friendly versions of interoceptive exposure activities. There are a few important differences relative to interoceptive exposure activities that have been designed for adolescents or adults. The first important difference is that we do not expect children to have access to or to be able to articulate feared beliefs about their bodies. Thus, we are not designing these interoceptive exposures to disprove an entrenched or impairing belief. Instead, we refer to interceptive exposure activities in FBI as "acceptance-based." What we mean by this is that we are nonjudgmental and inquisitive about anything that happens during the course of a body investigation – rather than trying to prove or disprove something. Body investigations in FBI are designed to provoke a variety of body sensations, some of which may have been previously viewed as threatening, and to perform such provocations in a playful context in which we learn something new about the body. The outcome of an FBI Body Investigation is akin to "Wow, I did not know my body did that, or Well, isn't that interesting." Instead of "Well, I guess that feared outcome that I believed would surely occur may not occur." Through this stance, children learn to meet uncertainty with curiosity and lightness rather than anxiety. They also learn that not only can they merely cope, but they even have superhuman powers!

Where possible, we do set up expectancy violations when designing our investigations. These expectancy violations showcase numerous (and seemingly limitless) examples of how wise the body is, how strong the body is, and how important it is to tune into your body to investigate all its mysteries. For example, it may be that a child runs faster than they thought they could, even when their gut was feeling uncomfortable (because they deliberately tightened a belt too tight as part of an interoceptive experiment); it may be investigating whether muscles get stronger with practice; it may be exploring what activities or circumstances bring out the most butterflies. While all FBI Body Investigations are designed to demonstrate the body's wisdom, some of these investigations will also be in the form of an expectancy violation if the child makes a prediction that is different from what actually occurs. Thus, at the beginning of a body investigation, we encourage the child to make a prediction about what they think their body will do – how many times their heart will speed up if they start running, whether they can do more push-ups with practice, etc. There is never a right or wrong answer. However, finding the answer demands an experience with the body, and via that experience, we learn something about the body.

To ensure that these messages of body wisdom are, in fact, being internalized as intended, we summarize what we learned from each body investigation on the child's Body Map. As you will learn more about in Session 1 (and was briefly introduced in Chapter 1), a Body Map is a silhouette of the child's body that is used to document all the body's wisdom that has been learned via Body Investigations and homework. This Body Map will serve as a concrete reminder of all that was learned throughout the course of the therapy. Table 4.1 lists the basic components of a Body Investigation conducted in FBI – Pain Division.

Table 4.1 Components of a Sample Body Investigation

1. Each session starts off with the ritual of a Henry Heartbeat Investigation (introduced in Session 1).
   a. In a Henry Heartbeat Investigation, everyone learns something about the wisdom of their heartbeat – how it is smart enough to adapt the strength of its pumping to help everyone manage a variety of situations. Children also learn that they can choose to engage in certain activities that raise or lower their heartbeat. One mystery that is often explored in a Henry Heartbeat Investigation is what those activities are.
   b. A typical investigation has the child choose two activities to compare – to see which one raises their heartbeat more and/or to see how accurate their predictions are about how much their heart will go up when they perform a certain activity.
   c. Investigations are conducted as "scientifically" as possible. In between heart-raising activities, the child will choose an activity that lowers the heartbeat. This is often an additional investigation that can be performed at the same time – seeing how long it takes the heartbeat to get back to baseline.
   d. Via any investigation, the child is practicing tuning into their body and listening to their body sensations with curiosity. Thus, it is crucial that the child (NOT the parent) do the counting. It is less important that they get the right answer. It is much more important that they practice listening. No devices should be used and whatever the child gives as the answer is the answer. It is their experience.
   e. In a typical heart rate experiment, the child will take their pulse to get a baseline (the parent and therapist can certainly help the child find their pulse) for a set increment of time (usually 10 seconds). Then, they perform activity number 1 for a set interval (e.g., one minute of jumping jacks). Then they take their pulse for 10 seconds. Then they bring their heartbeat back to baseline using the activity they choose (e.g., taking deep breaths and checking their pulse every 30 seconds to see how long it takes to get back down). They then repeat this with activity number 2.
   f. After an investigation, they will have learned a few things about their body. Each of those lessons need to be recorded on their Body Map. This is critical to help consolidate that new lesson about the wisdom of the body.
   g. To make sure this lesson is strongly stamped in memory, the family also comes up with a summary of what was learned about the wisdom of the body. For example, a lesson could be: My heart is smart. It adapts how hard it beats to help me get through any situation.
   h. We then add this lesson to the Body Map as well.
2. Typically, two to three investigations are performed each session, usually based on the new body sensations characters that were learned that session. In every session, we provide examples of investigations and body lessons.
3. Each investigation is designed to try to notice that sensation, often after some type of manipulation that is designed to bring on that sensation.
4. Because it is an investigation, there is typically a question or mystery we are exploring. Do I feel Gerda Gotta Go after I drink 5 ounces/ ml of water? 10 ounces/ml? What happens to Ricky the Rock if I apologize for something that I did? What makes my muscles more tired – doing push-ups for 30 seconds or staying in a plank position for 30 seconds?
5. What is learned is added to the Body Map and the relevant wisdom of the body is summarized.

Designing In-the-Moment Investigations

During a typical day of someone with sensory superpowers, there are numerous opportunities to design and engage in a variety of body investigations. Rather than intentionally provoking body sensations, these investigations take advantage of a sensation that is already being experienced; children would then proceed with an experiment and see what happens. For example, some children may have a diurnal pattern to their pain in which they get stomach aches in the mornings, pain that complicates school attendance. In this situation, we help parents and children design in-the-moment investigations that capitalize on the tenets of inhibitory learning. For this example, the child may identify all the different body sensations they are feeling on their Body Clues Worksheet. Then, the child may make predictions about what they expect to happen to these sensations by the time recess happens. They can bring along their Body Journal (the little notebook they are given during the first session to record the various wisdoms of the body) and document what happened. In this investigation, they are just watching what happens. On another day, they might try a manipulation: like counting the number of Betty Butterflies at the beginning of every class, taking a few deep breaths in between classes, doing some things to get Henry Heartbeat up at recess – and then seeing what happens to the body sensations they noticed before school. The lists are endless.

Applying an acceptance-based framework to these investigations means that we are non-judgmental and curious about what we learn. We do not have a set agenda or belief we are trying to disprove (e.g., like proving that Polly the Pain will get better at recess). That could be a question that we ask and that would be an interesting investigation. However, whatever happens will be interesting and will be added to the Body Map. One can imagine if every day the parents and children design a new investigation or keep repeating a prior investigation, there are a lot of new memory pathways and associations with morning abdominal sensations – they are not just threatening stimuli that necessitate retreating to the safety of one's room rather than going to school. These sensations can mean lots of interesting things. These new memories reinforce that the body is wicked smart.

Creating New Memories: Reflecting on Challenging Situations

There is one final strategy that we use to reinforce the parent and child's confidence and belief that their bodies are very wise: we reflect on big moments with big sensations and see what we can learn from them. As discussed in Chapter 3, we have learned that we can design a body investigation in which we intentionally provoke sensations. We can also create an investigation on-the-fly when we are faced with a situation that may be tough for the child to approach. We can also use the steps in our Body Clues Worksheet to review what happened, how our bodies were feeling when it was happening, what our bodies were trying to tell us, how we tried to listen to the messages our bodies were communicating, and how it went. Parents are instructed to pull out a worksheet and work through it with their child after they just had a big event or as a way to review their day. We remind everyone of this in this chapter because what we are doing via that review is putting our creative and investigative context around that intense moment so that what is remembered is not how intense that moment was, but rather how very very smart we are.

I have a very vivid memory of one of the first family sessions that I led with the FBI – Pain Division protocol. We were performing a Henry Heartbeat activity (the activity introduced in Table 4.1). It was the first time that this child had deliberately paid attention to their heartbeat, performed an activity, and counted how their heartbeat increased from the activity that they had chosen (running). They found this whole exercise, how they could choose to do certain activities, how they could observe the influence of these activities on their heart beat, how they had the power to actively manipulate their heart rate with their own actions – so exciting that they literally starting bouncing up and down with joy. As treatment progressed, they were able to notice their heartbeat and label what it was telling them (was it part of their excitement? nervousness?). After verifying what they felt in that moment, they selected an activity from their Body Clues Worksheet, a worksheet that helps you choose activities to try when you are feeling certain things. In this particular moment, they decided that Henry Heartbeat was telling them that they were feeling happy and excited. What activity can one do when one is already feeling happy and excited? Well, you dance, of course. So, this aspiring FBI agent chose to dance to further accentuate the excitement they were feeling and off we went into a dance routine. To get into the headspace of the body's amazing capacities, we need to inculcate the awe of a five-year-old.

References

1. LeDoux, J. (1996). *The Emotional Brain: The Mysterious Underpinnings of Emotional Life*. New York, NY: Simon & Schuster.

2. Méndez-Bértolo, C., Moratti, S., Toledano, R., et al. (2016). A fast pathway for fear in human amygdala. *Nat Neurosci 19*(8), 1041–1049. https://doi.org/10.1038/nn.4324

3. Lissek, S., Rabin, S.J., McDowell, D.J., et al. (2009). Impaired discriminative fear-conditioning resulting from elevated fear responding to learned safety cues among individuals with panic disorder. *Behav Res Ther 47*(2), 111–118. https://doi.org/10.1016/j.brat.2008.10.017

4. Dunsmoor, J.E., Ahs, F., Zielinski, D.J., et al. (2014). Extinction in multiple virtual reality contexts diminishes fear reinstatement in humans. *Neurobiol Learn Mem 113*, 157–164. https://doi.org/10.1016/j.nlm.2014.02.010

5. Craske, M.G., Treanor, M., Conway, C.C., et al. (2014). Maximizing exposure therapy: an inhibitory learning approach. *Behav Res Ther 58*, 10–23. https://doi.org/10.1016/j.brat.2014.04.006

6. Bouton, M.E. (1993). Context, time, and memory retrieval in the interference paradigms of Pavlovian learning. *Psychol Bull 114*(1), 80–99. https://doi.org/10.1037/0033-2909.114.1.80

7. Craske, M.G., Wolitzky-Taylor, K.B., Labus, J., et al. (2011). A cognitive-behavioral treatment for irritable bowel syndrome using interoceptive exposure to visceral sensations. *Behav Res Ther 49*(6–7), 413–421. https://doi.org/10.1016/j.brat.2011.04.001

8. LaBar, K.S., Phelps, E.A. (2005). Reinstatement of conditioned fear in humans is context-dependent and impaired in amnesia. *Behav Neurosci 119*(3), 677–686. https://doi.org/10.1037/0735-7044.119.3.677

9. Zucker, N., Mauro, C., Craske, M., et al. (2017). Acceptance-based interoceptive exposure for young children with functional abdominal pain. *Behav Res Ther 97*, 200–212. https://doi.org/10.1016/j.brat.2017.07.009

The Medical Evaluation of Abdominal Pain in Children – One General Pediatrician's Approach

Chapter 5

In my 35 years as a practicing pediatrician (MG), I saw many children for abdominal pain. This chapter provides a brief overview of my approach to evaluating abdominal pain in children aged 5 to 11 years old (pre-pubertal). This outline is not meant to be comprehensive or exhaustive, and it assumes its readers are clinical providers with training in the medical evaluation of children. We hope that its inclusion will help to provide a structure for excluding medical causes prior to starting the FBI treatment program. However, we include this caveat: your own clinical judgement must be your guide; no outline can substitute for your own evaluation of an individual patient.

Introduction

Children often complain of abdominal pain. Sometimes abdominal pain is the chief reason for a visit to the doctor; at other times, families bring it up in the context of the annual check-up. No matter how the pain presents, we need to be thorough and methodical in determining its cause.

Although arriving at the correct diagnosis is always our object, this goal is particularly important in the context of implementing the FBI treatment program. Why? Because the FBI program treats children whose pain does not stem from physical causes. We must exclude medical causes prior to starting the program, and we must also pay attention to any symptoms suggesting a new, medical cause of abdominal pain while implementing the FBI methods. Remember: even a child who has functional abdominal pain can develop appendicitis or constipation! Therefore, even after starting the FBI program, we must always keep our eyes and ears attuned to any new or different symptoms that children may develop.

Let's begin. Although the differential diagnosis of abdominal pain is quite broad, a systematic approach to making the diagnosis narrows down the cause to a few possibilities – even within the standard 15-minute outpatient visit.

The first thing I always try to establish is whether the pain is acute or chronic. Acute causes generally necessitate immediate action, whereas chronic problems often require a careful sequential work-up over time.

The History

As with any medical problem, a thorough history forms the foundation for making the diagnosis. Stick with the classic questions, as follows in Table 5.1.

The Physical Exam

Once you have gotten this history, you should have a pretty good image in your head of what this child's pain is like, and you will have determined whether it is an acute problem or a chronic one. Now it's time for the physical exam.

The most important thing to look at first is the growth chart. The appearance of the growth chart offers a fork in the road in your evaluation of any child: **you should be worried about any child who is falling off in weight or in height because such a child is much more likely to have a significant underlying medical problem.** Conversely, the preservation of linear growth and weight gain offers reassurance (although not certainty) regarding a serious underlying medical issue.

Next comes the actual physical exam. It is extremely important to do a thorough physical exam, because systemic problems can manifest as abdominal pain. For example, a child with fever and a stomach ache may actually have streptococcal pharyngitis, or a child with chronic pain and diarrhea may have anal fistulae that signify inflammatory bowel disease. Doing a cursory or perfunctory exam can rob you of important clues to your diagnosis.

Pay particular attention to the following features of the general physical exam (Table 5.2).

And now for the abdominal exam. Children are often apprehensive about abdominal exams, especially if they are having pain. They worry that you will make them hurt more. In addition, if you push down quickly and firmly on the abdomen, and there is any gas present, then you will actually cause pain by having the gas quickly distend the intestine after you lift your hand off; this can not only give you a false positive for pain but also make the child guard more during your exam. Therefore, take it easy with your exam. Make sure to warm your hands, ask the child where they hurt, start by pressing gently as far away as possible from the site of the pain, distract the child by making small talk, and work your way gently to the tender area. If pressing causes pain, confirm by pressing again once, gently, but don't press repeatedly. Another tip: if a child is just so anxious that he or she will not permit you to palpate the abdomen, put your stethoscope in your ears and use the stethoscope in your hand as the palpating instrument: children generally are not afraid of stethoscopes and you can often use this technique at least to determine whether a child has focal pain or not.

Table 5.1 Gathering a comprehensive history

1. The pain itself –
   - When did the pain start?
     - Has it changed since it started?
   - Where is the pain?
     - Does it move around?
   - Does it come and go, or is it constant?
   - How does it feel? (e.g., sharp, dull, burning, cramping)
   - How severe is the pain?
     - Does it wake the child from sleep? **Anything that awakens a child from sleep should be presumed to have a medical cause until proven otherwise.**
     - Does it interrupt activity? **If it does, this gives you a measure of the severity of the pain.**
   - What makes it better?
   - What makes it worse?
   - What things have you tried already?
   - Any association with any foods or activity?
2. "Fellow travelers" – a focused Review of Systems
   - Are there any other symptoms? (Fever, nausea, vomiting, diarrhea, constipation, urinary frequency, dysuria, rash, sore throat, decreased activity or energy, poor sleep).
   - Any change in appetite?
   - **Any weight loss** or weight gain?
   - Does anyone else at home have similar symptoms?
3. "The poop questions"
   - When was the last bowel movement, and what was it like (hard balls, lumpy logs, or smooth tubes)?
   - Is the stool brown, tan, white, green, or black?
   - Any blood in the stool?
4. Context
   - Any recent changes in this child's life? (School, home, pets, family)
   - Any environmental exposures? (Foreign travel, unsanitary water sources, e.g., rivers or streams, non-chlorinated water)
5. Past medical history
   - Any significant medical history? (Prematurity, illnesses severe enough to require hospitalization)
   - Any chronic medical problems?
   - Any past surgery?
6. Current medications
   - Is the child taking any medications or supplements that might cause abdominal pain?
7. Family history
   - Abdominal pain
   - Gastrointestinal disease
   - Chronic medical problems
   - Anxiety/depression
8. Things I haven't thought to ask –
   - "Is there anything else you and your child have noticed that you think is important?"
9. Things that have worried you –
   - "Is there something you want to make sure is NOT going on?"

Pay particular attention to the following on the abdominal exam:

Bloating/distention

Tenderness
   Generalized or focal?
   Make sure to distract the child during the exam to see if the tenderness resolves.

Hepatosplenomegaly

Mass(es)
   - Stool – firm balls or sausage-like masses in the LLQ; often you can actually break these up by pushing gently
   - Non-stool masses – masses elsewhere in the abdomen obviously raise the concern for malignancy; they require a prompt and extensive evaluation that is beyond the scope of our discussion here.

Table 5.2 Features to consider in a general physical exam

Vital signs
 - Fever
 - Hypertension
 - Tachycardia
 - Tachypnea
 - Abnormal pulse oximetry

General
 - Does the child look ill?
 - Can the child hop in place?
 - Can the child move around comfortably, getting on and off the exam table without pain?
 - Does the child look sad or anxious?

HEENT
 - Pharyngitis

Heart
 - New or changing murmur

Lungs
 - Wheezing, rales

Skin
 - Rashes

Ano-genital
 - Fistulae

Once you have taken a good history and done a good exam, you should have some ideas about the source of a child's abdominal pain. You will have determined if the problem is acute or chronic, and the physical findings (if any) should narrow the diagnosis down considerably. Let's walk through some of the most common diagnoses and how we arrive at them.

Acute Abdominal Pain: Differential Diagnosis

Here are some common causes of acute abdominal pain, with clinical features that I have found helpful.

Appendicitis
 - Appendicitis often begins as vague generalized pain that over the course of 24–48 hours localizes to the right lower quadrant; it is accompanied by fever, malaise, and lack of appetite but usually not by vomiting or diarrhea. On exam, these children are usually uncomfortable or may look quite ill. They have focal tenderness in the right lower quadrant. Keep in mind, however, that a perforated appendix will give generalized abdominal pain and often a diffusely tender abdomen on exam. It is important to be aware of BOTH presentations.

Mesenteric adenitis
 - Mimics the symptoms of appendicitis; may require CT scan or abdominal ultrasound to differentiate.

Gastroenteritis

- Can be bacterial dysentery or viral gastroenteritis. Vomiting, diarrhea, hematochezia, fever, pharyngitis, conjunctivitis, viral exanthems. Exam may show non-focal tenderness, pharyngitis, rash.

Streptococcal pharyngitis

- Generalized or epi-gastric abdominal pain, bright red throat, enlarged anterior cervical lymph nodes. May have scarlatina rash.

Urinary tract infection (UTI)

- Lower abdominal or flank pain, dysuria, frequency, foul-smelling urine, hematuria, +/− fever.

Type I diabetes mellitus

- Abdominal pain, polyuria, polydipsia, polyphagia, weight loss, malaise, nausea, vomiting. May or may not look ill.

Pancreatitis

- Epigastric pain, nausea, persistent vomiting.

Food poisoning

- Vomiting, diarrhea, +/− fever. Abdominal pain comes in cramping waves, often followed by vomiting and diarrhea.

Obstruction

- Acute onset of severe persistent vomiting, often bilious. No fever. Generalized abdominal tenderness and guarding. Child looks ill.

Ovarian torsion

- Although ovarian torsion is more common after puberty, it **can** occur in pre-pubertal girls. Torsion presents with acute onset of severe lower abdominal pain, nausea, and vomiting; there is unilateral focal tenderness on exam; a palpable mass may or may not be present.

Asthma flare or pneumonia

- Now you are probably wondering why I put this diagnosis in here and whether I did so mistakenly: I did not. Small children who cannot get enough air because of an asthma attack can present with a complaint of acute abdominal pain. Such children may look as if they are in no distress, but on exam they will be moving very little air; once they receive a nebulized beta-agonist, you will hear air movement as well as wheezes and rales; the abdominal pain will be gone. Children with pneumonia can also present with a complaint of abdominal pain. Pneumonia in the lower lobes causes diaphragmatic irritation, which can manifest as upper abdominal pain; these children will have focal rales present on exam, giving a clue to the true diagnosis.

Chronic Abdominal Pain: Differential Diagnosis

Just as we outlined some common causes of acute abdominal pain in children, we can also summarize some common causes of chronic abdominal pain with their associated clinical features, as follows:

Constipation

Constipation is one of the most common but also most over-looked causes of chronic abdominal pain. If you mention constipation as a possible cause, be prepared for the parents to dismiss this as a possibility. They will often say, "no, my child has a bowel movement every day." People do not realize that it is possible to be "regular" while still being quite backed up with stool. You must ask about the quality of the bowel movements. If they are quite large, quite firm, or even stopping up the toilet, then constipation is a real possibility. On occasion, you may have to order a plain film of the abdomen in order to prove or disprove the presence of large amounts of stool in the abdomen.

Lactose Intolerance

I again find that parents often immediately dismiss this diagnosis as a possibility. They typically tell me that their child eats something like pizza all the time without any problem. I then explain that lactose intolerance is not "all-or-nothing," that symptoms occur when children eat more lactose than their systems can digest. I then ask parents to stop all lactose for a week to see if the pain goes away. If it does, then we gradually add lactose back into the diet until symptoms return.

Gastroesophageal Reflux Disease

Children can have gastroesophageal reflux disease (GERD) symptoms for years without appreciating that what they are feeling is abnormal. You must specifically ask about excessive burping, tasting "throw-up" in the throat, and having epigastric pain – the latter especially at night when lying down. The pain may be triggered by acidic or spicy foods. GERD can also present with episodic vomiting.

Celiac Disease

Celiac most often presents with vague abdominal pain, sometimes accompanied by constipation or short stature. In addition to classic celiac disease (with positive antibodies) some children have antibody-negative gluten sensitivity; they may benefit from gluten-free diets.

Inflammatory Bowel Disease

Inflammatory bowel disease (IBD) presents with chronic abdominal pain that is often accompanied by diarrhea. Diarrhea may contain gross or occult blood. The physical exam may show weight loss, loss of linear height velocity, and/or peri-anal fistulae.

Irritable Bowel Syndrome

Irritable bowel syndrome (IBS) is one of the most common causes of chronic abdominal pain but unfortunately is a clinical diagnosis, without any specific physical findings or laboratory abnormalities. The pain is vague, non-focal, and non-specific. There can be different patterns of constipation, diarrhea, or both, often accompanied by bloating. Symptoms can worsen with different foods or with stress.

Abdominal Migraine

Recurrent distinct episodes of vague abdominal pain, with associated nausea, vomiting, headache, and/or pallor; often accompanied by a family history of migraine.

Giardia Infection

This parasite infection is not common but still must be considered in anyone with a history of foreign travel or of drinking unsanitary water; patients complain of vague chronic abdominal pain, sometimes triggered by lactose-containing products, with associated diarrhea and sometimes weight loss.

Peptic Ulcer Disease

Peptic ulcer disease (PUD) is uncommon in children but still important to bear in mind. It is typified by epigastric pain that is relieved by eating, and may be accompanied by melena.

The Diagnostic Work-Up

Now that you have completed a good history and physical exam, you should consider what testing, if any, would be appropriate. Your differential diagnosis should determine your specific testing.

Acute abdominal pain requires immediate action. Depending on your concerns, you may do a strep test, urinalysis, complete blood count, metabolic panel, flat plate of the abdomen, abdominal ultrasound, or abdominal CT scan.

Chronic abdominal pain generates a more step-wise approach that starts with some basic screening labs. If the history I have taken elicits no "red flags" that suggest an acute problem or a specific chronic cause, and the general physical exam is normal, I find the following screening labs useful.

Complete Blood Count with Differential

Look for anemia suggesting chronic blood loss, elevated white blood cell count suggesting infection or inflammation. Obviously, any other abnormalities such as abnormal platelet count or abnormal white blood cell pattern would force you to consider a much wider differential than we have discussed here.

Testing for Occult Blood in Stool

Guaiac testing (three samples obtained on three different days) is important to rule out occult blood loss. The presence of occult blood in the stool would necessitate further evaluation of possible organic causes, e.g., inflammatory bowel disease or peptic ulcer disease.

Complete Metabolic Panel

Elevated serum glucose indicates diabetes mellitus. Look as well for elevated liver function tests indicating occult liver dysfunction, or elevated creatinine from occult renal disease.

Urinalysis

Look for glycosuria, proteinuria, hematuria, pyuria, and bacteriuria.

C-reactive Protein (CRP) and Sedimentation Rates (ESR)

If either of these is elevated, you need to consider inflammatory bowel disease.

Tissue Transglutaminase IgA Antibodies (tTG IgA)

If these antibodies are positive, then you need to pursue a further evaluation for celiac disease. Make sure that your lab includes a total serum IgA level, since IgA deficiency can cause the tTG IgA antibodies to be falsely low and therefore mask the deficiency found in celiac disease.

Flat Plate of Abdomen (KUB)

Occasionally needed if you feel certain that constipation is playing a role but the family needs more evidence of increased stool burden.

Stool for Giardia Antigen

Useful if there has been any history of foreign travel or ingestion of unchlorinated water.

Summing It All Up

If your history generates no "red flags," growth chart is normal, exam is completely normal, and your screening labs are normal, then it is reasonable to make the diagnosis of functional abdominal pain and to begin the FBI program. If at any point in the initial work-up or during the treatment, a child's symptoms, growth, or exam changes, then you must ask yourself if the diagnosis should be re-considered or if a new source of abdominal pain has developed.

Further Reading

There are many excellent resources, including textbooks and journal articles, that discuss the medical evaluation of abdominal pain in children. The following review articles are ones I think particularly helpful to those in primary care.

Acute Abdominal Pain

The following article offers a comprehensive review of both common and uncommon causes of acute abdominal pain, broken down by age group and by clinical urgency.

Neuman, M.I. (2022). Causes of acute abdominal pain in children and adolescents. UpToDate. Literature review current through November 2022. This topic was last updated: April 8, 2022.

The following detailed review further breaks down the etiology of acute abdominal pain by age group and gives attention to what imaging studies are helpful in making diagnoses.

Baker, R.D. (2018). Acute abdominal pain. *Pediatr Rev 39*(3), 130–138

Chronic Abdominal Pain

The following text is a superb, comprehensive review of the etiology of chronic abdominal pain as well as of its multiple causes. It includes excellent tables delineating the symptoms and physical findings that would increase concern for underlying organic disease. It also discusses what lab tests might be helpful and when to order them.

Fishman, M.B., Aronson, M.D., & Chacko, M.R. Chronic abdominal pain in children and adolescents: Approach to the evaluation. UpToDate. Literature review current through November 2022. This topic was last updated: April 1, 2022.

In addition to reviewing organic causes and "red flags" for organic disease, the following article focuses on the pathophysiology of functional abdominal pain and its treatment.

Hyman, P.E. (2016). Chronic and recurrent abdominal pain. *Pediatr Rev 37*(9), 377–389

Session 1: Initiation into Feeling and Body Investigators

And may your limits be unknown
And may your efforts be your own
Be Still by The Killers

From here on out, all remaining chapters have a similar structure. We will explain and demonstrate how FBI – Pain Division is implemented session by session. This chapter will cover the following material:

1. A session outline
2. Recommended session materials
3. A discussion on therapist demeanor, attitude, and behavior
4. A step-by-step guide through the session with sample dialogues
5. A Q&A section with questions we have encountered from clinicians

This first session presents an overview of FBI to both the parent and child, and so contains more material than the sessions that follow. Accordingly, this session will also be a bit longer than the others. When we use the term FBI, we are referring to FBI – Pain Division.

Outline for Session 1

1. Introduce the parent to the rationale and framework of FBI: Their child as a sensitive human being with sensory superpowers (Chapter 2)
2. Discuss the parent's own experience with pain and sensory sensitivities, if applicable, and opportunities to "start over" as a parent, role model, and learner (Chapter 3)
3. Introduce the child to the concept of body detectives and sensory superpowers (Chapter 2)
4. Create a body map to consolidate the lessons learned in body investigations (Chapter 4)
5. Learn the body sensations for this session (an overview of a collection of different sensations without a specific theme to give everyone a jump start into the program) (Chapter 4)
6. Conduct your first body investigation (Chapter 4)
7. Complete your first Body Brainstorms worksheet (Chapter 1)
8. Home practice: Pick two body sensations to monitor over the next week for practice

Materials for Session 1

Large paper roll (such as butcher paper) to outline the child's body outline to create a body map

Markers to draw on the body map

A small journal for homework assignments

Workbook pages, Session 1 (Part III)

Body Brainstorms Worksheet 1 (Part III)

Optional Prizes: A detective hat, a bag to keep all supplies (https://fbikids.org for ordering information)

Optional Button: Gassy Gus (https://fbikids.org for Ordering Information)

Therapist Demeanor, Attitude, and Behavior

As in all interpersonal psychotherapies, there are several within-session, relationship-based channels through which a therapist can influence a client's behavior and encourage positive change. Simply, there is the content of what is said, the process by which it is said, and there are all the nonverbal behaviors and interactions between a client and a therapist. In FBI – Pain Division, the therapist has an additional mechanism: the therapist acts as a role model, reacting to both sensations that they experience in their own bodies and their client's reported sensory experiences in a manner that demonstrates the playful curiosity that we are trying to inculcate in parent and child. To the extent possible, the therapist joins with the parent and child in performing or facilitating somatically focused activities, demonstrates a willingness to be interviewed by the child about their own intense somatic experiences, and exhibits a calm and inquisitive demeanor when the child displays an intense emotion or somatic sensation.

When the child reports an intense sensation (including pain), some examples of leading sentence strings that illustrate this stance include:

Isn't that interesting!? I wonder what would happen if we did X or Y?

Wow! That was unexpected! Has that ever happened to you before? What did you do? What should we try?

Tell me more about it. Do we have a name for it yet? Do we need to think of a new character?

As you will see throughout the sample dialogues, the therapist capitalizes on all opportunities to model how a parent would respond to their child outside of sessions, and to shape a child's own internal dialogue about their somatic and emotional experiences. Essentially, the FBI therapist is always demonstrating how a body investigator behaves when faced with a complex clue.

The most critical element of this stance is having fun while being effective. If you are not, that is an excellent signal for you to do your own investigation about what your needs are in that moment (or prior to a session). In the spirit of self-parenting, it may be a good idea to tune in to what your body is telling you and address your needs so that you have the energy and vitality to be a fully engaged FBI agent. Our work can be exhausting. Role modeling how we key into our own needs and respond to them when those moments arise is an incredibly powerful learning opportunity for both the children and their parents. If you are personally having a low energy session, announce that and turn it into an investigation for everybody!

Session 1 Step-by-Step Content
Introduce the Parent to the Rationale and Framework for FBI

A strong predictor of the success of any intervention is whether the patient believes in the rationale of the intervention and has confidence in the person delivering it. To lay this foundation, FBI – Pain Division begins with a conversation with the parent alone.

Typically, the child plays or reads in view while the adults talk. (It is becoming easier and easier to get privacy given the number of children with headphones …)

The purpose of this conversation is the following:

1. To ensure that the therapist and parent have a shared understanding not only of the child's difficulties with pain, but also with sensory and interoceptive sensitivities more broadly;

2. To validate the parent about the challenges of parenting a child with these sensitivities;

3. To change the framework for the parent so that these sensitivities are viewed, in part, as a wondrous gift; and

4. To give the parents a chance for themselves be seen and heard in describing their own experiences with sensitivities. As FBI – Pain Division involves the parent–child dyad, it is an opportunity for both parents and children to learn and for parents, perhaps, to heal.

To start, we provide you with a sample conversation between an FBI therapist and a parent. Then, we break this dialogue down piece by piece so you understand the core elements that were communicated.

Key Take-Home Message

As you read these chapters about session content and format, what is important is that you understand the spirit of the messages being communicated and the overall principles and philosophy of FBI – Pain Division. Never be concerned about saying things in a certain way. The art of delivering this therapy is that you are also having fun while administering it. It is hard to have fun if you are worried about memorizing your lines.

Moment of Reflection

The first time you read through this dialogue, imagine that you are the parent of a child who has had recurrent episodes of abdominal pain that cause the child great distress. It is indescribable to see your child in pain and to feel helpless that you do not know what to do to help your child manage that pain. You may further imagine what it would be like to be a parent with their own history of pain and thus having the added distress of not wanting your child to go through what you have been through. Try to imagine how hearing this dialogue would make you feel. That will help you understand the essence of what we are trying to communicate to distressed parents in this situation.

Sample Dialogue 6.1: Introducing the Framework and Intention of FBI – Pain Division to Parents

THERAPIST:

Hi there. I'm Dr. Pain Therapist. I'm really looking forward to working with you and your child, Sam. I wanted to speak with you alone for a few minutes so I could give you a bit more information about the treatment and answer any questions you may have. Before I get started, are there any questions that you wanted to ask me?

– Address parent questions as an initial demonstration that we want parents to feel seen and heard.

So, I want to talk to you a bit about children with pain in general. Then, I want to hear from you about what aspects of what I describe sound like your child and which do not.

We think of children with pain as sensitive children and we mean that in a literal way and in a beautiful way. We mean that they are sensitive because they may notice sensations in their body at a level that other children may not notice, or may experience these things more intensely than other children may experience them. The formal name for this is 'visceral hypersensitivity'. Simply, what this means is children who experience frequent pain feel things strongly and deeply – and we suspect that this includes not only things in their body but things in the world around them. One way to think of this is that they are sensory and emotional sponges that soak up everything in the world around them. Quite frankly, this makes them wonderfully sweet and sensitive children – the future artists, scientists, and innovators of the world.

Rather than thinking about this sensitivity as a weakness or vulnerability, the purpose and goal of the FBI intervention is to appreciate this sensitivity as a gift – a beautiful gift that allows your children to feel things deeply, care about others deeply, and live life out loud! The world of a sensitive child has a level of richness and pizzazz that children without those sensitivities do not get to experience in the same way.

Which parts of this sound like your child and which parts are different?

– Allow the parent time to reflect on their own experience of their child and to think about and discuss this formulation as it relates to their child's sensitivity to experiences – including pain.

I wonder, do any of these descriptions sound like you or your child's other parent?

> Allow the parent time to reflect and share their own personal examples of this. As noted in Chapter 3, parents of children with frequent pain may have their own challenges and histories with pain. Thus, it is crucial that we witness and validate the parent's experiences as they take the opportunities provided by FBI to improve their own self-parenting. Doing so ensures that they are the best equipped to help their child. Give them the time they need. It is a critical investment.

Our goal for your child is that we want them to feel safe in their bodies. We want them to know and believe that their bodies are smart and tough. We want them to feel confident that they can listen to what their bodies are telling them and know what to do. Thus, when they notice something, such as pain, rather than being afraid or letting pain get in their way, they can be little investigators who ask: "Hmm? What is the pain telling me? What might be an interesting investigation to try?"

Children with pain often try to silence or ignore what their bodies are telling them (Figure 6.1). While this makes sense, this ignoring can also get in the way of learning important things about their body and learning to trust their body. Children are just figuring out what their bodies are trying to say. For example, if they notice a sensation in their gut, they have to figure out: is this a hunger pain? Is it butterflies in my tummy? Does my tummy have a knot in it? They then have to figure out what that sensation means. Am I hungry? Anxious? Dreading something? Ultimately, these important body messages let us know what is going on with ourselves so we can figure out what to do. If I am hungry, I should eat. If I am anxious, I may need to figure out what the problem is and get help if I need to. If I am dreading something, I may need to come up with a plan to make the thing more tolerable …

Imagine if a child with pain tried to ignore all these sensations and messages? What learning they would miss out on! Instead,

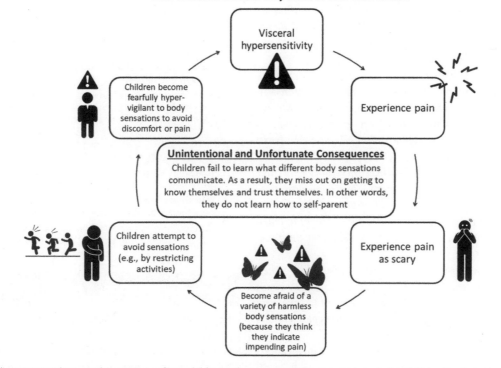

How Sensitive Children May Learn to Fear Their Bodies

Figure 6.1 This diagram provides a graphic summary of how children with sensory superpowers can learn to fear their bodies. It may be helpful to walk through these diagrams with the parent as you are describing the nature of pain sensitivity and the rationale for the FBI treatment. It is often even more helpful to draw out these diagrams as you talk to parents so they experience it as individualized and inclusive of their input. Either way, the diagram provides a concrete representation of your discussions, something they can take home to remind them of why we are doing what we are doing. We include this diagram as a worksheet in www.cambridge.org/fbi-clinical-guide. The workbook caption reads: Children with sensory superpowers feel things very strongly (a fancy name for this is visceral hypersensitivity). This includes both positive things like feeling really excited about things, but also uncomfortable things like pain. If children do not learn about their superpowers, they might become afraid of these intense feelings and may start to avoid doing things as a way to avoid feeling a variety of things. They may do this because they think all these different feelings in their body might be harmful. The end result is a child misses out on a lot of joyous activities. The child misses out on learning about themselves. They come to think they are weak instead of strong.

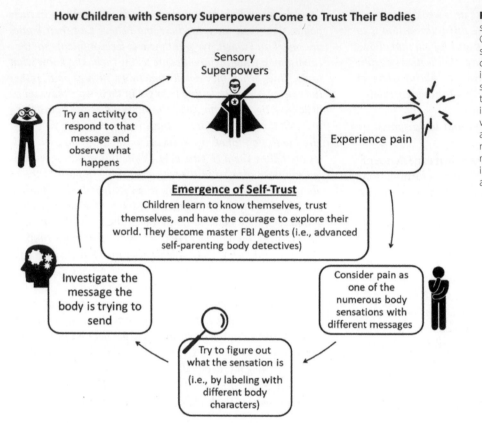

How Children with Sensory Superpowers Come to Trust Their Bodies

Figure 6.2 How children with sensory superpowers come to trust their bodies. Children with sensory superpowers notice something in their bodies – including pain or other uncomfortable sensations. They start investigating: trying to figure out what the sensation is and what the sensation is trying to tell them. They might even design a body investigation: they might pick an activity and see what happens to the body sensation both during and after the activity. If they learn something new, they will add it to their body map. The end result is that they will become master FBI agents – individuals who know themselves really well and are ready to explore the world.

helping your child to learn to tune in and decode what their body is telling them gives your child a powerful foundation for the rest of their lives: they know themselves, they trust themselves, and they feel powerful that they can figure things out and get through it when things get challenging.

So, the FBI treatment works in a very logical way. Each week we learn about the meaning of different body sensations. To make sure we can approach these sensations head-on, we do activities that intentionally bring on those sensations so we can practice figuring out what to do and so we can learn even more about the body (Figure 6.2). All of these activities are designed to show your child how incredibly wise their body already is. Not only that, though. Your bodies are constantly learning and getting smarter! Because we want you to do everything with your child, we hope that you get to learn how smart your body is (or that it is even smarter than you thought!)

There are about ten meetings that we will go through together. Typically, these meetings happen once per week. We say about ten because there may be a session that we want to take a bit more slowly if your child is having particular struggles with the things we are learning.

Do you have any questions about what we are going to do together?
– Allow the parent to ask questions.
Are you ready to get started? Now we are going to join your child and I'm going to give them a simpler and shorter explanation of what this treatment is about. Then we will start our first body investigations!

To summarize these points, let's take a look at the first page of the workbook that we will all work on together (Table 6.1).

Table 6.1 Welcome to the Feeling and Body Investigator Academy!

You and your child have been chosen to be part of a very special team of investigators. We are training to be experts in understanding the mysteries, power, and wisdom of the body. By the time this training is over, you and your child will have achieved the following goals:

1. **You and your child will be able to figure out what your bodies are trying to tell you.**

Pain can have many different messages. Your stomach has many different messages as well. Some common reasons children may notice sensations in their stomach are that they are feeling scared, hungry, guilty, or having other, different feelings. Your child (and you) will also be able to tell the difference between different types of pain (e.g., gas pain, hunger pain, injury pain, and emotional pain).

2. **Your child will not be as worried or afraid of sensations they are feeling in their body.**

3. **Your child will be less likely to let pain, or other body sensations, keep them from doing their normal day-to-day activities.**

The first section of this workbook will introduce you to what you can expect during our journey together through the FBI Academy.

Moment of Reflection

Now stop for a minute. You are still imagining that you are a parent of a child with pain. What was it like to hear all that? Were you skeptical because you have been to so many doctors and this sounds too good to be true? Or were we able to describe your child in such a way that you actually had the feeling that we understood your child's experience, and so you had some hope? Did we describe the situation so well that it made you sad, because it sounds a bit like yourself and you wished you had gotten this kind of care when you were young? Back to your clinician self … the point is, do not under-estimate the power of this conversation to set the stage for transformative change.

In this next section, we repeat this entire dialogue but with an explanation of what each section is intending to do. The goal of this section is to help you get the spirit of what is being communicated rather than worrying about memorizing a speech (see Table 6.2).

Table 6.2 Elements of a sample conversation introducing the FBI – Pain Intervention

Excerpt from therapist dialogue	Rationale for therapist dialogue
"Hi there. I'm Dr. Pain Therapist. I'm really looking forward to working with you and your child, Sam. I wanted to speak with you alone for a few minutes so I could give you a bit more information about the treatment and answer any questions you may have. Before I get started, are there any questions that you wanted to ask me?"	This introduction is intended to decrease uncertainty about exactly what will happen in the treatment sessions. It signals transparency on the part of the therapist. It also serves as reassurance that parents' wisdom is recognized and their opinion matters.
"So, I want to talk to you a bit about children with pain in general. Then, I want to hear from you about what aspects of what I describe sound like your child and which do not."	This is intended to reinforce that the parent is the expert on their child and a vital source of information about them. We are also aiming to increase the parent's confidence that we are knowledgeable about children with pain.
"We think of children with pain as sensitive children and we mean that in a literal way and in a beautiful way. We mean that they are sensitive because they may notice sensations in their body at a level that other children may not notice them or may experience these things more intensely than other children may notice them. The formal name for this is 'visceral hypersensitivity.' Simply, what this means is children who experience frequent pain feel things strongly and deeply – and we suspect that this includes not only things in their body but things in the world around them. One way to think of this is that they are like sensory and emotional sponges that soak up everything in the world around them. Quite frankly, this makes them wonderfully sweet and sensitive children – the future artists, scientists, and innovators of the world."	The intention of this introductory paragraph is to immediately give parents a mindset shift. They have been distressed about their child's vulnerability; in the new paradigm, we want parents to start viewing this vulnerability as an asset.
"Rather than thinking about this sensitivity as a weakness or vulnerability, the purpose and goal of the FBI intervention is to appreciate this sensitivity as a gift – a beautiful gift that allows your children to feel things deeply, care about others deeply, and live life out loud! The world of a sensitive child has a level of richness and pizzazz that children without those sensitivities do not get to experience in the same way."	This hammers that point home, but also conveys that the parent does not have to believe us right away – we are going to show them how to harness this sensitivity as an asset.
"Which parts of this sound like your child and which parts are different?"	It is really annoying to have a professional presume to know what you or your child is experiencing. Yet, we also want to build parent confidence that we know what we are talking about. Simple questions like this keep us humble.
"I wonder, do any of these descriptions sound like you or your child's other parent?"	While this treatment is focused on the child, all of us can stand to improve how we parent ourselves. In parents with a history of their own pain, this treatment is an important opportunity for them to "start over," regaining (or gaining) trust in their bodies after a lifetime of mistrust. While this may sound overly optimistic, optimism is a central tenet of FBI. In addition, "helping yourself to help your child" is an exceedingly powerful incentive for parents to make changes in themselves that they otherwise would not have.
"Our goal for your children is that we want them to feel safe in their bodies: that they know their bodies are smart and tough and that they feel really confident that they can listen to what their bodies are telling them and know what to do. Thus, when they notice something, such as pain, rather than being afraid or letting pain get in their way, they can be little investigators who ask: 'hmm? What is the pain telling me? What might be an interesting investigation to try?' *Children with pain often try to silence or ignore what their bodies are telling them. While this makes sense, this ignoring can also get in the way of learning important things about their body and learning to trust their body. Children are just figuring out what their bodies are trying to say. For example, if they notice a sensation in their gut, they have to figure out: is this a hunger pain? Is it butterflies in my tummy? Does my tummy have a knot in it? They then have to figure out what that sensation means. Am I hungry? Anxious? Dreading something? Ultimately, these important body messages let us know what is going on with ourselves so we can figure out what to do. If I am hungry, I should eat. If I am anxious, I may need to figure out what the problem is and get help if I need to. If I am dreading something, I may need to come up with a plan to make the thing more tolerable …* *Imagine if a child with pain tried to ignore all these sensations and messages? What learning they would miss out on! Instead, helping your child to learn to tune in and decode what their body is telling them gives your child a powerful foundation for the rest of their lives: they know themselves, they trust themselves, and they feel powerful that they can figure things out and get through it when things get challenging."*	This is the big pitch. This is where we try to explain, in a lay-friendly way, the lessons of Chapters 2 and 3 about the powerful foundation for self-awareness and emotion awareness that comes with self-parenting. It is not unusual for parents to feel very moved by this discussion for complicated reasons: they may experience hope, relief, and perhaps a little sadness that they did not receive this kind of care when they were young. That is why it is important that we keep emphasizing the strength of the dyad and the family and how every family member will grow from learning to be an FBI agent.

Table 6.2 (cont.)

"So, the FBI treatment works in a very logical way. Each week we learn about the meaning of different body sensations. To make sure we can approach these sensations head-on, we do activities that intentionally bring on those sensations so we can practice figuring out what to do and so we can learn even more about the body. All of these activities are designed to show your children how incredibly wise their body is and it is constantly learning and getting smarter! Because we want you to do everything with your child, we hope that you get to learn how smart your body is (or that it is even smarter than you thought!)	Here, we give a broad overview; in a few minutes we are going to demonstrate exactly what we mean by doing our first investigation.
There are about ten meetings that we will go through together. Typically, these meetings happen once per week. We say about ten because there may be a session that we want to take a bit more slowly if your child is having particular struggles with the things we are learning."	
"Do you have any questions about what we are going to do together?"	Parents should leave this meeting feeling confident about what you are doing. Give them the time they need to ask questions.

Sample Dialogue 6.2: Introducing the Framework and Intention of FBI – Pain Division to Children

And off we go!

Note: Throughout this book, we will switch off whether we are talking with or about moms or dads. In all cases, we are using these terms just as place-holders to represent any caregiver that is assisting the child through this intervention.

THERAPIST: *Hi there! I'm Dr. Pain Therapist. You are Sam, right?*

SAM: Yup.

THERAPIST: *Sam, I am really glad you are here. You, your mom, and I are going to have a lot of fun together. In fact, if you and your mom want to, you can bring your brothers and sisters to this so we are all doing this fun stuff together. I will let you and your mom decide that.*

Let me tell you a little bit about why you are here. I work with children who get stomach aches a lot. After getting to know these kids for a long time, I have learned something about them, and I have figured out some ways to help them. Some of these things may sound like you. You will have to let me know the parts that may sound like you, the parts that may not sound like you, and the parts that you are not sure about.

These kids are REALLY good at noticing things. They are really good at noticing what is going on in their bodies. They can also be really good at noticing things that are going on in the world around them. In fact, they may be better at noticing things than children without pain! Does any of this sound like you?

CHILD RESPONDS: I don't know.

(to the child's response) That is really interesting to know! We will have to pay attention and keep learning about the things that you notice!

Now, while noticing things can be annoying because that means you notice when your stomach hurts, there are also some really cool things about that.

By noticing all these things, it may make the world more beautiful and exciting! Think about that! It is like for other people, things are good. But for children who have stomach pain, things can be amazing!! That is because they feel things so deeply.

So, what we are going to do together is to help you so that you can feel really strong and so you can learn more about all the really

smart things your body does. We are also going to help you so you can get really good at figuring out what your body is telling you.

Have you ever watched a movie about a super hero who was just learning about their superpower and they were not really good at using those powers yet?

– Let the child respond.

Well, at first, they do not know how to use their superpowers. They have to practice. That is exactly what we will be doing.

Do you know what a detective is?

– Let the child respond. If they do not know what a detective is, ask them what a police officer is.

What is a detective/police officer's job?

– Let the child respond.

That is right! Detectives/police officers have to gather clues to solve crimes! That is exactly what we are going to do! We are going to do all kinds of investigations to learn more about your body!

It is important that we figure out a way to keep track of all the clues and all the things we learn about your body. A detective sometimes makes a map. If they are investigating some crimes in a city, maybe they will have a map of the city and mark down everything they have learned on that map. We are going to do the same thing, except we are going to make a map of your body!

Creating the Child's Body Map to Keep Track of New Wisdom Learned About the Body

– This is where the therapist will need the butcher paper. Spread the paper out on the floor so that there is enough paper to fit the child's body. You will need to weight it down on the corners with some books or other objects so that the paper does not curl up. Then the parent will trace the outline of the child's body. (The children get pretty interested by this).

We are going to trace your whole body on a big sheet of paper and make a body map. Come and help me lay out this sheet of paper!

– Starting with the next session, finding the child's sheet of paper with their body map becomes part of the opening rituals of the FBI session. My office (NZ) typically has a collection of rolled-up maps leaning in the corner. The butcher paper curls up, so I have the children write their first name or codename on the outside of the roll so that it's easy to find. At the beginning of the session, the child goes to find their body map and gets a bunch of books to help lay it out on the floor. We think that it is neat for them to see all the other maps so that they know other children are doing this too. I'm sure this will immediately make you think, why don't you do this in a group? We get to that issue in our last chapter. The answer: it's a lot of fun in a group.

Sam, do you want to pick your favorite color marker that your mom will use to trace your body?

– Like any child therapist, ready art supplies are a must. We always make sure to have a tin of colored markers ready for any art emergency.

Okay Sam, now lay down on the sheet of paper on your back. Now your mom is going to trace you so no giggling! Sam's mom, do not worry if you are not an artist, anything that you do will be great.

– The parent proceeds to trace the child's outline on the paper. Remember the spirit of encouragement and confidence building: there is no wrong way to trace your child on a sheet of paper. This is your first chance to demonstrate how playful FBI therapy will be.

Sam, you look terrific! I like how because of the way you are lying on the paper it looks like you have a teeny tiny little foot. Do you want to go ahead and draw in your face and write your name and date on the sheet of paper?

So, what we are going to do with this body map is that every time we learn something new about your body, we are going to add it to this map. For example, we may draw a picture of what we learned on the map of your body or around the body. This sheet will help us keep track of all that we do together. When our treatment is over, you will get to take this paper home with you and you can hang it on your wall in your bedroom if you want.

– The children usually enjoy decorating their bodies, but don't worry if they do not. Just go onto the next thing.

Learning About the First Body Characters

For the next part of this first session, we will pull out our workbook and read the pages together aloud. The first pages describe the new body sensation characters and what some of the messages of these sensations may be. We typically ask the parents to read to get them as involved as possible. However, if you get the impression that they are not comfortable reading, then, by all means, the therapist will read through the workbook pages. If older siblings attend the sessions who are fluent readers, then they are your golden ticket! Have them read the workbook pages out loud to get them involved immediately as a role model.

You may be thinking at this point that the first FBI session has a lot in it to cover, even considering that it is meant to be longer than the others. Think of it like the initial pilot for a television series: you really need to hook the audience in!

More characters are introduced in this session than in most of the remaining sessions. We wanted to introduce many characters in the first session to get everyone excited about what we are going to be doing together and to introduce some of the various meanings that body sensations can take, including emotional experience, pain, or digestive functions. The workbook presents a picture of each character and describes what that body sensation might signal or the situations in which it might arise.

You can go through this section quickly reading through the characters, stopping at every character and talking a bit about it, or choosing a few characters to discuss more in-depth. Your decision will depend on the interest and energy levels of the child; if you do a deep dive into all of them, you may lose the child's attention, and yet some children just adore such an in-depth look at every character. When you are exploring a body sensation further with a child, ask the family questions about whether, when, and where they experience that sensation. We will then summarize some of those observations in our Body Brainstorms worksheet toward the end of the session.

Black and white session materials for Sessions 1 through 3 are in Part III of this handbook. Color versions of all the materials for all the sessions are available for free download at www.cambridge.org/fbi-clinical-guide. To better ease the flow of the session format, we put necessary excerpts from these workbook pages embedded in the text here.

THERAPIST: *Okay, great job everybody. Now let's move on to the next part of our session – learning our first body sensation characters!*

Sam's mom, would you like to start reading about these new body sensation characters?

Gassy Gus

Gassy Gus is a character that represents the sensation of having to pass gas, or as children like to say, "farting." We start off with Gassy Gus as our first character because, let's face it, children love to talk about farting. There is no better rapport builder with children.

In the workbook, Gassy Gus describes itself with the following quote:

> "Hi! I'm Gassy Gus!
> I sometimes cause sharp pains in your stomach that you can get rid of by doing guess what?? FARTING."

As you can see, these are playful introductions to sensations. These introductions and descriptions are written to build interest and curiosity and not to read like precise textbook descriptions of anatomy and function.

Questions that the therapist may use to encourage discussion of the various body sensations may look something like the following.

THERAPIST: *Does that ever happen to you? Does your stomach sometimes hurt, and then you fart, and you are like, "Ah, that feels a lot better!" How about you, mom? Does that ever happen to you? In a few sessions, we will do some fun experiments to see who can have the smelliest farts!*

Polly the Pain

We are going to have many characters for different types of pain. Polly is our generic pain character. We make her look a little sneaky as pain sometimes communicates things in ways that can be tricky to understand, but these messages are no match for a talented FBI agent!

Parent reads the following from the workbook:

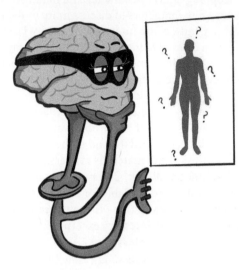

"Hi! I'm <u>Polly the Pain</u>.
I'm here to help you. I let you know when there is something in your body that you need to pay attention to. Sometimes, in fact, a lot of the time, you may not need to do anything. Your body is really smart and can figure out how to take care of a lot of things on its own. But if you are unsure, we can always do an investigation together to figure out what I am trying to tell you!"

> Polly the Pain is our first introduction to the core lesson of the entire FBI program – that children's bodies are really smart and are always getting smarter.

We are going to be learning a lot about different types of pain together.

Betty the Butterfly

Betty the Butterfly is a fluttering sensation that one may experience when one is feeling excited or nervous about something. The fancy fact about butterflies is that the experience may result from changes in gut permeability that occur when an individual is aroused due to an emotional or stressful circumstance (Chapter 2). We will learn a lot more about Betty the Butterfly in Session 4.

A quote from Betty from the workbook:

"Hi! I'm <u>Betty the Butterfly</u>.
I cause a fluttering in your stomach when you feel scared or worried about something."

THERAPIST: *Isn't she cute!! Has that ever happened to you? You might be scared about something that is happening, like maybe you are watching a scary movie, and you feel some feelings in your stomach? [The therapist might want to flutter their fingers around their stomach to demonstrate what they mean.] How about you, mom, has that ever happened to you?*

Ricky the Rock

Ricky the Rock is our sensation for the pit of guilt or dread. Ricky the Rock is a pretty advanced sensation. When a five-year old identifies with Ricky the Rock right away, you know you have a precocious kid on your hands.

"Hi! I'm <u>Ricky the Rock</u>!
I sometimes make you feel like you have a tight knot or heavy stone in your tummy. I usually come around when you are feeling guilty or sad about something that has happened."

THERAPIST: *This is like when you feel "uh-oh! I shouldn't have done that …" Can you remember the last time you felt like that?*

Samantha Sweat

We put Samantha Sweat in this first session just because that is a relatively easy sensation for children to recognize and a great way to warm them up to what we are trying to do. We will visit Samantha again in Session 4 when we discuss high arousal emotions, part 1.

"Hello! I'm <u>Samantha Sweat</u> – Sam for short.
I like to visit you when your body is preparing for a challenge (like when you are going to take a difficult test or run a race). I help keep your body cool so you can face the challenge."

Henry the Heartbeat

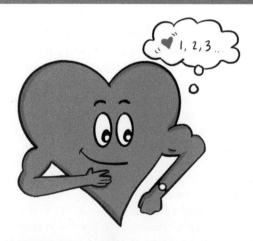

"Hello! I'm <u>Henry the Heartbeat</u>!
I am a very powerful machine that pumps blood to all of the parts of your body. The harder you work, the more I pump. I am

like a secret decoder ring. You might be able to tell by how fast and how slow I am beating whether there is something important or relaxing going on. The speed and strength of my beats are the secret to the code."

Spend a minute having everyone list some situations or activities that make their hearts beat faster. We will add these to our Body Brainstorms worksheet later in the session.

We are going to spend some time learning about Henry the Heartbeat in just a few minutes!

As noted, you can go through this section quickly reading through the characters, stopping at every character and talking a bit about it, or choosing a few characters to discuss more in-depth. Your decision really depends on the attention and energy of the child. Now go ahead and read through the remaining characters: Gerda Gotta Go, the urge to pee; Gordon Gotta Go, the urge to poop; and Patricia the Poop Pain, the feeling of discomfort you may get when you have a particularly hard poop.

The First Body Investigation – Henry the Heartbeat

Every FBI session will begin with a Henry the Heartbeat investigation. This is for several reasons. First, we are working with energized children and it is good to have them run around and get their energy out. Second, it starts off the session with something fun. Third, it is a great way for children to practice the emotion regulation capacity of raising and lowering their arousal. The focus of these investigations is to demonstrate how smart your heart is – your heart knows how to adapt the amount of blood and oxygen you need depending on the activity that

you are doing, and it does that completely on its own! Pretty amazing.

Okay! It is time to do our first body investigation! Are you ready?! We are going to learn a bit more about Henry the Heartbeat. So, let's think of two different things that we can do right here and now that you think are going to make your heart beat faster.

– Have everyone agree on two activities.

Now, let's come up with one thing that we can do to lower our heart rate.

Now here's what we are going to do. First, we are going to see how much our heart is beating to start with. Then we are going to do one of the activities that we've picked out for a specific amount of time. How does one minute sound? (Everyone agrees to a time). Then, we are going to measure your heartbeat again and see if the number of heartbeats changed after you did that activity. Then we are going to try to lower our heart beat back to where it started from. We will do the heartbeat raising and heartbeat lowering activities for the same amount of time to see whether it takes longer to get our heartbeat to raise or lower. Then we will do the same thing all over again with the second activity. What should we do to try to lower our heart rate?

The suggested steps for a Henry the Heartbeat activity appear in Table 6.3. These are just suggestions. There are many types of Henry the Heartbeat activities.

> A central lesson of a Henry the Heartbeat investigation: Your heart is smart. It knows how to adapt how hard it beats to help you to get through any situation.

Table 6.3 Henry the Heartbeat Body Investigation

1. Choose two activities that may raise your heartbeat that you are going to compare.
2. Choose one activity to try to lower your heartbeat.
3. Decide on how long you are going to perform each activity. To be more scientific, you should do each activity for the same amount of time.
4. Have the child find their heartbeat. It is important that they sense their heartbeat by taking their own pulse rather than have a parent do it for them or using some kind of gadget. The essential component of this exercise is the child tuning in and listening to their body. The parent may need to help the child find their heartbeat initially. Sometimes, when a heartbeat seems particularly tricky to find, we have the child jump up and down for a few seconds to make the heartbeat easier to detect. What is also important is that whatever the child counts as their heartbeat, even if that number seems illogical, we stick with it. The point here is that we are getting the child, perhaps for the first time, to tune into their body, sense something, and describe it. That is the important point – not getting the right answer.
5. If possible, it is ideal that every member of the family that is attending the session join the activity. So have everyone try to find their pulse at this point.
6. Find a stopwatch. The therapist is going to time everyone for ten seconds while everyone counts their pulse. This will serve as the baseline heartbeat measure.
7. The therapist says "on your marks, get set, count!" After ten seconds, the therapist says "stop!"
8. The therapist asks everyone how many beats they have counted and records this on a piece of paper.
9. Therapist: *Okay. Now that we know where our starting point is, what are people's guesses as to how many beats your heart is going to go up to after each of the activities?* [The therapist writes down these guesses.]
10. Therapist: *Ok, I'm going to set my timer for XX seconds [whatever was agreed upon] and then you are going to do Activity #1 (for example, doing jumping jacks). When I say stop, you will stop and we will count your heartbeats and see whose guess is the closest.*
11. The therapist times the activity and all participants take their heart rate. Everyone should write down what they got or the therapist can keep track.
12. Therapist: *OK, now for the next minute, we are going to do the activity that we picked to bring our heart rate back down. On your marks, get set, slow down your heart beat!*
13. After the minute, the therapist once again directs everyone to count their heart beat. If it is back to baseline, you continue with the next activity. If not, you perform the heartbeat reduction activity for another minute.
14. Repeat these steps for the second heart beat raising activity and then repeat the heart reduction activity.
15. At the end of this activity everyone will have learned the following: which activity causes the heart to beat faster; how long (approximately) it takes to bring the heart rate back down to baseline; and who had the best guess.
16. Therapist: *Now, let's add what we learned to our body map! (See below) Wow! We learned so much about your heart today.*

Adding What Is Learned to the Body Map

While adding something to the body map is a straightforward task, it is also complex and important therapeutically. We are contextualizing a memory and ensuring that what children stamp in about the experience is what we hope they will remember – that the body is smart and powerful. By writing this on their body map, we give them a permanent memento of this investigation. Chapter 4 describes more of the logic of this approach.

What goes on the child's body sheet contains two elements. The first is whatever the child wants to put on the sheet. This is usually quite literal. For example, in the exercise that we just did, we know the number of beats that their heart went up by when they were doing, for example, jumping jacks versus running. So, children can add to their body sheet the following: my heart beats 22 times when I run and 18 times when I do jumping jacks.

The second element that is added to the body map is the lesson that was learned. For today, that lesson can be as simple as "My heart sure is smart." To learn that lesson, the therapist initially makes an observation about what they have just seen. However, as time goes on, the parent and child will get better at making these observations on their own. It could look something like this:

"Wow! How did your heart know to do that? To beat faster when you are running? That is pretty cool. Your heart just knows a lot of things."

Then, when it is time to add what we learned to the body map, the therapist could ask "Do you think we should add that your heart is smart to the body map?" If the child says no, just go with that. It is their body map. You will have plenty of opportunity to add to the body map later.

The First Body Brainstorm Worksheet

The final exercise of Session 1 is the Body Brainstorms worksheet. This worksheet is designed to help the child generalize what they have learned in the session to activities outside of the session. This worksheet contains a few questions, some of which we have already been answered earlier in the session. For this first session we ask the following:

What are some things that make your heart beat faster? Try to come up with three things!

What are some things that make your heart beat slower? Try to come up with three things!

What are some things that make you sweat? Try to come up with three things!

What are some things that make you have to pee? Try to come up with three things!

As you ask these questions, make sure to reinforce what you have already talked about. You can say things like *"Oh we already know this! Remember we listed some things already. Do you remember what they were?"*

Prizes

Finally, because we work with children, we are big on prizes. We have designed the FBI intervention so that participation is fun and thus, hopefully, rewarding for children. We do not think prizes are needed to keep a child wanting to participate. However, we have given out selective prizes that keep with the spirit of becoming a trained FBI agent. Throughout the intervention, children can earn parts of their detective costume (e.g., a magnifying glass) or tools that help in their role as an agent (e.g., a journal). These are optional, but certainly fun.

Because these children are training to be FBI agents, prizes for Session 1 are suitable for that. They get a mini journal to keep track of all their observations, a pen, a plastic detective hat, and a three-ring binder to keep all of their session worksheets. If that were not enough, we usually give the kids a button of one of the characters they have learned. On our book website, we provide some ordering information for in-session prizes.

The First Body Investigation Assignment (Home-Based Practice)

For Session 1, the home assignment is for the children to pick two of the characters that they have learned about that day. When they notice themselves feeling either of these characters, their instruction is to pull out their little journal and to draw a picture of what they were doing when they noticed it. We also give children coloring pages of the FBI characters. We give them only a few coloring pages after Session 1, as they will get the remainder of the characters' pages throughout the intervention.

Reminder for things to bring for Session 2: Have the parent and child bring in a snack that has lots of little pieces – like crackers or fruit snacks. Also, children should bring their journal with them.

Then you schedule the next session! Congratulations, you've just finished Session 1.

Take-Home Materials from Session 1

Here is a summary of what families get from Session 1.

1. A worksheet that summarizes the characters that they have learned so far.
2. Coloring pages
3. Session 1 Workbook Pages
4. The Body Brainstorms worksheet they completed
5. Optional: PRIZES! A detective hat, a bag, a three-ring binder, a journal, a pen
6. Optional: A Gassy Gus button

Therapist Reminders for Session 1

Do not forget to write down what characters they are tracking in their journal to review them at the start of next session.

A Final Reflection for Session 1

As a final reflection for this session, we want you to think about what it would be like to be the child who just had this therapy experience. They may have visited several doctors about their pain. They may be worried that something is wrong with them – that things do not come as easy for them as for other children. Today, they have been told that not only is nothing wrong with them, but also, the fact that they have had stomach aches frequently is an indication of a superpower. They have done investigations where they learned that their body is a bit smarter, perhaps, than they thought, and they got to talk about farting. It does not get much better than that!

Questions and Answers for Session 1

Q: The initial conversation with the parent seems like it could take a long time. Do you ever schedule that as a separate session?

A: Absolutely, you could do that. Particularly if you are aware that a parent has had their own significant history of pain, trauma, and/or mental illness, it might be very wise to schedule that session separately so you can take all the time that you need to really build up the case for the child's treatment and how the parent is a necessary component who may also benefit.

Q: You mentioned that during the body investigations, the child is correct about counting their heartbeats even if the number does not seem logical. What should I do if the parent keeps correcting them?

A: In the moment, I would say something neutral like, "We all feel all kinds of different things" or "Interesting point! It's ok; we're interested in each person's experience of change in heartbeat from one activity to another rather than medical accuracy. Remember that everyone is the expert on their own experiences!" However, if you feel like the parent is not picking up on the spirit of what you are trying to do in terms of inculcating curiosity towards body sensations, then I would grab the parent's attention for a minute, privately, at the beginning of the next session and just remind them of what the purpose is. While it may seem minor that the parent is correcting the child's experience of their body, this is actually a big deal. As well-intended as it may be, it is actually a form of invalidation (see Chapter 3). Only the child knows what is going on in their body …

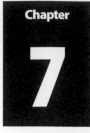

Chapter

7

Session 2: The Eats

Cheeseburger in paradise
Heaven on Earth with an onion slice
Cheeseburger in Paradise, by Jimmy Buffett

Overview of Session 2

Welcome back. You may notice that this is the first session organized by theme. Session 2 is "formally" referred to as *The Eats* as we will focus on learning the body sensations associated with hunger, fullness, food deliciousness, and thirst. In this session, we will start to establish the routines that organize each session for the remainder of the program. We provide you with a session outline, a list of suggested materials, and necessary background information about the session. We will then go through the session step-by-step and will end with a Q&A. While the workbook material for Session 1 was primarily focused on teaching the FBI characters, the workbook pages in Session 2 contain additional instructional content designed to help children think about what their bodies feel like when hungry and thirsty.

Session Outline

1. Perform a Henry Heartbeat warm-up activity
2. Review homework and add new concepts about the body to the Body Map
3. Learn new characters related to hunger, fullness, food enjoyment, and thirst
4. Perform a Body Investigation (or two or three if time permits)
5. Complete a Body Brainstorms worksheet
6. Learn the first two steps of the Body Clues Worksheet for home-based practice
7. Give out coloring pages
8. Optional: give out prizes

Session Materials

1. The child's Body Map from last session
2. Workbook, worksheets, and coloring pages for Session 2, Appendix B, FBI – Pain Division Session 2
3. A snack the child brings or that you have on hand. Note: this activity can be performed with any snack but works best if you have a snack that is already in small pieces (like cheese crackers, goldfish, or fruit snacks etc.)
4. Optional Prizes (sunglasses, invisible ink pen, Georgia the Gut Growler Button (see https://efbi-kids.org)

Background Information for Session 2: Food as Delicious Fuel

This session focuses on body sensations related to hunger, fullness, perceived food deliciousness, and thirst. In addition to information about new characters, workbook pages in this section include several self-exploration exercises related to hunger, fullness, and deliciousness that we will work through together (Part III, Session 2: The Eats). Because of our emphasis on the body (rather than food), we naturally focus on how food makes our bodies feel. It would have been very easy to go down a rabbit hole of "good foods" make your body feel good while "junk foods" make your body feel bad – and we definitely did not want to do that. As our background is in eating disorder research and our passion is helping children experience joy and pleasure with eating, we focus here on the most fundamental, useful, and experiential metric: food gives us energy and thus makes us feel energetic and peppy. Food is also scrumptious. Children can learn through trial, error, and curiosity which foods give them a bigger spring in their step, rather than by being told how various foods *should* make them feel. Categorizing foods as "healthy" versus "unhealthy" actually decreases the consumption of nutritious foods. Conversely, focusing on how tasty a food is has been found to increase vegetable consumption – and the expectations that vegetables will be delicious.[1]

Children can develop nuanced and sophisticated tastes by exploring how foods make them feel right after they eat and examining how long these feelings last. For example, do certain foods give them a lot of energy right away, but then they feel like their energy crashes an hour later? Do some foods give them a peppy feeling that lasts till the next snack or meal? There are numerous energy-focused investigations that we can implement to encourage experiential learning that facilitates body knowledge and trust.

To increase children's pleasure with eating and their awareness of how food makes their bodies feel, we introduce metaphors, new characters, and an energy meter. We pay attention to their energy levels and help them notice how delicious a food is as they eat. Children with gastrointestinal pain can fall into an obsessive trap of worrying about food. They (or their parents) may try to be vigilant about everything they eat in an attempt to avoid painful GI sensations. We try to strike a balance by maintaining a curious awareness of the body while eating, seeing what happens to our energy as we eat, and learning from experience.

Many health professionals are concerned about pediatric obesity. Perhaps our focus on the energy that food provides has raised alarm bells. Are we just training children to prefer candy and other high-energy foods? Our intention and experience indicate the opposite. By teaching children to notice hunger and fullness cues and to enjoy the taste of foods, we intend for children to eat slowly enough that they can listen to what their body needs. Some children will eat more if they were undereating before treatment and some will eat less if they were not tuning in to fullness cues. Becoming attuned to the body and its signals will improve our ability to notice what are bodies are trying to tell us.

Off we go.

The Experience of Hunger

As summarized in Table 7.1, we will use a five-point scale to teach about the different phases of hunger and fullness. As you will see, we use child-friendly definitions rather than strict biological definitions. Our goals are for children to tune into their bodies as they are eating, increasingly learn the nourishing effects of food, and enjoy the delicious tastes of food: we want to help these children develop an ongoing awareness and appreciation of the pleasure of eating and the gift of feeling fueled.

There are many different scales that have been created to help adults recognize different stages of hunger (e.g., intuitive eating scales) with some indicating as many as 12 different graduations of various stages of hunger and fullness. While these may be very helpful for adults, they can be very complicated for children (and even for some adults). Instead, we developed a five-point scale, in collaboration with our dear friend and colleague, Dr. Linda Craighead at Emory University. She uses this as part of an Appetite Awareness Training Program.[2]

Table 7.1 Feelings of hunger and fullness

Phase of hunger and fullness	Definition for FBI – Pain Division purposes
Starving/Uncomfortably Hungry (Harold the Hunger Pain) Of course, this does not mean literally starving but rather "uncomfortably hungry." Your stomach may hurt, you may have a headache, you are low in energy, you may have difficulty concentrating, and you would never want to sign an important document in this condition or reply to an irritating email. 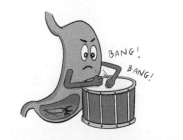	**Hungry (Georgia the Gut Growler)** This is a gentle but noticeable hunger: your stomach is growling, your energy is lowering, your concentration is turning toward the lunch menu. 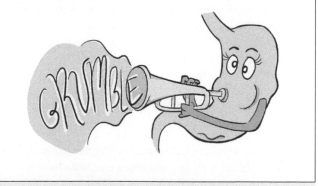
Getting energized	
We use this label to describe what your body feels like as you are eating, i.e., during the process of fueling your body. This is the feeling you get when you have taken the edge off of your hunger, but you are not satisfied yet. If you were at a restaurant and finished your meal, you would feel like you did not quite get your money's worth. To appreciate the feeling of becoming energized, it is important to pause throughout the eating episode and check in with how your body is feeling. We will be practicing this with our energy meter in our body investigation this session and when we eat our snacks during every session.	

Table 7.1 (cont.)

Satisfied (Solomon Satisfied)	Stuffed (Sabrina Stuffed)
Your body is fueled so that you feel fully energized and ready to go. You feel bouncy and exuberant. You may feel like dancing. 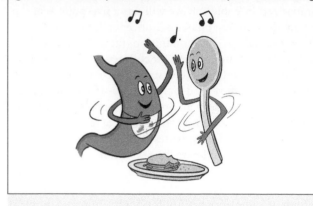	You have gone past the stage of feeling energized and might feel a bit sleepy or uncomfortable. If you were a bear, you would be heading to a cave to hibernate. 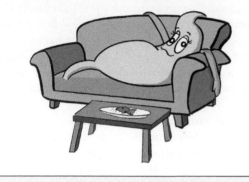

Step-by-Step Guide to Session 2
Henry Heartbeat Warm-Up Activity

From now on, every session will start with a Henry Heartbeat warm-up investigation. As noted in Session 1, we do this for several reasons. First, children may have been sitting around all day at school; thus, they may be tired of concentrating. We want to get their blood flowing and activate their attention. Second, we want them to feel confident raising and lowering their heartbeat. Our heartbeat is one index of our level of arousal, and we want the children to be masters at noticing their heartbeat and using techniques to raise or lower it, depending on whether they need to calm themselves down or rev themselves up.

You can conduct Henry Heartbeat activities the same way as described in Table 6.3 of Chapter 6, or you can get creative! Table 7.2 lists some ideas for Henry Heartbeat warm-up activities. We will also learn a lot more about him in Session 4 when we discuss high-arousal emotions.

Review Homework and Add New Things to the Body Map

So begins the ritual of finding and laying out the child's body map. As we mentioned last session, we usually have rolled up papers of each patient's body map tucked in a corner of the office. The child has written their name on the outside of it (or codename for confidentiality). Finding their map among all the other children's maps can be a subtle and lovely way for the children to learn that they are not the only child doing these activities. Seeing their body map amongst the body

Table 7.2 Ideas for Henry Heartbeat investigations

What makes your heart beat faster; watching a scary movie clip (G-rated or child appropriate, of course) or running down the hall?
What slows your heart down more; taking slow deep breaths or doing a stretch (like sitting on the floor and bending over to have your hands touch as far away from you on the floor as you can – a great back and shoulder stretch!)?
How long does it take to slow your heartbeat down after doing jumping jacks for 30 seconds? How about after you do jumping jacks for 60 seconds?
If you practice jumping jacks every day for seven days, does your heart starting beating more slowly than it did when we measured it before? What about if you do it for 14 days? If it does, why do you think this is?
Does your heart beat faster when you are excited about something? Let's see!

maps of other children can help the child feel like they are not alone.

After the child has laid out their map, we proceed with homework review. This will typically involve working backward, first asking if the child learned anything new during the Henry Heartbeat investigation they just completed. This is followed by a review of the child's journal from last week. As a reminder, their assignment was to choose two of the new characters they met and to draw a picture or write about what they were doing when they noticed the sensation conveyed by that character.

Checking in on homework requires sensitive therapeutic skill. On the one hand, we do not want parents to feel discouraged or ashamed if they did not practice with their child outside of the session; on the other hand, we want them to understand the importance of practice.

If children and parents fail to bring any completed homework, our response will be to do the assignment immediately while in the session. We do not want them to miss out on the exercise! This demonstrates that there is no avoiding practice (because we will do it right there if they were not able to at home). We will then reinforce the importance of new things that the child learned about their body by adding it to the body map.

Homework Review Tip

It is essential that the therapist always reviews homework that was assigned. Otherwise, the child and parent will get the message that the homework was not really that important.

THERAPIST: *First of all, is there anything that we just learned from our Henry Heartbeat investigation that we should add to the map?*

– We have already learned that the heart is smart, but we can keep adding evidence of this as much as the child wants to. There are many nuances to the heart's intelligence.

THERAPIST: *Last week, you chose two body sensation characters to focus on: X and Y. Every time you felt one of those sensations, you were going to draw a picture of what you were doing in your journal. Let's take a look at your journal!*

If the child and parent did their homework:

THERAPIST: *Oh terrific! Show me what you did! [Review homework] Is there something that you think we should add to your body map?* [If so, have the child draw a picture on their body map.]

Homework Review Tip

Make sure to write a caption under each thing that the child draws. Otherwise, you will not remember what the drawing was supposed to be (some children are abstract artists!).

If the child and parent did NOT do their homework:

THERAPIST: *That happens sometimes. Weeks can be crazy! Let's go ahead and do it together right now. So, one of the characters that you were going to focus on was Samantha Sweat (as an example). Do either of you remember a time this past week when you started sweating? What was going on? Mom, should we make a miniature body map for you so we can add it?*

Parent Body Map tip

Parents are more than welcome to have their own body traced on butcher paper. Alternatively, what they can do instead is draw a body silhouette on a piece of paper and add whatever they have learned about themselves to that sheet. This is great role-modeling for their child.

Session 2 Read the Workbook: Hunger and Fullness

The Workbook Routines

Every session, the family will go through the workbook pages together and someone will be chosen to read the week's material out loud. The format of the workbook review will be similar every week. There will be investigative questions that prompt family members to think and talk about the body's wisdom. The workbook also introduces new body sensations (and therefore new characters) in each session. In some sessions, there will be additional educational material for everyone about the body; in other sessions, there will be information geared to parents.

Food as Fuel

The workbook for Session 2 begins with some questions to get the whole family thinking. As always, the intention of these questions is not to elicit the "right" answer at that moment (we will be discussing more information related to hunger during the session), but more to spark curiosity and ideas.

The Session 2 workbook questions read:

Why do you think people have hunger pains?

What might happen if you notice a hunger pain and then you ignore it?

How do you feel if you are eating a food that tastes so good that even though you feel full, you keep eating it?

To any response the child has, the therapist can reinforce and probe further with various follow-up questions (just as suggestions):

That is interesting! So, what do you think would happen then if the person with hunger pains ate some food?

Has that ever happened to you?

Then have the parent (or other volunteer like an older sibling) read through the workbook pages. Just as a car needs gas, we emphasize to the child that food provides the energy that the body needs to run properly. Figures 7.1 and 7.2 show images of

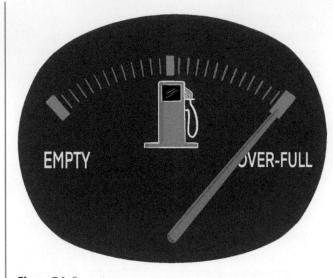

Figure 7.1 Gas meter.

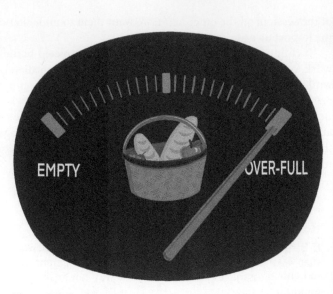

Figure 7.2 Food meter.

a gas meter and food meter from the workbook pages. These meters expand on the car metaphor and are used to illustrate the different benefits and consequences of energy derived from food.

Questions to pose after reading:

What do you think happens to your body when it does not get enough energy? Has this ever happened to you?

Noticing Hunger

After a brief discussion, continue reading the workbook pages which introduce the child to two characters related to hunger: Harold the Hunger Pain and Georgia the Gut Growler. Harold the Hunger Pain is a sensation that a child might experience if they let themselves get too hungry – something you might feel if you labeled yourself as "starving" – whereas Georgia the Gut Growler is a gentler gut-rumbling sensation you feel when you are hungry.

Have the child and parent think about what starving and hungry feels like for them and add those descriptions to the hunger/fullness descriptions in the workbook.

Throughout the workbook, there are some illustrations about what happens when children have difficulty noticing subtle signs of hunger (hint: Georgia the Gut Growler feels a bit ignored). These children may only register hunger at extreme levels of discomfort (as in Harold the Hunger Pain). It may take practice for children to become adept at detecting mild hunger, and that is a fun investigation to keep working on! For example, if children do not know what Georgia the Gut Growler feels like, they may start to notice

Georgia once they start paying attention. When they do, they can draw what Georgia the Gut Growler feels like in their body journal. This can be a powerful way of showing children that they can get better at listening to their bodies. This can be a great investigation for parents to perform at home. We provide more details about home-based investigations toward the end of this session.

Is "hangry" a sensation? A feeling? In FBI – Pain Division, children learn to notice and label different body sensations. Over time, they figure out what these sensations might be communicating. As you will learn, Hangry, a term that was invented to characterize the irritable feeling you get when you let yourself get too hungry, is what happens when you feel Harold the Hunger Pain and Tommy Thunderbolt. Very exciting! So, we decided to include Hangry as one of the emotional labels on our Body Clues Worksheet that is first introduced in this session.

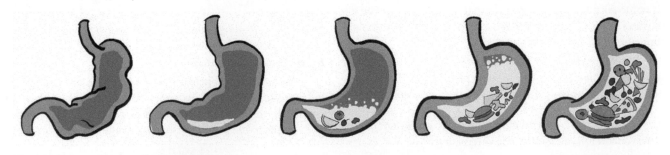

Figure 7.3 Image of stages of hunger/fullness.

Noticing Fullness

Solomon Satisfied and Sabrina Stuffed are the body sensation characters that signal that our body has been fueled up and we can stop eating. We use the term "satisfied" rather than "full" because we feel that satisfied more precisely conveys the dual experience of food sufficiency (which would equate to feeling "full") and taste satiety: feeling satisfied means you have had enough delicious food.

Time for Reflection

Spend a minute or two thinking about how you would optimally like to feel after a meal. Perhaps sensations such as invigorated and content come to mind. Have you ever eaten a sufficient quantity of blah-tasting food? You may feel full, but there may be a part of you that feels cheated, like you need a delicious taste to be truly satisfied. You can think of this as two different kinds of satiety: energy satiety and taste satiety. Thinking about how you want your body to feel after a meal and tuning in to the energy and flavors that your body needs can be a great way to make decisions about food. Exploring how different foods provide energy and flavor can provide really great ideas for body investigations.

The introduction to Sabrina Stuffed reads:

"Hello. I am Sabrina Stuffed! I have trouble stopping things that I am doing – especially when it is something that I really like to do – like eat! I really love food, so I have a hard time stopping myself from eating, until, you guessed it – I AM STUFFED! I guess that is where I got my name from. Everyone gets stuffed every once in a while. However, if you find that I am hanging around all the time, it may be time to start listening for Solomon Satisfied."

THERAPIST: *Has that ever happened to you? You were eating something and it tasted so good that you had a hard time stopping*

eating it even though you knew you already felt satisfied? How about you, Mom? That happens to me when I eat French Fries. I just love them. I guess we should meet Solomon Satisfied. (NZ has trouble stopping eating French Fries. For KL the food is homemade challah, and for MG it is really good key lime pie).

The introduction to Solomon Satisfied reads (from whomever is reading the workbook aloud):

"Why, hello. I am Mr. Satisfied, Solomon Satisfied, that is. I am always peppy, energized, and ready to go because I always have just the right amount of food that I need to fuel my body. My only problem is that I can be a bit quiet at times (I am rather shy). When the food tastes really good and Sabrina is getting excited because she doesn't want you to stop, it can be really hard to hear me. Once we get to know each other better, you will find that I have a lot of interesting things to say and it will be easier to notice me!"

THERAPIST: *Do you think that is true? Do you think that you can get better at noticing when you feel satisfied if you practice? Let's try practicing right now. To help you become an expert at noticing when your energy is changing, let's try another body investigation! I want to introduce you to the Energy Meter.*

Body Investigation: The Energy Meter

A page in the child's workbook illustrates the energy meter. The purpose of this meter is for a child to practice tuning in to how food makes them feel and to have a concrete way to index those changes. To do so, we use our hands and the space between our hands to indicate our increasing energy as we nourish our bodies with food (or with any other activity that causes our energy to rise and fall). The energy meter works like this: palms together indicates someone has zero energy or is "starving." As the child's energy increases, they move their hands farther and farther apart. Once they are fully satisfied, they flex their arms into two big muscles to indicate they are full and energized. If they get to the point where they are stuffed, they can dramatically take their flexed muscles and let them droop down to reflect the decrease in energy that comes from being overly full (see Figure 7.4).

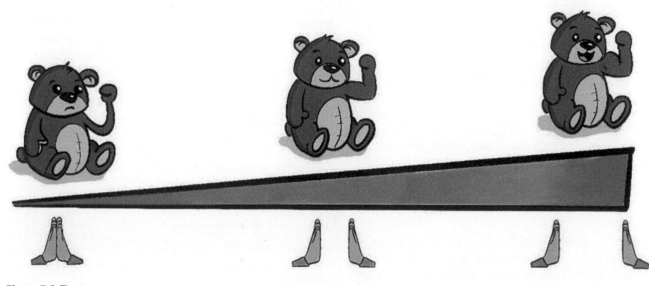

Figure 7.4 The energy meter.

Table 7.3 An example of a hunger investigation

1. Pick out a food that you are going to use to investigate hunger.
2. The child indicates their current level of energy using the distance between their hands on their energy meter (hands closed is equal to no energy, hands the widest they can be with muscles flexed is equal to feeling fully energized).
3. The child makes a prediction about how much food it will take to get fully energized. The parent can also make a prediction about how much food they think it will take for the child to become fully energized (in this way it is like a contest to see who is more accurate). Ideally, the parent will also do the investigation and make their own guesses about how much of the snack food it will take to get themselves fully fueled up. Similarly, the child can make a guess about how much it will take the parent.
4. Divide the food up into piles. This way it is easy to remember to check in with everybody's energy level after consuming each pile.
5. Have parent and child consume a small pile of food. Then have them pause, check in with how their body is feeling in terms of their energy levels, and indicate their energy levels with their hands.
6. Continue this until everyone feels fully energized.
7. See whose guess was the closest.

Note: As with all investigations, these are just suggestions. Children can be encouraged to come up with their own investigations and that may happen increasingly over time.

To practice using the energy meter, we will complete the following exercise as our body investigation. Table 7.3 summarizes these steps.

Ask every family member in attendance to participate in this investigation. First, explain the way the energy meter works.

THERAPIST: *I'm going to introduce you to our energy meter. We use this energy meter to indicate how much energy we are feeling. This energy can be from the food that we eat and from other things. I will show you how to do it. If I am feeling really low in energy, like I am starving, I put my hands together in front of my chest like this. That means I am empty.*

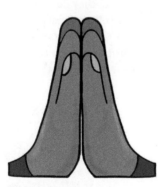

Figure 7.5 Hands together = very low energy.

Now let's say I started to eat a snack, and I could feel my energy increasing. I will move my hands farther and farther as my energy level keeps getting bigger and bigger. When I feel like I'm fully energized, my hands go to the widest apart that they can be and I flex my muscles because I have so much power and energy.

Does anybody have any questions about that? Let's all try it together. Let's take a minute and tune into our bodies and see what our energy feels like. When you think you've got it, show me with your hands.

Guide the family members in pausing, turning their attention to their energy level, and then indicating it with their hands.

THERAPIST: *Now, we are going to take out our snacks. Let's guess how many crackers/chips/fruit snacks it will take to get fully energized. After you tell me your guess, go ahead and count out the number of snacks (the snack could be anything but ideally is something in a lot of little pieces).*

Each person makes a guess and then counts out that number and makes a pile with their snacks.

THERAPIST: *Now, we are going to do a couple more things. Mom/Dad, I want you to guess how many snacks it will take Sam to get fully energized. I'm going to write everybody's guess down. Now Sam, you guess how many you think it will take your parents to get fully energized. [Therapist writes everything down, ideally where everyone can see.]. Now here is what we are going to go. I want everyone to take your pile of snacks and divide it into three small piles. We are going to eat a pile of snacks and then check in with our energy to see if we need to keep eating or whether we are already fully energized.*

The addition of the parent and child guessing what the other person needs to eat is a powerful demonstration that only the child knows what their hunger is and how much they need to eat. Thus, when we are eating with a group of people, we want to train these children with sensory superpowers to tune into their own bodies and get what they need rather than eating in accordance with the intake of those around them. This demonstration tends to "work" because the child makes sure they always win (that their guess about how much they need to eat is more accurate than their parent's guess).

The parent/child/family proceeds to eat their small pile of snacks.

THERAPIST: *Ok everybody. Now tune in and see what your energy feels like. When you are ready, show me where you are on the energy meter with your hands.*

If individuals are not fully energized yet, the therapist could say:

THERAPIST: *Ok, I guess we have to keep going. Go ahead and eat as much of the next pile as you need until you feel fully energized. [This proceeds until everyone is fully energized]. Great job everybody. Let's review our guesses and what happened. [Therapist reviews guesses and number of snack pieces actually consumed.] Hmmm, it looks like everyone's guess was a little off, but tuning into your body and your energy really helped you to give you the energy your body needed. It also looks like you were each better at knowing what your body needed than the other person who tried to guess for you. I guess that makes sense. We know our own bodies best!*

Body Lesson #1 from The Eats (May Be Added to the Child's Body Map)

My body can tell me that I need energy and when I'm fully energized.

Adding Things to the Body Map

The next step is to add what the child learned to the Body Map. As a reminder, this can be both the specific details of what happened (e.g., I thought I needed to eat 15 crackers to get fully energized, but I only needed to eat ten to fill me up) as well as the smart new body skills that were learned (e.g., my body can let me know when I need energy; I can get better at listening to my body's energy levels with practice, etc.).

Body Lesson #2 from The Eats

I can get better at listening to my body's energy levels with practice.

THERAPIST: *Ok! That was terrific! Should we add what we learned to your body map? What do you think we should put on there? Mom/brother/sister/Dad, is there anything you want to add to your body map?*

Noticing Thirst

Thirsty Theo is the feeling that lets us know that we need to fill our bodies up with some thirst-quenching liquids – like water. When your mouth and sometimes even your throat feels dry, it is time to explore the best ways to bring moisture back to your mouth and quench Thirsty Theo! Here are some investigations to learn a bit more about your thirst (Table 7.4).

Table 7.4 Investigations for Thirsty Theo

1. Investigate how long it takes you to get thirsty when you are playing a sport. Does it differ if you are playing the sport outside? Based on what you learn, how much water should you be sure to bring to a sporting event?
2. What beverage has the best thirst-quenching properties?
3. If when you get too hungry you might feel hangry (a combination of hungry and irritated), what does it feel like when you get too thirsty? What is a good name for that?
4. Does watching a commercial of a refreshing drink make your mouth dry and thirsty or does it just make you think you are thirsty?

Body Lesson #3 from The Eats

Feeling thirsty is a very unique sensation. It must be an important message.

Enjoying Food

The last body sensation that we will learn about in this session is that of food enjoyment. This relates to experiencing a moment of utter food deliciousness in your mouth. Umm-ma Uma is that overwhelmingly positive feeling of tastiness that you get when you have had a delicious bite and you cannot resist the urge to give an "Umm-ma" kiss of perfection (Figure 7.6). We will ask about this in our Body Brainstorms worksheet this week and use it as a part of our home-based practice.

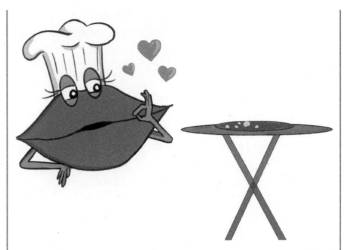

Figure 7.6 Umm-ma Uma when you experience a moment of food deliciousness.

THERAPIST: *We have one last character that we are going to learn today: Umm-ma Uma. This is the feeling of pure deliciousness that we feel when we eat a yummy bite. There are lots of fun investigations we can try with Umm-ma Uma (Table 7.5). Maybe there is one that you would like to try at home this week.*

Table 7.5 Fun investigations we can try with Umm-ma Uma

1. Investigate if foods taste more delicious when you eat it slowly versus quickly.
2. Investigate if foods taste more delicious if you are not doing anything but eating versus watching television while eating.
3. Do a taste comparison of your top five foods and see which one brings on the most Umm-ma Uma.
4. Try making a new recipe. Guess how Umm-ma Uma you think it will be and see what happens.

Body Lesson #4 from The Eats

Delicious food tastes even more delicious when you pay close attention to how the food tastes.

Summarizing the Body Lesson Learned

In FBI – Pain Division, new learning is generated primarily through lived experiences. That said, the therapist facilitates synthesis and consolidation of the material and lessons learned in each session through targeted questions at the end of the visit. By answering these questions, families can summarize and better remember the main points of their experiences (see Chapter 4 for more information about the logic of this as it relates to consolidating new learning). These lessons are added to the Body Map to make sure they are not forgotten.

THERAPIST: *OK everybody. Let's think for a bit about what just happened. We keep learning more and more about how smart your body is and how it keeps getting smarter. Is there anything that we learned today that shows how smart your body is that we can add to your body maps? [If they have trouble coming up with something, the therapist could ask something like:] "Do you think that it is pretty cool that your body sends you a message when you need more energy? Should we add that to our body map?"*

Body Brainstorms

As in the prior session, many of the answers to the Body Brainstorms worksheet were learned throughout the session. To help generalize what was learned in the session to daily life, we ask everyone to think about the following questions and answer them.

Can you remember the last time you heard your stomach growl? Can your mom or dad?

Have you ever felt Harold the Hunger Pain? Do you remember what happened that you got that hungry?

Is there a certain time of day when you notice Georgia the Gut Growler the most?

When was the last meal when you felt perfectly satisfied afterwards?

What is one food that is really hard to stop eating? Do you usually eat it until you are stuffed?

Can you think of the most delicious bite to eat?

What is your favorite thing to drink when you are really thirsty?

Introduction to the FBI Body Clues Worksheet

In this session, we begin to learn the steps of our Body Clues Worksheet. Last week, the children picked two sensations to focus on and then wrote or drew a picture when they noticed those sensations. This week, we introduce the first two steps of the Body Clues Worksheet. We will use this worksheet throughout treatment to help children learn the meaning of different body sensations. Children will then develop ideas of behaviors that they can perform in response to those body sensations to either meet the need or respond to the message that their body is communicating.

These worksheets are an important crux of this intervention as they are a guide to self-parenting (Chapter 3). Unlike a cognitive behavioral therapy intervention for older children, which is rooted in the content of one's thoughts and patterns of behavior, the FBI – Pain Division is sensation-based (as you well know by now). There are several cues that may prompt the parent or child to start completing a Body Clues Worksheet between sessions: the child may notice a sensation that they are confused about and want to think through what their body is telling them; the parent may have just helped the child get through a difficult moment; the parent and child may be figuring out what just happened after a difficult moment; and/or the parent and child may be reviewing the most intense moments of the day to reflect on what happened and what they can do differently next time. Table 7.6 lists the myriad ways that these worksheets can be used. However, we want to create some rituals and habits: these sheets will become the basis of all home-based practice and will guide the homework review at the beginning of each session from the next visit (Session 3) forward. In this session, the children are introduced to Steps 1 and 2 of the Body Clues Worksheet.

Table 7.6 Suggested ways in which the Body Clues worksheets can be used

Parents are encouraged to use this worksheet, in particular, in the following circumstances:
– After their child has had a big sensation moment, such as a pain moment, to help figure out what is going on
– When their child is having trouble figuring out what is going on in a given moment
– At the end of the day, as a way to review important moments during the day
– As a way to design and plan a new investigation

Parents and children can use this worksheet whenever:
– The child is having a sensation that they don't understand
– As a review of the biggest sensation moment of the day
– As an investigation game, a chance to practice interviewing a "witness" or to figure out what the other is feeling at a given moment
– As a way to design an investigation to help the child approach something challenging
– After a big moment to figure out what happened and what one might try next time
– However the parent wants to use it
– However the child wants to use it

The FBI Body Clues Worksheet Step 1

Circle all the sensations you are feeling. You can draw a few circles if you are feeling the sensations intensely. You can draw part of a circle if you are feeling them a little bit.

To help parents keep track of the characters (the children usually master the characters quickly), parent and child will receive a worksheet that summarizes the characters that they have learned so far. Similarly, the Body Clues Worksheet for each session will show only the characters that the child has learned so far. Step 1 of the Body Clues Worksheet is the initial assessment phase in which the child indicates what sensations they are feeling (Table 7.7). To help families practice using this worksheet, the therapist first establishes whether the child and parent are going to fill it out based on how they are feeling at the present moment or based on an event that happened in the recent past.

The following dialogue walks you through how we typically go through a Body Clues Worksheet.

THERAPIST: *Okay! It is time to fill out our first Body Clues Worksheet. Here is how it's going to go. First, I'm going to interview you about how you are feeling. Next, I'm going to have you interview your mom/dad/brother/sister about how they are feeling. The first thing that we need to decide is whether we want to focus on how you are feeling right now or whether we want to focus on something that happened to you earlier today or earlier in the week.*

If the child or parent requests to explore something that happened earlier in the day or earlier in the week, ask them the following:

THERAPIST: *Okay, since we are talking about something that happened earlier, I want you to take a minute and really picture the thing that happened in your mind. Go ahead and close your eyes and just really picture what was going on and what you were feeling. Try to imagine yourself in that moment just like it is happening right now. (The therapist waits a minute or two). Have you got it? Okay, let's proceed.*

STEP 1: LISTEN TO YOUR BODY.

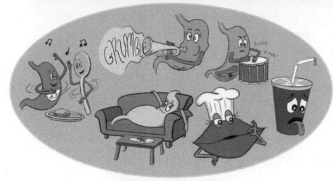

THE EATS

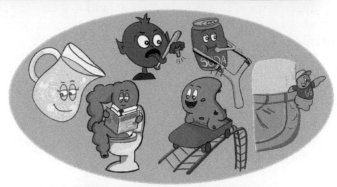

THE EXPLOSIONS

Figure 7.7 Diagram of the Body Clues Worksheet, Step 1. We demonstrate two of the session topics, The Eats and The Explosions. Children go through each character and circle what they are feeling.

Table 7.7 Instructions for completing a Body Clues Worksheet (Steps 1 and 2)

1. Determine whether you are focusing on the current moment or on an event in the recent past. If the latter, make sure to give the child and parent time to think about the event that happened and get a vivid picture of it in their memory so they can answer the questions.
2. The therapist will then go through each and every character, asking the child if they are experiencing that sensation in the moment (or when the event happened) and how much they were experiencing it. We circle the sensations that the child endorses. A fun way that the children learn to express the intensity of that sensation is by the degree to which the circle is completed around the character. So, they could answer a quarter circle if they are feeling it a little bit, a half circle if there feeling it moderately, etc. The therapist can be helpful by saying things like: Did you feel Henry Heartbeat a full circle? a half circle? a quarter circle? Whatever the child says is right. The important thing is that the child is turning their attention to their body with curiosity and trying to figure out what is going on in there.
3. In Step 2, the therapist asks the child to draw or write what they were doing when they noticed that sensation.

To make this exercise more playful, we typically pretend like we're a detective interviewing a witness. we'll adopt the tone of voice that someone would use in an overly dramatic television crime drama. Imagine the tone a detective would use when they're asking a suspect "where were you the night of X?" So, we'll say in a similar tone (but not in an accusatory tone, of course), "Were you feeling Henry Heartbeat?"

THERAPIST: *Now let's go through all the body sensations that we have learned so far and see what you are feeling. Were you feeling Henry Heartbeat?*

CHILD: Yes!

THERAPIST: *Okay! I'm going to circle Henry Heartbeat. Now if you are feeling Henry Heartbeat a lot, I'll put a whole circle around Henry. If you were REALLY feeling Henry Heartbeat a lot we can even put two circles around him. If you are just feeling Henry Heartbeat a little bit, I can just draw part of a circle – like a half circle – and if you are feeling Henry Heartbeat just a teensy bit we can draw just a teensy bit of a circle. Do you want to draw a circle around Henry Heartbeat? There is no right answer. You are going to get better and better at listening to Henry Heartbeat.*

CHILD: Okay. I'm going to draw a half circle.

THERAPIST: *That's great! Were you feeling Betty the Butterfly?*

CHILD: Yes!

THERAPIST: *Okay! What are you going to draw?*

CHILD: Just a little bit, like this (the child proceeds to draw approximately a quarter circle around Betty the Butterfly).

THERAPIST: *Were you feeling Gerda Gotta Go, the feeling like you had to pee?*

CHILD: No.

The therapist continues with this until they have gone through all the characters. They then move on to Step 2 of the Body Clues Worksheet.

The FBI Body Clues Worksheet Step 2

Step 2 is important because we want the children and parents to learn that different sensations can mean different things depending on the context.

THERAPIST: *You did a great job with that. For Step 2, we have to think about what you are doing or what was happening when you felt those sensations. Can you tell me what you were doing?*

STEP 2: CONDUCT AN INVESTIGATION.
What were you doing? What was going on?

Figure 7.8 Step 2 of the Body Clues Investigation. By thinking about what they were doing when they felt a given body sensation, they can better figure out what their bodies are trying to tell them.

CHILD: I was going to a birthday party.

THERAPIST: *Okay! Do you want me to write that here, or do you want to write it? Do you just want to draw a picture of it?*

CHILD: I will write it.

THERAPIST: *You really did a great job with that. Now it's your turn. How about you go ahead and interview your mom about how they are feeling right now or about something that happened to them this week.*

The child then proceeds to interview the mom (or other parent, sibling, etc.) For this first time, the therapist can offer gentle coaching questions, e.g., *"Should we ask your mom to picture what happened before she starts answering?"*

> Note: In Session 2, only Steps 1 and 2 of the Body Clues Worksheet will be learned and practiced. At this point in the intervention, the Body Clues Worksheet is just used to observe and describe what is going on.

Your Second Body Investigation Assignment (Home-Based Practice)

For Session 2, the home assignment is for the children and their parents to complete a Body Clues Worksheet – ideally once a day (or as often as is reasonable). The parent and child will go through the same steps that we went through in the session: the parent interviews the child, and then the child interviews the parent (of course, the child will most likely determine who goes first). As noted, the family can fill out the sheets in response to an event that just happened and/or as a review of their day. Eventually, families will also be trained to use Body Clues Worksheets to plan a future body investigation.

It is important that parents complete the Body Clues Worksheets about their own experiences and that they do so in a manner that their child can observe. Parent role modeling of self-awareness is critical so children can learn how important it is. In addition, if we think back to our conversations with parents in Session 1 and discussed in Chapter 3, the journey through the FBI intervention is part of their own journey as well.

Body Investigation Journal

In the child's body investigation journal this week, they can be on the lookout for Umm-ma Uma moments: moments when they have such a delicious bite of something that they feel compelled to give an Umm-ma Uma kiss.

Materials Families Take Home from Session 2

Below is a summary of what families take home from Session 2:

1. The Body Clues Worksheet which summarizes the characters that the child has learned so far and guides them in a mapping exercise of their body awareness
2. The Body Characters Worksheet which provides a key to who all the characters are
3. Coloring pages

4. The workbook pages for their binder which includes a summary of some of the Body Investigations we may have practiced and some ideas for other investigations
5. The Body Brainstorms worksheet they completed
6. Optional: Prizes! An invisible ink pen and a pair of sunglasses
7. Optional: A Georgia the Gut Growler button

Information on getting prizes and buttons and color worksheets and coloring pages can be found at: www.cambridge.org/fbi-clinical-guide.

Body Investigations to Practice at Home

In our web-based community and online resources for therapists (www.cambridge.org/fbi-clinical-guide) we provide ongoing and frequently updated ideas for various body investigations that you can perform with your families in session. As the intervention progresses, the families will become comfortable with and excited about designing their own investigations to explore at home and as they go about their days. Here are some ideas to get everybody started!

1. Family members can monitor their energy levels during a meal.
2. Children can try to slow down their eating and see what happens to the deliciousness of the food (they can do ratings of food deliciousness before slowing down eating and afterward).
3. If they feel extra full after a meal, the child can investigate what happens to Sabrina Stuffed if they go on a walk.
4. They can investigate how long the energy lasts from different meals.: for example, if they had a fruit or vegetable with their meal, what is their energy like? How long does their energy last?

Then you can schedule the next session! Congratulations, you've just finished Session 2!

Therapist Reminders for Session 2

Remind the parents and children to bring in the homework sheets they completed. From here on out, checking in on our energy and having a snack to get fueled up will be part of the ritual that begins our session. Thus, you may want to have a snack stash on hand or remind parents to bring in a snack in small pieces for the session.

A Final Reflection for Session 2

As a final reflection for this session, we want you to think about how a patient's relationship with food can change when they have been diagnosed with a gastrointestinal problem. Constant hypervigilance to post-ingestion symptoms, elimination diets, anxiety about eating out ... these are just some examples of the negative and fearful relationships to food that a patient can develop. Different foods have different effects on our system, but the fundamental role of food is to energize our bodies to meet our basic needs. In this chapter, we really tried to get the children and their families to adopt (or strengthen) this framework surrounding the energy that food brings us and to view body changes that occur after eating with curiosity rather than with fear. It may be a very informative exercise for you as a therapist to go through the next week focusing in on your own energy and its changes as you eat. Of course, we would also love for you to have some Umm-Ma Uma moments of your own!

Questions and Answers for Session 2

Q: What if the child does not want to eat or is already full?

A: No worries. Just have them use the energy meter and assess their energy in a different context. For example, the investigation you could do is to have them assess their energy before they do a Henry Heartbeat activity and see if their energy goes up or down after a few selected activities.

Q: Would you change anything if you are working with a patient who is overweight?

A: Nope. Body awareness is the way to help all children feel connected to their bodies and to develop a responsive relationship with food. Umm-Ma Uma moments help everyone to eat more slowly, enjoy what they eat more, and perhaps further tune in to when they feel satisfied.

References

1. Turnwald, B.P., Bertoldo, J.D., Perry, M.A., et al. (2019). Increasing vegetable intake by emphasizing tasty and enjoyable attributes: a randomized controlled multisite intervention for taste-focused labeling. *Psychol Sci 30*(11), 1603–1615. https://doi.org/10.1177/09567976198721912

2. Craighead, L. (2006). *Appetite Awareness Workbook*. Oakland, CA: Harbinger

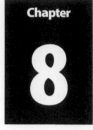

Chapter

8

Session 3: The Explosions

Overview of Session 3

Greetings. At this point in the treatment, we have learned all the rituals that begin the session: performing our Henry Heartbeat Warm-Up Exercise, reviewing our homework and adding new things we have learned about the body to our Body Map, and checking in with our energy and fueling up with a snack. Then, it is on to new things! This session is called "The Explosions." We learn about body sensations that we notice when we eat and digest food. The Explosions includes some impressive ways in which our bodies protects us from harm (like vomiting). We also learn two more steps of our Body Clues worksheet. These steps help to solidify the concept of self-parenting: learning how and why the body communicates and how to listen and decode those messages so that we feel safe in our bodies. Once everyone has learned these four steps, mastery of self-parenting will be underway. Insider tip: this session is known for having the best prizes (if you decide to give prizes).

Session Outline

1. Perform a Warm-Up Henry Heartbeat exercise
2. Review homework and add new things to the Body Map
3. Check in with your energy and fuel up with a snack
4. Learn new characters related to eating and digesting food – Gaggy Greg, Victor Vomit, and Burpy Bernie – by going over the workbook pages
5. Perform some Body Investigations
6. Complete a Body Brainstorms Worksheet
7. Learn steps 3 and 4 of the Body Clues Worksheet
8. Review the plan for the week
9. Give out prizes and coloring pages

Session Materials

1. Workbook, worksheets, and coloring pages for Session 3, Part 3
2. A snack the child brings or that you have on hand that is in small pieces for sensing our energy and fueling up
3. A tongue depressor and disgusting jelly beans for our body investigations (optional)
4. Barf bags, a Whoopee Cushion, and a Victor Vomit Button for Session Prizes (optional)

Background Information for Session 3
Lots of Weird Things Happen When Our Body Digests Food

Many gastrointestinal (GI) sensations are intertwined with the processes of eating and digesting food. Other GI sensations help the body to eliminate potentially threatening pathogens. Gassy foods, constipating foods, high-residue foods – nuances of foods can impact the experiences in our bodies. For example, some (but not all) children with sensory superpowers may have oral sensitivities: they are precisely aware of the way in which certain foods feel in their mouths. They may be very sensitive to the way foods smell or even the way they look (see Some Thoughts on Nausea, Vomiting, Gagging, and the Experience of Disgust for more information). Other children may be very sensitive to the consequences of eating: the sensations of gas or fullness that occur during the process of digesting food. For children with sensory super-powers, these experiences may be louder and more intense and thus carry with them the potential to interfere with daily functioning. Warning signals such as nausea and protective processes such as gagging and vomiting can become feared in and of themselves. Children can start to avoid activities or stimuli that they think have a possibility, no matter how small, of making them gag, vomit, or feel nauseated. This is consistent with the fear-avoidance model of pain that we have been discussing. When it comes to eating and digesting food, this can result in broad food avoidance. Let's consider an example.

A child is eating some yogurt and takes a bite that has an unexpected lumpy texture, prompting a gag response. The child, not liking the unexpectedness of that texture and the sensation of gagging, decides not only to stop eating that particular yogurt in that moment but, as a precaution, the child decides to avoid yogurt from now on. This is an example of maladaptive fear generalization that we discussed in Chapters 2 and 4. It is not hard to imagine that this sensitivity, and the learning processes that may accompany that sensitivity, could lead to a path of food avoidance and decreased food enjoyment as children become hypervigilant towards the effects of food on their bodies.

Consider the same scenario with a child trained as an elite FBI agent. They are eating some yogurt and POW! – they come across a lumpy texture and gag. "Whoa! I just had Gaggy Greg!

This calls for an investigation! If I keep eating the yogurt, will Gaggy Greg keeping coming? Get stronger? Get quieter? What other yogurts make me feel Gaggy Greg? Which ones make the biggest gag?" The investigations are endless …

As you are learning, in FBI, part of the enjoyment of eating is inculcating curiosity about the effects that food can have as you eat and while your body is digesting. For many young children, a clear path to pleasure is to "seriously" investigate what foods make you gag or pass gas the most. Becoming a strategic farter, one who can intentionally pass gas at key moments that add humor or awkwardness (and stench) to a given situation, is a skill only the most highly trained FBI agents have mastered and can use judiciously!

This approach is related to, yet also differs from, some exposure-based approaches that are utilized in cognitive-behavioral therapy. For example, in exposures designed to facilitate habituation or desensitization, a child may make a list of the various stimuli that provoke (or that they believe provoke) a sensation such as gagging or vomiting. The child may then be systematically presented with those stimuli to demonstrate that over time and with practice the sensation becomes less intense or that their beliefs about the negative implications of such sensations were not supported. The approach of FBI – Pain Division is similar but different in that we focus on the sensation (gagging, vomiting), change the context of experiencing that sensation such that it is "no big deal," and demonstrate that when the sensation occurs, the child can handle it. As you (and your clients) are increasingly understanding by Session 3, the premise of FBI – Pain Division is to interfere with this cycle by altering the perception of these sensations as threatening. Rather, these sensations are old friends, here to assist us as needed. Some of the lessons that we learn in The Explosions are: my body has some very noisy ways to protect me; my body gives me lots of helpful warning signs; and my body can get used to unexpected things with practice!

Some Thoughts on Nausea, Vomiting, Gagging, and the Experience of Disgust

The sensations of nausea and the experiences of gagging and vomiting may be part of the emotional experience of disgust. Disgust is an emotion that is designed to protect the body from potential pathogens. A pathogen exerts its effect when it crosses a body barrier (absorption through the skin, ingestion via the mouth, inhalation via nasal passages, etc.). The body has many cool sensory systems designed to detect irregularities and prevent the passage of pathogens into the body. Irregular visual features such as discoloration of food or more extreme examples such as mold on bread, slightly softer feelings of a piece of fruit, an irregular smell – these are all warning signs of potential contamination. One way to think about children with sensory superpowers is that they have lower thresholds for noticing these irregularities. Given that these children have a history of pain, it is not hard to imagine that this system will become even more sensitized as it tries to protect the body from harm by attempting to detect potential problems well in advance of food ingestion.

What we are trying to circumvent is anxious hypervigilance and avoidance. For example, children could become hypervigilant in their attempt to track which foods cause what symptoms. Such attention could totally sap the joy out of eating and elicit a fear of eating outside of the house. Moreover, if children are embarrassed by their bowel habits, they can become worried about going to the bathroom in public places. These fears may greatly limit their life experiences. From an FBI – Pain Division perspective, there is only one way out of this dilemma. We have to make these body experiences hysterically funny. We create characters about these sensations, acknowledge that we all have them, and embrace them. That said, it is great if children are curious about how various lifestyle behaviors affect their body. Consistent with our approach, however, we want this to be from the perspective of curiosity. Instead of "Oh my gosh! I can't poop." We are shooting for "Hmmm. I seem to be having trouble pooping. What investigation shall I try to relax my butt muscles or make my poops squishy?"

It should not be surprising that this is one of the most fun sessions.

Step-by-Step Guide to Session 3
Warm-Up Henry Heartbeat Activity

Since conducting Henry Heartbeat activities is probably familiar by now, we will not repeat all the steps here. In our experience, by Session 3 the children are coming in with their own Henry Heartbeat investigations that they have designed. If they do, we strongly advise that therapists participate in these child-created exercises to serve as excellent role models for openness to new experiences. Table 8.1 provides one idea for a Henry Heartbeat investigation. Our ongoing list of creative investigations can be found on the community website associated with this training program at https://eatingdisorders.dukehealth.org/functional-abdominal-pain.

Review Homework and Add New Things to Their Body Map

Table 8.2 reviews the steps for reviewing homework with the Body Map. Since we go through these steps in detail in Chapter 7, we only briefly review them here.

Table 8.1 Ideas for Henry Heartbeat investigations

How much can you slow down your heart beat?

First, measure how fast is it beating now. Then, choose an activity that you think will lower your heartbeat.

Decide how long you will perform the activity. For example, you could decide that reading a book will lower your heartbeat and you plan to read the book for two minutes.

Before you get started, take a guess by how many beats you think you can slow down your heart beat from reading. Will you slow it down by two beats? Ten beats? Have the parent and therapist do this too in regard to their own heartbeat.

Perform the activity that you chose and see how close you were in your predictions. If you want, you could compare it to a different activity and see if it works any better at slowing down your heart.

After the activity is over, think about some situations where slowing your heartbeat down may come in handy. Add all of what you just learned to your Body Map.

Table 8.2 Steps for reviewing homework and summarizing new body sensation experiences

1. The child finds their Body Map and lays it on the ground (and weights it with objects so it stays flat). The parent pulls out their Body Map (most likely on a sheet of paper in their FBI folder).
2. If anything new was learned in the Henry Heartbeat activity, this is added to the map.
3. Last week, the children and parents were instructed in the first two steps of the Body Clues Worksheet. The therapist will review these (see dialogue below).
4. Anything new about the body that was learned from the Body Clues worksheet is added to the Body Map.
5. If the children and parents did not complete any Body Clues worksheets, the therapist will work on completing it with them right then and there in the session.

THERAPIST: *We keep learning more and more about the things that make your heart beat faster and slower. Is there anything that we just learned from our Henry Heartbeat investigation that we should add to your Body Map?*

Last week, we learned the first two steps of our Body Clues Worksheet. Were you able to fill out any sheets that we can look at together?

If Parent and Child Brought in Homework

THERAPIST: *That is so terrific that you both filled out some sheets. Let's see what you learned!*

The therapist has the child go through each sheet. The child tells what body sensations were circled and what they were doing during that time. The therapist's job at this point is just to summarize and nudge them to add new things to their Body Map.

THERAPIST: *OK. So let me make sure I got this. You had a little bit of Betty Butterfly, your heart was beating a half circle, you had a quarter circle of Samantha Sweat, and you had Georgia the Gut Growler, full circle. Do I have that right?*

CHILD: Yeah. I was going to the first day of baseball.

THERAPIST: *I wonder what your body was trying to tell you? We are going to figure out what that means as we become smarter and smarter FBI agents. Should we add that the first day of practice gives you Betty Butterfly, Henry Heartbeat, and Samantha Sweat to your Body Map?*

CHILD: OK.

THERAPIST: *What do you think Georgia the Gut Growler was telling you?*

CHILD: That I was hungry.

THERAPIST: *That makes sense. Nice detective work!*

If the Child and Parent Did Not Do Their Homework

The therapist will have the parents and child complete a homework sheet at that moment. They can fill out a sheet either according to how they are feeling at that moment or they can think about a time previously in the week that they can remember well, when they were having a really big sensation moment.

THERAPIST: *Sounds like everybody had a really busy week. I sure hope you are able to fill them out together next week. We get so much better at these things with practice. Let's go ahead and do it together right now. Do you want to fill out a sheet about how we are feeling right now or should we think of a big moment that happened earlier in the week?*

MOM: Remember when we had that tough time getting to school? Let's do it about that.

CHILD: Ok.

THERAPIST: *Sari, do you remember the morning your mom is talking about?*

CHILD: Yes.

THERAPIST: *OK. I want you both to take a minute and close your eyes and picture that moment. Try to think about what was happening and how your body was feeling. Let me know when you have a good picture of it in your mind.*

CHILD: I'm ready.

MOM: Me too.

THERAPIST: *OK, Sari. I'll start with you. Were you feeling Henry Heartbeat? …*

The therapist proceeds to review the sheet and do a "witness/criminal investigation" as described in the past session.

THERAPIST: *Great job, Sari. Do you want to interview your mom now? [After the review] Is there anything we should add to our Body Maps?*

Assessing Your Energy and Fueling Up

The ritual added to the beginning of every session is checking in with your energy using our energy meter and fueling up till everyone participating feels satisfied. We perform this activity so children get better at detecting hunger and fullness and so that everyone's brains are ready to take in new information. The child can be fueling up while you read the workbook pages, however, if you do this, be sure to stop reading throughout to do an energy check.

THERAPIST: *We have one more thing to do before we start learning about new characters. Let's check in with our energy and see if we need to fuel up before we learn new things. We want to make sure our brains get enough energy to learn.*

Session 2 Workbook: The Explosions

As part of the ritual and routine of the session, the therapist can make a habit of asking who wants to do the reading today. One goal for all sessions is for the child and the child's family to read things together and talk about them. While we give you some ideas of things the therapist could ask during these readings, these are merely suggestions. The spirit of this part of the session is further inculcating that spirit of playful curiosity towards all the things the body does, so any question is a great question.

This week's investigative questions ask families to think about the following body mysteries.

Session 3: Body Mystery Questions

Why do you think that bodies are designed so that they throw up?

Why do you think that we pass gas?

The therapist's job is to get the children and parents thinking about these things. So, if the child immediately says "I don't know," the therapist can encourage them to spend a minute or two just thinking about it and making a guess. The goal here is not to get the right answer. Instead, the goal is to warm people up to get them thinking about the body in a curious way. To whatever the family says, the therapist just offers encouragement (e.g., Those are some really interesting thoughts! … I never thought about that. That's a really cool idea … That makes a lot of sense. The therapist can also be a role model by describing a related experience.)

Gaggy Greg

Gaggy Greg is the sensation you have when you feel like you might gag or when you actually gag. Children learn in the workbook pages that gagging is designed to protect you from things that could make you sick or as a reaction to things that are unexpected. Children with sensory superpowers have extremely high-tech, precise systems for detecting potential threats. In other words, when we talk about sensory superpowers, we often describe these children as feeling things that others do not feel, seeing things that others do not see, smelling things that others do not smell, and tasting things that others do not taste. Every child has different sensory superpowers so your patient may only endorse some of these features.

This is really cool. However, it can also mean that the system can have some false alarms. A powerful investigation that can be done is noticing what happens to a gag reflex when an individual is eating something for the second, third, or fourth time, as the food becomes more and more familiar. Does the gag get weaker because Gaggy Greg is smart enough to know what to expect and learn that things are safe? Does it get stronger because Gaggy Greg associated that food with gagging? Is the pattern the same for every food? Pretty interesting to find out …

The workbook attempts to explain these fascinating but complicated concepts in child-friendly terms (Part III – Session 3: The Explosions).

THERAPIST: *Let's see what Gaggy Greg has to say.*

GAGGY GREG: *I'm a reflex. Did you ever have a doctor hit your knee with a hammer and your foot flies up? That is kind of like me. If I sense something that feels a bit unexpected or unfamiliar, I may get activated and I try to protect you by gagging.*

Once I get used to something, I stop. For kids with sensory superpowers, it just may take me a bit longer to get used to stuff. But I can and I will!

THERAPIST: *Has that ever happened to you? You go to the doctor and she hits your knee with a hammer and your foot flies up? Imagine that you had a really sensitive knee reflex. Your foot would just randomly fly up when your knee felt the slightest thing and pretty soon you're just kicking everybody. That might be a bit annoying! Sometimes people's gag reflexes are like that and they get activated pretty easily. That is cool. We can learn more about it and see what sets it off and see how it gets used to things.*

There is a page in the workbook that shows Gaggy Greg getting used to a new taste. Questions the therapist can ask while the family reads this page include:

Have you ever eaten something that made you gag the first time you tried it? How about you, dad?

Did you try it again? What happened?

Victor Vomit

FBI agents are not afraid of vomit. Vomiting is intense. It is jolting. It is gross. It is fast. It is messy. It smells disgusting. It has all the features that children may love. We prepare for vomit, we get excited when it happens, and disappointed when it does not. In the child's workbook, Victor Vomit introduces himself like this:

Victor Vomit

Hi FBI agents and chiefs! It's me, Victor (Figure 8.1)! I know it might be hard to see me hidden underneath all of this barfed up food! I love action and adventure! For me, every time you throw up, I get to go on a super-speed roller coaster ride!! Whoo-eeee!! That is what vomiting is. There are sensors throughout your body on the look-out for harmful substances. If the sensors detect something dangerous, the muscles of your stomach use ALL THEIR POWER, and with great FORCE and SPEED, force the bad things out of your stomach, back up your throat, and out of your mouth! Whammo!!!! Vomit time!!! For me, it is a super fun ride – but it may not be as fun for you!

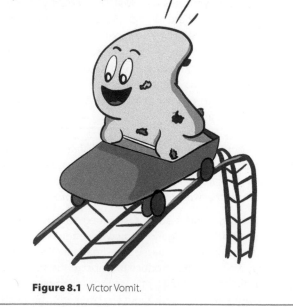

Figure 8.1 Victor Vomit.

THERAPIST QUESTIONS: *Have you ever thrown up before? What happened before? What happened afterwards? Dad, how about you?*

The goal with this questioning is to normalize the experience, to demonstrate the adaptive qualities of vomiting, and to show that often, a person feels a bit better after throwing up. These conversations can all help to make throwing up less scary. In addition, how we behave in our body investigations towards nausea and vomiting will really drive this point home.

What Happens to Food When You Eat It?

Let's spend a brief moment thinking through the processes that take place when you eat a piece of food. We present just a brief, over-simplified diagram of digesting food to reduce the uncertainty about what occurs. However, a diagram can only do so much. It might be helpful to pull up one of the numerous educational videos about digestion to help normalize all the myriad visceral experiences that accompany chewing, swallowing, and digesting food. Initially, the child or parent can just follow the arrows and explain what happens to food according to the diagram.

THERAPIST: *So, you just ate a snack a few minutes ago. Do you want to show me what happened to it?*

Gassy Gus

Gassy Gus is back. This gives us more permission to talk about a favorite topic among children: passing gas. In the spirit of curiosity and fun, we give individuals who pass gas the most the highest status in the family…

Gassy Gus

I'm back! It's good ole Gassy Gus (Figure 8.2)! You may be wondering why you pass gas. Well, I'm so glad you asked! Some foods are too hard for your digestive system to break down. These food parts travel to your large intestine. There, the healthy bacteria that lines your intestine turns these food products into – you guessed it – <u>Gassy Gus</u>!

Certain foods may cause a lot more of me than other foods. What foods give you gas? I love beans! Beans really love good ole' Gassy Gus!!

THERAPIST: *So, are there any foods that you eat that you have noticed give you a lot of gas? Who passes the most gas in your family? Do you think it is what they eat or are they just a super gas-passer? I wonder what foods make farts the smelliest?*

All of this generates some fascinating conversations. For home-based Body Investigations this week, suggested activities include performing some gassy investigations. These include examining the foods that produce the most or the smelliest gas and determining who in the family is the gas champion. While all these activities may seem ridiculous (and they are), the intention

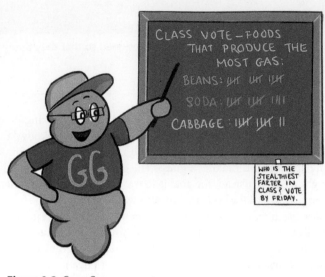

Figure 8.2 Gassy Gus

is important: we are creating a context in which bodily events which can be pain-inducing, such as gas, are experienced with curiosity rather than fear. We are also trying to create a framework in which a child can investigate these events without obsessiveness or hypervigilance. So, if you are feeling ridiculous during a session, that is confirmation that you are being a true FBI agent.

Burpy Bernie

Belching, burping, or eructation (if you want a fancy word) is another way in which your body protects you by providing relief from gas pressure. Burps can be noisy or silent so it is particularly fun for a family to identify the stealthy burpers. Some suspected contributions to burping can be eating really fast (and accidentally swallowing lots of air) or drinking carbonated beverages. But does talking really fast lead to burping? Do different types of carbonated beverages lead to different degrees of burping? Does being at a fancy dinner where you are expected to be polite and not burp actually make it harder to keep from burping? These are all very important investigations to try.

Gordon Gotta Go

Our final sensation of the week is Gordon Gotta Go, the sensation that you feel when you have to make a bowel movement. Bowel movements can be a great example of how the body learns patterns and develops routines. For example, some people are very regular in their bowel habits and go to the bathroom around the same time every day. Yet, at other times it can be quite an emergent situation. In the workbook, we refer to this as Gordon REALLY Gotta Go (and you can extrapolate from there). Children can have fun with the point at which sensing Gordon is so strong that they almost do not make it to the bathroom (e.g., Gordon

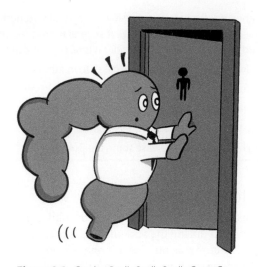

Figure 8.3 Gordon Really Really Really Gotta Go

REALLY REALLY REALLY Gotta Go, Figure 8.3). We get the children and parents to think about their individual patterns in our Body Brainstorms worksheet this week.

Body Investigation: Getting to Know Your Gag Reflex

As with all our Body Investigations, there is much room for creativity. We provide you with some examples here, and our web-based community provides a forum for therapists to contribute new ideas. The home-based body investigations are usually saved for those activities that would be harder to accomplish within the time limits of a session, but feel free to experiment.

A Gaggy Greg Novel Taste/Texture Investigation

If you have a child that is sensitive to new tastes or textures, the first taste of a new food can result in activation of the gag reflex. Remember what we discussed earlier about disgust, an emotion that protects us from pathogens. Children who are disgust-sensitive may also have a sensitive gag reflex that gets activated whenever their mouth tastes an unexpected taste or texture. This makes sense. The child's gag is being very cautious with new things.

Body Investigation: Eating Something Gross

There is no better way to experience Gaggy Greg or Victor Vomit than to just dive in and eat something gross. We go "all in" for this. Whenever we are conducting an investigation that has the possibility of evoking Gaggy Greg or Victor Vomit, we are prepared in the event that we do, in fact, throw-up. We have our garbage cans or fancy vomit bags (we have found some with the vomit emoji on it) ready. If a child is a super-gagger or an extra-sensitive vomiter, we might really ham it up and all wear bibs. As with any body investigation, there are many lessons to

be learned. In the case of Gaggy Greg and Victor Vomit, important lessons can be that our body has automatic mechanisms to protect us.

It is interesting to think about situations in which you may get used to something and not vomit with practice, versus those in which a stimulus may perpetually make you a bit sick. There may be some things that it is not in your body's best interest to get used to. For example, you would not want to make friends with the mosquito carrying malaria and have it hang around as your pet. An additional important lesson, however, can be that sometimes our body is overprotective at first and needs to get to know something before concluding that it is safe. There might be a new flavor profile that your mouth is not at all used to. Because the taste or texture is unexpected, Gaggy Greg may show up at first and then go away as your mouth gets used to the taste and texture with practice. All these are rife for investigations. We outline the protective response of the body by playing a fun game, the BeanBoozled jellybean game produced by the company Jelly Belly® at the time of this writing. We outline this game and investigation in Table 8.3.

Of course, this investigation can be done with any challenging food – not just gross jelly beans! Have parents and children each pick a food that is manageable but challenging – ideally a food that they have not had before. For children who have sensory superpowers to new tastes or textures, this may be a new food. For those children who try new foods quite easily, family members can try this with a food from a highly unfamiliar cuisine.

Decide what your investigative approach is going to be: are you going to go all in and just take a bite, or are you going to design baby steps to approach the food gradually? Either way, we observe whether Gaggy Greg shows up.

If Gaggy Greg shows up, perhaps design another investigation: come up with a routine that may help to shake it off. Maybe wiggle your body from your head to your toes? Once you have wiggled for a while and Gaggy Greg is off doing other things, approach the food again and see what happens to Gaggy Greg. Does Gaggy Greg get quieter? Louder? Remember: as an FBI agent, we are just curious about what happens. An investigation does not succeed or fail. We just learn something new.

Table 8.3 What does your body do when something is super gross?

1. In the Jelly Belly BeanBoozled® game, children combine both the experience of tasting something that is unexpected with the possibility of tasting something really disgusting.
2. Prior to starting this game, we get ready for the potential that everyone who plays might throw up. We get our garbage cans ready along with some napkins and Kleenex just in case.
3. Everyone takes turns and spins the spinner that comes with this game. The way the game is set up is that each color jellybean can have one of two flavors. One of these flavors is delicious and one is utterly disgusting. The player does not know which they are going to get until they taste it. Examples of disgusting flavors include barf, dog food, and stinky socks etc. You get the picture.

Playing this game is a great example about how your body protects you from things that you are not supposed to ingest. Furthermore, it does so in a funny way so that responses like our gag reflex can be viewed with awe rather than fear.

Body Investigation: Gaggy Greg and Surprises (Tables 8.4 and 8.5)

Table 8.4 Embracing the unexpected

What happens to something unexpected when you expect the unexpected? Does it become expected? We can have a lot of fun with this with Gaggy Greg.

1. Pick a new or challenging food.
2. Make a guess at what it will taste and feel like. Crunchy? Salty? Creamy? Sweet?
3. Make a plan for the unexpected: if you are way off in your predictions, is it time for celebration (Figure 8.4)? Time to wipe off your tongue with a napkin?
4. Take a taste and see how off your predictions were. Then compare your strategies to embrace the unexpected. Did Gaggy Greg show up with one strategy more than another?

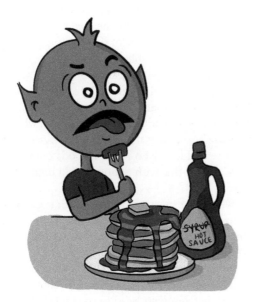

Figure 8.4 Embracing the unexpected.

Table 8.5 Slurping and burping

1. Do certain drinks or foods cause more burping than others? This question might be a great one to answer in our home-based body investigations because it is best conducted over a few days.
2. Decide on at least two things that you are going to compare. Let's say lemonade versus a carbonated lemon drink. On one day, drink a glass of lemonade. Record how many burps you have for the next 60 (or whatever time you choose) minutes.
3. On the next day, pour yourself the same amount of drink #2. Record your burps. See which drink wins!

Possible Body Lessons from The Explosions

My body has some very noisy ways to protect me.

My body gives me lots of helpful warning signs.

My body can get used to unexpected things with practice.

My body has a lot of automatic things that it does that try to protect me from harm.

Sometimes my body is oversensitive and thinks something is harmful. At those times, I can give it several more tries and see if my body gets used to it and decides it is not harmful after all.

Certain foods may make me more gassy than others.

Certain foods may make my gas smellier.

Eating things fast may make me burp.

Drinking things with bubbles may make me burp.

Burping helps my body release some pressure.

Adding to the Body Map

Do not forget this critical step to help consolidate the memory that was formed during the session. This is particularly important during intense sessions like this one. We want to make sure the child remembers how smart, protective, and powerful their body is – rather than focusing on the fact that they vomited, gagged, etc. The context in which that happened is key – their body was doing that to help them adjust to changes. Background about the learning and memory principles that guide this intervention can be found in Chapter 4.

Body Brainstorms

Throughout the session, we discovered many answers to the questions on our Body Brainstorm worksheet. The therapist should review what was already discovered and ask about any unknowns that are remaining. Questions on our Body Brainstorms worksheet this week include the following:

What are some foods that make you have gas?

What are some things that make you burp?

Is anyone in your family a stealthy farter – one who can fart undetected?

Is anyone in your family a stealthy burper – one who can burp undetected?

Does anyone in your family weaponize farting? They can fart on command when it is least expected or most unwanted?

Are there any things that have made you gag in the past? Do they still make you gag?

What is the time of day when you're most likely to poop?

Step 3 of the FBI Body Clues Worksheet

We reviewed Steps 1 and 2 at the beginning of the session as part of our homework review. We then added what we learned about the body from the homework to the child's and parent's Body Maps. In Session 3, we get a bit more advanced. This is one of our most important sessions. In this session, we first introduce the concept that our bodies communicate messages, telling us what we need. We can then use these messages to guide our behavior to get those needs met. This is a pretty complex concept. We do not need the children to understand this abstract principle. Rather, we have them learn this directly from their actions as mapped out in Steps 3 and 4 of the Body Clues Worksheets.

We do hope the parents are taught this overriding principle. We remind parents of these principles in their workbook pages. We discuss some of the evidence and theories behind this view of emotional experience in Chapter 2.

> Steps 3 and 4 of the Body Clues Worksheets help children and parents to learn that the sensations in their bodies communicate messages about what their bodies need. These messages help an individual organize their behavior to get those needs met.

Remember that when we are reviewing these Body Clues Worksheets in session, we often pretend we are detectives interviewing a witness to keep it playful. Step 1 reviews the body sensations that the child is experiencing during the event being reviewed. Step 2 helps the child figure out what the body might be communicating by contextualizing those sensations (Figure 8.5). While the child is merely describing what they were doing, they are learning through repeated practice that the same sensation might mean something different depending on the situation, an observation the therapist can make with the child.

In Step 3, we try to figure out what our bodies are trying to tell us. Much like in Step 1, the therapist will go through the entire list with the "witness" to learn what the child thinks might be going on. Reading through this whole list is very important because it teaches children how to label the meanings of diverse body sensations. Step 3 is organized as a list of different emotions the child may be experiencing, different types of pain (that they will learn more about in Session 6), and diverse body states like hunger and fatigue.

The following is an example dialogue after the therapist, parent, and child have identified a current or previous event that they are going to complete a worksheet about. In this example, the therapist has already completed Steps 1 and 2 with the child.

THERAPIST: *Now we are ready to learn some more steps so we can figure out what your body is trying to tell you. Now let's see. You've told me that you are feeling Ricky the Rock – full circle, Harold the Hunger Pain – full circle, and Betty the Butterfly – half circle. Did I get that right? In Step 2, we learned that you got into a fight with your friend at lunch time and that you did not have time to finish your lunch. Did I get that part right? Okay. Now I'm going to go through some options with Step 3 and see if we can figure out what your body might be trying to tell you.*

Prior to reading the options for Step 3, it is a good idea for the therapist to repeat what was identified in Steps 1 and 2 so that the child learns to connect the sensations with the meanings that are listed in Step 3.

THERAPIST: *Do you think your body was telling you that you were feeling happy? Excited? Sad? Angry? … And so on …*

> To emphasize that the body communicates needs that we have, we often have the therapist ask about Step 3 by using phrases such as "Do you think your body was telling you that you were … "Or "What was your body telling you was happening?" The important emphasis is that it is the body that is doing the communicating.

For every body meaning that the child endorses, the therapist should mark that in some way on the worksheet (e.g., underline, star, or circle that on the worksheet).

> It is important to read through all the options in Step 3 to help the child learn to label the diverse body sensations they are experiencing by increasing their descriptive vocabulary.

Step 4 of the FBI Body Clues Worksheet

For every body meaning that is listed in Step 3, there are suggestions about ways to get those needs met in Step 4. Therapists and families first take each state (e.g., of emotion, pain, etc.) that was labeled in Step 3 and find the suggestions for that state in Step 4. The therapist then goes through and reads the different suggestions for each state. The child then decides what they will try at that moment and/or the next time they experience that sensation. Figure 8.6 illustrates the connection between Steps 3 and 4.

These worksheets can be completed as an event is unfolding or after the fact. Because of this, they are written so that they can help the child or parent decide what to do in that moment or to plan for what to do the next time a similar situation arises. The wording of Step 4 provides options for each of these scenarios. When the therapist is reviewing the worksheet with the child, if the situation is going on at that moment, the therapist would be eliciting strategies that the child might want to try right then. Then, the child will employ the strategy, which constitutes another in-session Body Investigation. Alternatively, if the child is describing an event that occurred in the past, the purpose of Step 4 is to see what they tried, to be curious about what happened, and to make a plan for what to try next time.

Here is an example of a dialogue and worksheet that is being reviewed about a situation that is occurring at that moment. See also Figure 8.7.

THERAPIST: *In Step 3, you said that you were feeling guilty, sad, and had some hunger pains. Let's see what some of the suggestions are in Step 4 to see what we might try.*

The therapist deliberately circles the suggestions in Step 4 for guilty, sad, and hunger pains.

THERAPIST: *Let's see. Let's start with guilty. It says see if there is a problem that needs fixing. You might need to apologize, fix something, or have a good talk with someone. Do any of those sound like a good idea?*

CHILD: Yeah, when I have a fight with my friend I might need to apologize.

THERAPIST: *That's a good idea. So, is this a fight that is going on right now?*

CHILD: Yeah. It happened today at school.

THERAPIST: *Well, is this something we should do right now then? Maybe we could practice it or maybe we could write down what you would say in a text to your friend? I could pretend to be your friend and you could say something to me?*

CHILD: That is weird. I like the idea of writing down what I will say in a text to my friend.

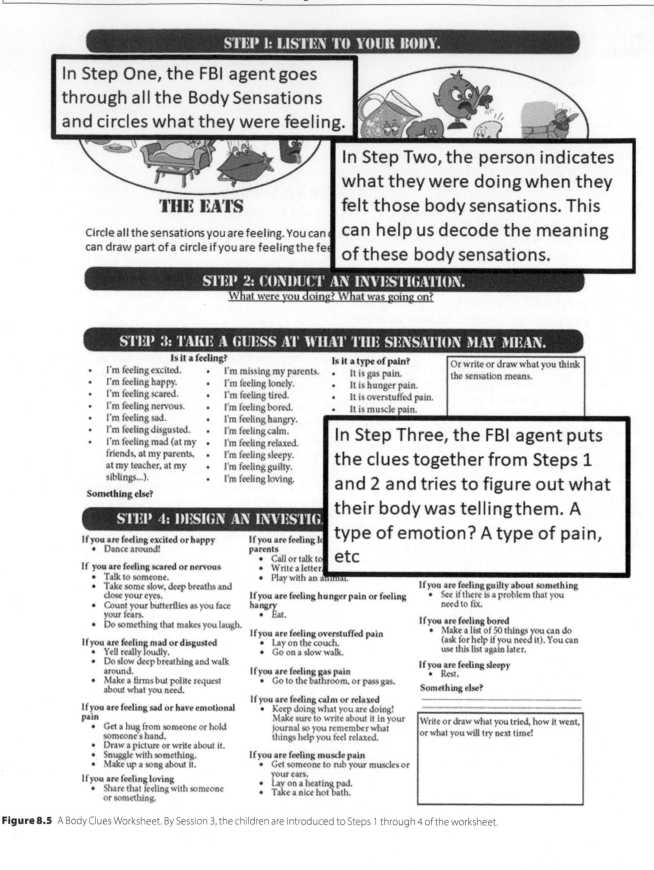

STEP 1: LISTEN TO YOUR BODY.

In Step One, the FBI agent goes through all the Body Sensations and circles what they were feeling.

THE EATS

Circle all the sensations you are feeling. You can [...]
can draw part of a circle if you are feeling the fee[...]

In Step Two, the person indicates what they were doing when they felt those body sensations. This can help us decode the meaning of these body sensations.

STEP 2: CONDUCT AN INVESTIGATION.
What were you doing? What was going on?

STEP 3: TAKE A GUESS AT WHAT THE SENSATION MAY MEAN.

Is it a feeling?
- I'm feeling excited.
- I'm feeling happy.
- I'm feeling scared.
- I'm feeling nervous.
- I'm feeling sad.
- I'm feeling disgusted.
- I'm feeling mad (at my friends, at my parents, at my teacher, at my siblings...).

- I'm missing my parents.
- I'm feeling lonely.
- I'm feeling tired.
- I'm feeling bored.
- I'm feeling hangry.
- I'm feeling calm.
- I'm feeling relaxed.
- I'm feeling sleepy.
- I'm feeling guilty.
- I'm feeling loving.

Is it a type of pain?
- It is gas pain.
- It is hunger pain.
- It is overstuffed pain.
- It is muscle pain.

Or write or draw what you think the sensation means.

Something else?

In Step Three, the FBI agent puts the clues together from Steps 1 and 2 and tries to figure out what their body was telling them. A type of emotion? A type of pain, etc

STEP 4: DESIGN AN INVESTIG[...]

If you are feeling excited or happy
- Dance around!

If you are feeling scared or nervous
- Talk to someone.
- Take some slow, deep breaths and close your eyes.
- Count your butterflies as you face your fears.
- Do something that makes you laugh.

If you are feeling mad or disgusted
- Yell really loudly.
- Do slow deep breathing and walk around.
- Make a firms but polite request about what you need.

If you are feeling sad or have emotional pain
- Get a hug from someone or hold someone's hand.
- Draw a picture or write about it.
- Snuggle with something.
- Make up a song about it.

If you are feeling loving
- Share that feeling with someone or something.

If you are feeling l[...]
parents
- Call or talk to[...]
- Write a letter[...]
- Play with an animal.

If you are feeling hunger pain or feeling hangry
- Eat.

If you are feeling overstuffed pain
- Lay on the couch.
- Go on a slow walk.

If you are feeling gas pain
- Go to the bathroom, or pass gas.

If you are feeling calm or relaxed
- Keep doing what you are doing! Make sure to write about it in your journal so you remember what things help you feel relaxed.

If you are feeling muscle pain
- Get someone to rub your muscles or your ears.
- Lay on a heating pad.
- Take a nice hot bath.

If you are feeling guilty about something
- See if there is a problem that you need to fix.

If you are feeling bored
- Make a list of 50 things you can do (ask for help if you need it). You can use this list again later.

If you are feeling sleepy
- Rest.

Something else?
_____

Write or draw what you tried, how it went, or what you will try next time!

Figure 8.5 A Body Clues Worksheet. By Session 3, the children are introduced to Steps 1 through 4 of the worksheet.

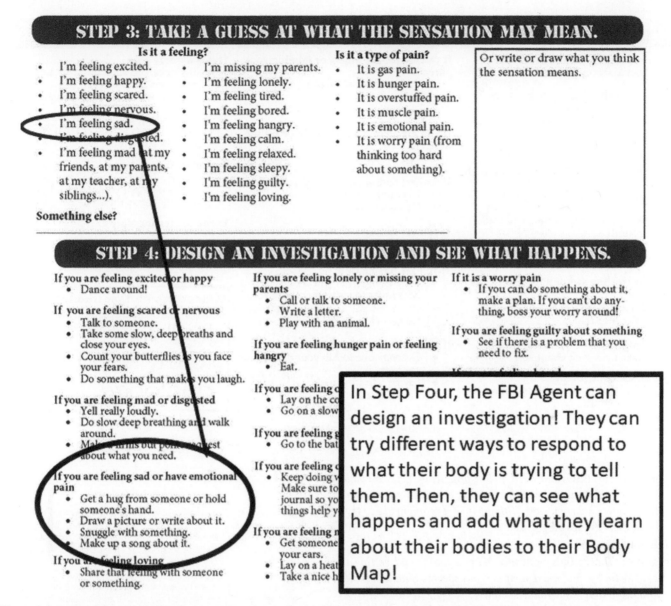

STEP 3: TAKE A GUESS AT WHAT THE SENSATION MAY MEAN.

Is it a feeling?
- I'm feeling excited.
- I'm feeling happy.
- I'm feeling scared.
- I'm feeling nervous.
- I'm feeling sad.
- I'm feeling disgusted.
- I'm feeling mad (at my friends, at my parents, at my teacher, at my siblings...).

- I'm missing my parents.
- I'm feeling lonely.
- I'm feeling tired.
- I'm feeling bored.
- I'm feeling hangry.
- I'm feeling calm.
- I'm feeling relaxed.
- I'm feeling sleepy.
- I'm feeling guilty.
- I'm feeling loving.

Something else?

Is it a type of pain?
- It is gas pain.
- It is hunger pain.
- It is overstuffed pain.
- It is muscle pain.
- It is emotional pain.
- It is worry pain (from thinking too hard about something).

Or write or draw what you think the sensation means.

STEP 4: DESIGN AN INVESTIGATION AND SEE WHAT HAPPENS.

If you are feeling excited or happy
- Dance around!

If you are feeling scared or nervous
- Talk to someone.
- Take some slow, deep breaths and close your eyes.
- Count your butterflies as you face your fears.
- Do something that makes you laugh.

If you are feeling mad or disgusted
- Yell really loudly.
- Do slow deep breathing and walk around.
- Make affirms but politely request about what you need.

If you are feeling sad or have emotional pain
- Get a hug from someone or hold someone's hand.
- Draw a picture or write about it.
- Snuggle with something.
- Make up a song about it.

If you are feeling loving
- Share that feeling with someone or something.

If you are feeling lonely or missing your parents
- Call or talk to someone.
- Write a letter.
- Play with an animal.

If you are feeling hunger pain or feeling hangry
- Eat.

If it is a worry pain
- If you can do something about it, make a plan. If you can't do anything, boss your worry around!

If you are feeling guilty about something
- See if there is a problem that you need to fix.

In Step Four, the FBI Agent can design an investigation! They can try different ways to respond to what their body is trying to tell them. Then, they can see what happens and add what they learn about their bodies to their Body Map!

Figure 8.6 Body investigations designed in response to what your body is feeling. For every sensation listed in Step 3, there are some ideas for investigations in Step 4. However, it is great if clever FBI agents design their own investigations as well. As with in-session investigations, anything new that we learn about our bodies as a result of these investigations gets added to the Body Map!

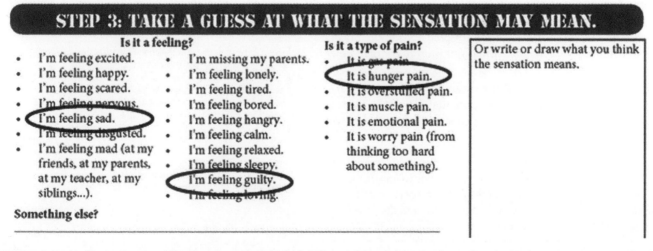

STEP 3: TAKE A GUESS AT WHAT THE SENSATION MAY MEAN.

Is it a feeling?
- I'm feeling excited.
- I'm feeling happy.
- I'm feeling scared.
- I'm feeling nervous.
- I'm feeling sad.
- I'm feeling disgusted.
- I'm feeling mad (at my friends, at my parents, at my teacher, at my siblings...).

- I'm missing my parents.
- I'm feeling lonely.
- I'm feeling tired.
- I'm feeling bored.
- I'm feeling hangry.
- I'm feeling calm.
- I'm feeling relaxed.
- I'm feeling sleepy.
- I'm feeling guilty.
- I'm feeling loving.

Something else?

Is it a type of pain?
- It is gas pain.
- It is hunger pain.
- It is overstuffed pain.
- It is muscle pain.
- It is emotional pain.
- It is worry pain (from thinking too hard about something).

Or write or draw what you think the sensation means.

Figure 8.7 Example of Step 3 Completed. The therapist, parent, and child go through the worksheet together. In this case, the therapist is interviewing the child and the child has determined that they are feeling guilty, sad, and have some hunger pains.

STEP 4: DESIGN AN INVESTIGATION AND SEE WHAT HAPPENS.

If you are feeling excited or happy
- Dance around!

If you are feeling scared or nervous
- Talk to someone.
- Take some slow, deep breaths and close your eyes.
- Count your butterflies as you face your fears.
- Do something that makes you laugh.

If you are feeling mad or disgusted
- Yell really loudly.
- Do slow deep breathing and walk around.
- Make a firms but polite request about what you need.

If you are feeling sad or have emotional pain
- Get a hug from someone or hold someone's hand.
- Draw a picture or write about it.
- Snuggle with something.
- Make up a song about it.

If you are feeling loving
- Share that feeling with someone or something.

If you are feeling lonely or missing your parents
- Call or talk to someone.
- Write a letter.
- Play with an animal.

If you are feeling hunger pain or feeling hangry
- Eat.

If you are feeling overstuffed pain
- Lay on the couch.
- Go on a slow walk.

If you are feeling gas pain
- Go to the bathroom, or pass gas.

If you are feeling calm or relaxed
- Keep doing what you are doing! Make sure to write about it in your journal so you remember what things help you feel relaxed.

If you are feeling muscle pain
- Get someone to rub your muscles or your ears.
- Lay on a heating pad.
- Take a nice hot bath.

If it is a worry pain
- If you can do something about it, make a plan. If you can't do anything, boss your worry around!

If you are feeling guilty about something
- See if there is a problem that you need to fix.

If you are feeling bored
- Make a list of 50 things you can do (ask for help if you need it). You can use this list again later.

If you are feeling sleepy
- Rest.

Something else?

Write or draw what you tried, how it went, or what you are planning to try!

I will write a text to my friend to apologize.

Figure 8.8 An in-the-moment investigation is being planned to address a fight with a friend.

THERAPIST: *Ha. It is weird but I do like practicing. Let's do what you said and write it down instead. I'm going to write that in this box here, where it says "Things you did or might like to try next time."*(Figure 8.8)

Child drafts the text.

THERAPIST: *That sounds really nice. If I was your friend, getting a text like that would make me feel really special. Should we ask your mom to remind you to send it?*

MOM: I would be happy to do that.

THERAPIST. *Let's move on to the next thing that you circled in Step 3. You said you were feeling sad. Under things you can do when you are feeling sad, it says "Write about what happened, talk to someone, get a hug, go snuggle on the couch with an animal or person, listen to some music." Do any of these things sound like something you want to try right now or later today …*

This review proceeds until all the meanings that were underlined in Step 3 are mapped onto potential actions in Step 4 (Table 8.6). If there is enough time, you would repeat this activity with the parent.

If you ever have a child who is not able or not willing at that moment to participate, move to the parent and perform all the activities you would have done with the child with the parent. Believe us, the child is watching.

Table 8.6 Instructions for completing a Body Clues Worksheet Steps 1 through 4

1. Determine whether you are focusing on the current moment or on an event in the recent past. If the latter, make sure to give the child and parent time to think about the event that happened and get a vivid picture of it in their minds so they can answer the questions that will follow.

2. The therapist will then go through each and every character, asking the child if they are experiencing that sensation in the moment (or when the event happened) and how much they were experiencing it. Because we circle the sensations that the child endorses, a fun way that children learn to express the intensity of that sensation is by the amount of the circle. So, they could answer a quarter circle if they are feeling it a little bit, a half circle if there feeling it moderately, etc. Do not worry about precision. Use whatever metric the child wants to use. The important thing is that they are turning their attention to their body with curiosity and trying to figure out what is going on in there.

3. In Step 2, the therapist asks the child to draw or write what they were doing when they noticed those sensations.

4. In Step 3, the therapist will review what was circled in Step 1, what the child was doing in Step 2, and ask the child what they think their body was trying to tell them. The therapist will then read through all the options in Step 3 and mark what the child indicated.

5. In Step 4, the therapist will first go through and find the things the child indicated in Step 3 and underline them in Step 4. The therapist will then go through each meaning and think through what the plan is to get that need met (the suggestions offered in Step 4). If the event is going on right then, the child may try the strategy immediately and see what happens. The result of this investigation can then be added to the Body Map.

Once the parent and child have been through all four steps of this worksheet a few times, things start to really click, like an "ah-ha" moment.

> The idea that you can listen to what your body is telling you and respond to it is an incredibly powerful feeling. It makes you feel safe. It makes you feel like you really know yourself.

Your Third Body Investigation Assignment (Home-based Practice)

For Session 3, the home assignment is the same as the last session and will continue for the remainder of the treatment. The parent and child should fill out the worksheet as often as is reasonable, but ideally once per day. They can complete a worksheet to help understand what is going on in a given moment, right after an intense moment to figure out what to do next time, to plan an investigation for the future (we will discuss this more in later sessions) and/or as a summary of the most intense events or highs and lows of the day. Completed worksheets should be brought to the session so everyone can review what was learned about the body, and this information is added to the Body Map.

Body Investigation Journal

In the child's body investigation journal this week, they can be on the lookout for smelly farts and stealthy burps.

Materials Families Take Home from Session 3

Here is a summary of what families get from Session 3.
1. A worksheet that summarizes the characters that they have learned so far
2. The Body Clues Worksheets
3. Coloring pages
4. The workbook pages for their binder that includes ideas for home-based body investigations
5. The Body Brainstorms worksheet they completed
6. Optional: Prizes! Some cute vomit bags and a whoopee cushion
7. Optional: A Victor Vomit button

Information on getting prizes and buttons can be found at https://www.fbi-kids.org

Body Investigations to Practice at Home

In our web-based community and online resources for therapists (https://eatingdisorders.dukehealth.org/functional-abdominal-pain), we provide ongoing and frequently updated ideas for various body investigations that you can perform with your families in session. It is also a great idea for families to design their own investigations and practice them at home. Here are some ideas to get everybody started! If helpful, jot down what the family plans to try in the child's Body Investigation Journal.
1. Come up with your own scale to measure the intensity of passing gas. Family members can post a chart on the refrigerator and everyone can mark their own intensity to determine who is the gas champion.

2. Children can try to add or subtract some foods that are supposed to be gassy and see whether that really effects the frequency, intensity, or smelliness of their farts.
3. If the children have a sensitive gag reflex to new tastes, they could see what happens to the intensity of their gag after they have had that food one time, two times, three times, etc.

Then you schedule the next session! Congratulations, you've just finished Session 3!

Therapist Reminders for Session 3

Remind the parents and children to bring in the homework sheets they completed. From here on out, checking in on our energy and having a snack to get fueled up will be part of the ritual that begins our session. Thus, you may want to remind parents to bring in a snack in small pieces and also have a backup snack stash on hand.

A Final Reflection for Session 3

Gagging and vomiting are not pleasant sensations. You may have your own intense memories of experiencing these sensations. For some individuals, these memories can be quite embarrassing and even humiliating. It may be quite powerful for you to take a step back and think about these situations as moments when your body was protecting you. Even if these events happened because of sub-optimal decision-making on our parts (e.g., we drank too much at a party), our bodies were trying to defend us from our own behavior. Our bodies are always there for us, trying to do their best job even if sometimes they are over-vigilant. Like a caring parent, they are looking out for us. It can be a powerful and overwhelmingly positive feeling to truly inculcate that relationship with your physical body.

Questions and Answers for Session 3

Q: Do you really want the child to throw up?

A: **What we really want is for everybody to not be afraid of throwing up. What that means is that we are prepared that throwing up can happen, and, if it does happen, it is no big deal. Imagine the change in experience that a child who is a cyclical vomiter has when the room is cheering them on and commenting on how powerful that was. That change in response can help shift the child's emotional reaction to sensations that may predict future vomiting such as nausea and actually circumvent the vomiting from happening in the future. Chapter 4 describes more about these counterconditioning processes.**

Q: **What if the family seems uncomfortable about the use of informal terms like farting?**

A: **It is important that we remain culturally sensitive to the norms of the family while not losing sight of the playful curiosity that we are trying to impart. Ask the family for the words they use to describe passing gas and use those.**

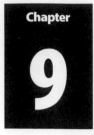

Chapter 9

Session 4: The Zoomies and the Shakies, Part 1

I wrapped my fear around me like a blanket.
Closer to Fine by the Indigo Girls

Overview of Session 4

The routines and rituals of the sessions are now set. From here on out, we are embellishing the framework that we have developed by meeting new characters and performing additional body investigations to learn more about the wisdom of the body. All sessions will now start off in the same way, and will incorporate all four steps on the Body Clues Worksheet that we learned about last session. Several sessions will focus on emotional experience. Session 4, the Zoomies and the Shakies, Part 1, addresses high-arousal emotions with negative valence (more about this below). Unlike most other sessions, however, we spend some focused time with parents to better understand their comfort and challenges with their own, and their children's, emotional experiences. Have fun!

Session Outline

1. Perform a warm-up Henry Heartbeat exercise
2. Review homework and add new things to the Body Map
3. Check in with everyone's energy and fuel up with a snack
4. Revisit some characters we have met and learn new characters related to high arousal and negatively valenced emotions: Henry the Heartbeat, Betty the Butterfly, Julie Jitters, Tommy Thunderbolt, Stressed-Out Stella, and Mind-Racing Mikella, by going over the workbook pages
5. Perform some Body Investigations
6. Complete a Body Brainstorms Worksheet
7. Time with Caregivers/Parents: The Emotional Wave
8. Review the plan for the week
9. Give out prizes and coloring pages

Session Materials

1. Workbook, worksheets, and coloring pages for Session 4 (downloadable at www.cambridge.org/fbi-clinical-guide)
2. A snack the child brings or that you have on hand that is in small pieces for sensing our energy and fueling up
3. Optional: A stress ball, and Betty Butterfly button for session prizes

Background Information for Session 4

> Emotions help us understand how we feel about things, rapidly communicate to us and others what is going on in the world, and help guide us in what to do.

Chapter 2 provided a detailed discussion about a functionalist framework for understanding emotional experience. To briefly review, emotions communicate to ourselves and others what is happening in a given situation. More specifically, they communicate what is needed to help manage a given situation. Emotions are also complex, full-body experiences. The body changes that accompany an emotional experience assist us in getting these needs met. For instance, an individual experiences fear. Fear communicates that there is danger. The bodily changes that accompany fear – a beating heart, changes in digestive function, profuse sweating, etc. – are all designed to give that individual the energy and power to escape from danger. Emotions are therefore our allies. They are the partners that travel along with us throughout life, helping us to take care of ourselves. When we are proficient at decoding our emotional experiences, we learn to know and trust ourselves. The back and forth of tuning in to our bodies, figuring what our bodies are communicating, and acting on those needs helps us to feel safe. And safety is the foundation and springboard from which vitality, joy, and adventure launch.

It is a crucial and profound undertaking for us to help young children begin to view emotions as their helpers rather than as experiences to be feared and avoided. Many of the most intransigent psychiatric disorders have a fear of emotional experience as an essential element. Individuals with major depressive disorder may come to dread and fear signs of sadness, individuals with obsessive-compulsive disorder can come to dread and fear signs of anxiety. By starting young and creating a framework in which emotions are helpers and messengers, we hope to protect children from the emergence or exacerbation of psychopathology as well as give children vital tools to manage pain and distress. This is particularly crucial as recurrent pain and psychiatric disorders often co-occur.

A Hypothetical Organizational Framework of Emotional Experience

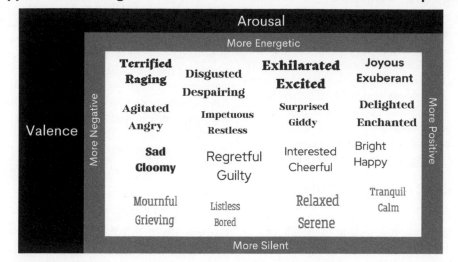

Figure 9.1 An organizational framework of emotional experience. We provide a simplified categorization of emotions based on how they feel: the level of arousal one feels when experiencing a given emotion. For ease, we cross arousal with valence which helps us organize our chapters. Negatively valenced emotions often communicate that we may want to try doing something different, whereas positively valenced emotions encourage us to keep doing what we are doing.

There are many ways of organizing and categorizing emotions. Here we choose an oversimplified two-dimensional framework, that of arousal and valence. We further classify the arousal dimension as high or low, and the valence dimension as positive or negative. Figure 9.1 illustrates this framework.

We provide this to help you understand how sessions are organized. However, we do not present this to the children because we want to encourage them to regard their emotions as informative rather than label them as negative or positive. That said, this session and the next focus on what are thought of as negative emotions. Session 4 addresses the sensations that may constitute high-arousal negative emotions such as anger, fear, anxiety, and worry. Worry is a little complicated because it is associated with decreased autonomic arousal. We include it in Session 4 because it often does not feel that way, and respecting the child's subjective experience is central to our work. Worry can be experienced as racing thoughts, so that is what we attend to with our character Mind-Racing Mikella. Onward!

Step-by-Step Guide to Session 4
Warm-Up Henry Heartbeat Activity

We will quickly review instructions for our opening routines, starting with Henry Heartbeat, because by Session 4, therapists have the gist of how the initiation of each session proceeds. We will slow down again in Session 6 when we introduce pain experiences.

A reminder that it is more than OK to repeat Henry Heartbeat Investigations. A child can learn many things by doing the same thing over again. Repetition may provide an opportunity to demonstrate that their heart keeps getting

stronger, for example, as when their heart needs less and less time across multiple sessions to return to its baseline rate after an activity.

Review Homework and Add New Things to Their Body Map

This is our first session in which parents and child had Steps 1 through 4 of the Body Clues Worksheet to complete for homework. As in previous sessions, we will have the child lay out their Body Map and add anything new that was learned about the wisdom of their body. Here are a few important reminders about homework review. If the parents and children have not completed any Body Clues Worksheets in between sessions as practice, make sure to complete one right then and there. At this point in the treatment, we would continue to recommend that the therapist interview the child and then the child interview the parent. Once you feel the parent has mastered the worksheet, you as the therapist can step out of this altogether and have parents and child interview each other. Also remember that we are trying to take a step back from the experience that the child wrote about and consider what that experience demonstrates about the body's wisdom and to add that wisdom to the Body Map.

At the end of the intervention, the child should have a powerful summary of many of the wise things the body does. The belief that their body is wise and tough is made stronger by juxtaposing the child's narrative account of what the body did with statements that explain the body's wisdom in that moment. Together, these strategies may potentiate our young FBI agents' learning.

Assessing Your Energy and Fueling Up

The ritual of checking in with one's energy using the energy meter and fueling up is hopefully becoming more familiar at this point. As a brief reminder, everyone uses the distance between their hands as an indication of their increasing energy. When individuals are fully fueled up, they flex their arm muscles. If individuals were completely empty of fuel, their hands would be together. The child should check in with their energy level as they are eating their snack. This helps to remind them that fueling your body up with food is an interactive process that involves repeatedly tuning in to how the body feels.

Session 4 Workbook: The Zoomies and the Shakies, Part 1

We go quickly through the workbook section in this chapter as we want to spend more time on Body Investigations. As usual, as a group you will read through all the new body characters. If the child seems particularly interested in a given character, that is a good window of opportunity to dig in and have a discussion about the situations in which the child has experienced that body sensation. We will note that meeting the new characters is generally a very exciting part of the session.

This session – and the next few – have an extra bonus in that the therapist spends some time with the parent alone. This session we discuss the Emotional Wave and how to use worksheets most effectively in high-intensity situations. We introduced the Emotional Wave in Chapter 3 as a metaphor to index the intensity of someone's emotional experience. Parents can then use the intensity of their child's emotional experience to guide the appropriateness of various responsive parenting strategies. We promised in that earlier chapter to provide more details about the wave, and we do so later in this description of Session 4. This week's investigative questions ask families to think about the following body mysteries.

Session 4: Body Mystery Questions

Take two minutes with your FBI agent and list as many emotions as you can think of. Ready … go!

Why do you think that people have emotions?

What do you think would happen if emotions did not exist?

Why do you think that people get angry?

Why do you think that people get scared?

Try to have every family member answer these questions if possible.

Table 9.1 summarizes the characters that are reviewed or introduced in this session.

Table 9.1 Body sensations characters for the Zoomies and the Shakies, Squad 1

Henry the Heartbeat

The feeling of your heart pounding in your chest like the pounding of a drum.

Do any scary things make your heart beat really fast?

Have you ever had your heart beat really fast in school?

What about when you were playing sports?

Do you remember what happened in those situations and what you did?

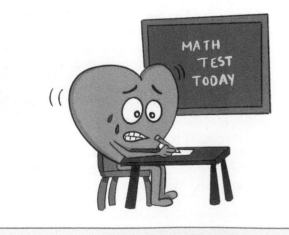

Julie Jitters

A feeling of shakiness: your hands may shake or your whole body may shake. You may feel Julie Jitters when you are nervous or scared about something that is about to happen.

Have you ever been so scared about something that you started shaking? Do you remember what happened and what you did?

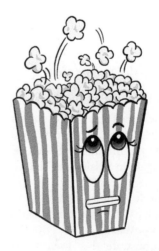

Table 9.1 (cont.)

Betty the Butterfly

Betty the Butterfly is a fluttering feeling you get in your gut or maybe even your chest. It can feel like there are a bunch of fluttering wings flapping about.

Let's imagine what a swarm of butterflies looks and sounds like. Now imagine that a swarm of butterflies has decided to make their home inside your stomach and they are just flying around in there, fluttering their wings. Have you ever had a feeling like that? Like there was a fluttering in your stomach that seemed like it could be a swarm of butterflies?

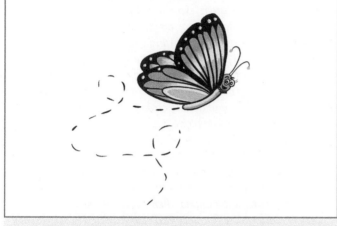

Tommy Thunderbolt

Tommy Thunderbolt is a feeling of building up pressure and heat, like a volcano in which lava is building up and is about to explode.

Have you ever had the feeling like you were just about to explode? Do you remember or do you know the types of things that make you feel that way?

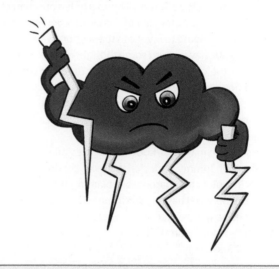

Mind-Racing Mikella

Mind-Racing Mikella is the feeling of a whirring or spinning inside your head – like things are moving so fast that everything is just a rapid blur.

Imagine that there is a Merry-Go-Round that is spinning so fast that you cannot even tell what the different characters are on it! It is moving so fast that it just looks like a blur. When people are nervous or worried about something, sometimes the thoughts in their head feel that way – like everything is moving very, very fast so they can't even tell exactly what they are thinking. Has that ever happened to you? Can you think of situations that may make you feel that way?

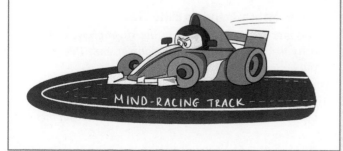

Stressed-Out Stella

The feeling you have when you have too much to do and do not have enough time, brain power, or energy to do those things. Stressed-Out Stella can feel like you are just stuck – like you are holding on by a thread and do not know how to even start.

Have you ever had too much to do? Maybe in the morning when everyone is rushing around to get ready for school? What did you do about that?

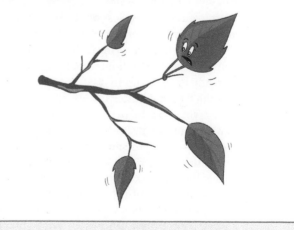

Zoomie and Shaky Characters and Body Investigations

Tommy Thunderbolt

What does it feel like as your anger is increasing? If you can imagine moving from mildly irritated to frustrated to angry and then to rageful, what do you notice in your body as your mood shifts? We think of these changes as feeling like an impending storm in our bodies: a buildup of tension and heat to a point where we feel like we are about to explode. Tommy Thunderbolt is our character that reflects this increased intensity of sensations. Some of these sensations are challenging to invoke in the session. We address this in several ways. We have added some thought exercises in the workbook to get the children to think about different scenarios and how their body might feel in those scenarios. We also can perform "dramatic enactments." These are not interoceptive exposures. Instead, they are more like role-playing but with a focus on how one is feeling at a given moment.

The scenario in the workbook that is designed to bring about discussions of Tommy Thunderbolt asks children to imagine a situation in which their parents are blaming them for something they did not do. What happens to Tommy Thunderbolt in that situation? Does he get weaker or stronger? What should we do with that energy from Tommy Thunderbolt so we can get our mind back and think clearly?

Body Investigation/Dramatic Enactment: Feeling Some Heat

THERAPIST: *So, you've decided that you want to do an investigation about Tommy Thunderbolt. Let's think about some situations that make you really mad.*

CHILD: When my sister takes my stuff without asking and then I can't find it. Sometimes she even wrecks it.

THERAPIST: *Yeah, I definitely would be feeling Tommy Thunderbolt in that situation. What about you mom? What are some things that make you really mad?*

MOM: Well, I get annoyed a lot of the time by little things. For example, I get annoyed when I have to ask the kids to do something three times in order to get them to listen. I don't get really mad about that though. I would get really mad if someone did something that hurt my children's feelings.

THERAPIST: *These are great examples. Let's read about Tommy Thunderbolt again here to remind ourselves what our bodies may feel like as we are starting to get mad. So, let's try this. It's really hard to just get mad on the spot. So, what if we pretend that these things are happening right now. Then you can imagine and act how it would feel to have Tommy Thunderbolt slowly increasing and getting stronger up to the point where you are just about to explode. Just when you get to that point, let's think of some investigations we can do to figure out where to put all that energy. So, let's pretend that you just walked into your room and your sister broke one of your things. Then you act out Tommy Thunderbolt getting stronger and stronger and you're just about to explode when … you decide to put all that energy somewhere so you don't do something that you will feel bad about later. What do you want to do with that energy when you feel it?*

CHILD: How about if I do karate kicks in the air?

THERAPIST: *Wow. That sounds perfect. Why don't you show me a couple of kicks right now? …*

Revisiting Characters from Session 1: Betty the Butterfly, Henry Heartbeat, and Samantha Sweat

We met all these characters in Session 1. We know Henry Heartbeat really well given all of our Henry Heartbeat activities. Betty the Butterfly is that fluttering feeling in your stomach when you're feeling a bit nervous about something such as when you are getting ready to speak up in class or begin a hard test. We capitalize on the fact that butterflies are cute and beautiful and seem like they would be the perfect companions when we are having an anxious moment. Body investigations related to Betty the Butterfly are some of the most fun. One type of Henry Heartbeat Investigation is when you compare any two activities to demonstrate that the heart is smart enough to adapt how hard it beats to meet the demands of those situations. Similarly, as Betty the Butterfly is a little helper, we can see how many of her team we need when we compare different activities that might bring on some butterflies. If you remember, in the last session, we were disappointed if we did not see Victor Vomit. We tried to set up a context in which the occurrence of vomiting was exciting and powerful rather than dreaded and scary. So it is with

dear Betty the Butterfly. We are excited to see her and her gang and we are disappointed when fewer butterflies come to the party than were expected. Often, we set up these investigations with an initial activity that is designed to evoke butterflies. Then we just keep trying to up the ante to see if we can add more and more butterflies.

Body Investigation: Gathering Butterflies

THERAPIST: *OK, let's think of an investigation we can do with Betty the Butterfly. Should we think of some things that give you butterflies or should I tell you my idea?*

CHILD: Tell me your idea.

THERAPIST: *What about if we all turn off all the lights and sit in the dark. Do you think the butterflies will come out then?*

CHILD: Yes!

THERAPIST: *Should we all try that? How many butterflies do you think will come out if we do that?*

CHILD: A hundred.

THERAPIST: *Oh wow! This is going to be really exciting!*

Therapist and child and family members all sit in the dark.

THERAPIST: *Ok. I'm going to set my timer for two minutes and then we can all count the butterflies.*

Can children (or adults) really count the number of butterflies in their stomach? Probably not, though they certainly may notice the sensations of fluttering and can count that. Does it matter? No. Think about what is happening here. We are taking an emotion, fear, and creating a context in which children are curious about the way their bodies feel and think of those sensations as signals that they are ready to face whatever challenge lies ahead.

CHILD: I count five.

PARENT: I count ten.

THERAPIST: *Oh wow! We were thinking we were going to get 100! What can we do to bring on more butterflies?*

CHILD: We could block the light from under the door.

THERAPIST: *Great idea! Let's see if that works to bring on more butterflies!*

Ideas to Bring on Butterflies

1. Create a timed math test.
2. Make everyone prepare a speech that they have to give to the family.
3. Tell a scary story in the dark.
4. Play Hide and Seek.
5. Find some child-friendly but scary film clips to watch.

Body Investigation: Making Your Thoughts Race

As noted in Chapter 1, FBI – Pain Division is unlike cognitive behavior therapy interventions for children because we do not focus on the contents of a child's mind. We do, however, focus on the experience of thinking. Mind-Racing Mikella is the experience a person can have when they are worried. Thoughts can feel like they are racing so fast that the mind is a blur and one cannot focus. It is certainly not an experience that is conducive to problem-solving so we can have a lot of fun with that. Interestingly, from the body experience perspective, research has shown that worrying is often accompanied by decreased autonomic arousal. It is as if the racing thoughts actually dampen one's experience of the anxious arousal that accompanies worry. One theory is that racing thoughts are a form of avoidance that prevent you from facing and mastering the details of your fears! However, it certainly does not feel like one is in a state of decreased arousal when one's mind is racing. That is why we decided to put Mind-Racing Mikella in this chapter. Of course, as with all body investigations, we are not afraid to face sensations head-on so we look forward to making Mind-Racing Mikella race as fast as she can!

THERAPIST: *We just read about Mind-Racing Mikella. Has that ever happened to you? Where your mind was spinning? Maybe because there were things that you were so afraid were going to happen that your mind did not even want to slow down and*

think about them? How about you mom? Does that ever happen to you?

CHILD AND MOM: Yep

THERAPIST: *Okay. Let's do an investigation. I'll give you a minute to just think. And then when I say on your marks, get set, and go, I want you to shout out all the things that you worry about as fast as you can. I'll try to write them down as fast as I can. You ready? On your marks, get set, and go!*

The child proceeds to say the things that are going on in their mind as fast as they can.

THERAPIST: *Okay stop! Now what happened to the speed of your thoughts? Is your mind still racing?*

CHILD: Yep

THERAPIST: *I guess Mind-Racing Mikella is going to do what she wants to do, huh?*

CHILD: Yep, I think she is.

THERAPIST: Do you think we can get her to go even faster?

CHILD: I think I can. (The child proceeds to say all the worries all over again, but this time even faster).

THERAPIST: *Wow! Mind-Racing Mikella has a lot of ideas!*

Ideas to Bring on Mind-Racing Mikella

1. Have a child start listing all the things they are worried about as fast as they can. Then, have them run in a circle at the speed that their thoughts are racing. Have the parent or therapist randomly call "Freeze" – just like in the game freeze dance – and see what happens to the speed of their thoughts. You can help them imagine the words of their thoughts racing around like cars and when the child stops suddenly, they hit the car in front of them, swerve around it, and keep going. One powerful lesson of this exercise: My mind has a mind of its own. I cannot just turn it off, but I can have fun with it.
2. Have the child repeat the exercise in which they shout out the content of their mind. However, this time, they shout out the contents of their mind at a really slow speed. Have them notice whether Mind-Racing Mikella gets slower or faster.
3. See what happens to Mind-Racing Mikella if the child takes the energy from her racing thoughts and channels it into some kind of movement like a spinning and jumping dance or racing down the hall. Does Mind-Racing Mikella get slower? Faster? Stay the same?
4. What if you do an activity that tries to slow down Henry Heartbeat? What happens to the speed of Mind-Racing Mikella then?

Keep in mind the premise of acceptance-based body investigations. We are **not** performing these investigations to demonstrate that a certain outcome occurs: like our thoughts slow down if we say them slowly. We are just curious about what happens and eager to learn more about how Mind-Racing Mikella operates. This stance competes with and eventually overtakes the experience of worry as a burden.

Getting the Jitters!

Julie Jitters is that jittery, trembling feeling that can happen for many reasons, but often because you are scared about something. If you have ever forgotten to dress properly for a really cold day and started shaking from the cold, then you may be familiar with Julie Jitters.

What are some ways to get the Jitters? Maybe listening to a spooky story, watching a child-friendly but still scary film-clip, sitting in the dark while individuals take turns sneaking up on each other – Julie Jitters is a big fan of anticipation so Julie Jitters likes to come out when one is expecting something scary and your body is getting ready to run, run, run! In fact, that is the theory behind shaking when you are scared: that it is due to the flood of adrenaline to your muscle fibers that are over-firing as they are getting you ready to escape. This theory leads us to some very interesting investigations for Julie Jitters ….

Body Investigations with Julie Jitters

What happens to Julie Jitters when you move around a lot?

When someone has Julie Jitters, their body is shaking like a leaf! It may seem the opposite of what you might think, but what if moving more actually quieted down Julie Jitters? If you are ever in a situation in which you are shaking because you are so nervous or scared about something, what happens if you:

– Do jumping jacks for a minute?
– Breathe deeply for a minute?
– Scream?
– Dance?
– Jump up and down like a jumping bean?
– Try moving very, very slowly ….

For investigations with Stressed-Out Stella, check out the workbook!

Possible Body Lessons from the Zoomies and Shakies, Part 1

Butterflies are my little helpers. They keep me company and make sure I can handle any challenge.

Tommy the Thunderbolt gives me the energy I need to look out for myself and protect myself.

Julie Jitters helps me get ready to move if I need to make a quick exit.

Mind-Racing Mikella makes sure I have lots of options!

Stressed-Out Stella reminds me that I need to slow down and make a plan.

Scenario of a Child on Top of the Emotional Wave

The child has just experienced an extremely upsetting event and it is clear that Tommy Thunderbolt is in full force.

Parent: C'mon. Let's go race around the block as fast as we can and see what happens to Tommy Thunderbolt. I bet I can beat you.

Time with Parents/Caregivers: The Emotional Wave and the Body Clues Worksheet

We have spent the first three sessions teaching parents and children a lot of material. They are starting to get accustomed to the routines and rituals of FBI sessions and the between-session home practice. We will spend some time alone with the parents over these next few sessions so we can make sure they feel confident in implementing the strategies we have taught them. We often have the children working on their coloring page just outside the door while we have these conversations.

This first conversation introduces parents to the concept of the emotional wave, depicted in Figure 9.2. As we noted in the beginning of this chapter, we are organizing emotions across two dimensions – the intensity of the arousal and whether it has a negative or positive valence. The emotional wave is our representation of the level of arousal of an emotion. We teach the emotional wave to parents because we want them to understand some optimal times to use a Body Clues Worksheet with their child, and how to use high-arousal moments as an opportunity to design Body Investigations. We also hope that this metaphor will be useful for their own self-parenting, helping parents match optimal responses to their own emotional intensity.

The first principle of the emotional wave is that the more intense the emotional experience, the higher the wave. As we have talked about in Chapter 2, emotions communicate needs and guide our behavior to get those needs met. It stands to reason then that the message being communicated, the urgency of that message, and the strategies that we have available to us will differ depending on the intensity of the situation. As we travel up the emotional wave, our arousal and other body sensations, and the emotions that are made up of those body sensations, get stronger. When the intensity of an emotion is at its highest level, what we like to call the "top of the wave," it is certainly a situation that is important to us, maybe even an emergency. It may be a situation that demands immediate action. Strategies that may be challenging to do at the top of the wave are those that involve thinking slowly and systematically about a problem. For example, it might be hard for your child to be interviewed about all the different sensations that they are feeling when they are "on top of the wave" – in the middle of an intense moment. Strategies that are well-suited to the top of the wave are body-focused – physical and sensory strategies – basically, doing stuff – including performing a Body Investigation! Being on top of the wave is the perfect time to design an in-the-moment Body Investigation (Step 3 of Figure 9.2)! Here is what a scenario could look like.

Being on top of the wave is a great time to plan and perform a Body Investigation right then and there – see what you can learn about the wisdom of the body in high intensity moments.

Because there is a lot of energy at the top of the wave, and because many Body Investigations require a lot of energy, the top of the wave presents an opportunity for experiential learning when we cannot connect to cognitive logic. Top-of-the-wave strategies often help a child get through a difficult moment. However, as FBI agents we go beyond this; we investigate mysteries. In doing so, we feel masterful and safe even when our arousal is very, very high.

> After a child is down from the top of the wave, we can learn even more. It is the perfect time for parent and child to work through a Body Clues Worksheet to figure out what we just learned from our Body Investigation. If we are super-sleuths, we can go one step further and use our Body Clues Worksheet to learn what put us on the top of the wave in the first place!

As such, once we get down from the top of the wave there is still work to be done. What just happened was a Body Investigation!

We have to use what just happened to learn something about ourselves and grow wiser. Now is a perfect time to pull out a Body Clues Worksheet (Step 4 of Figure 9.2). First, we have to figure out what we learned from the Body Investigation that we just performed. However, for really advanced parents and children, there is another question we need to investigate. We have to try to figure out what got us to the top of the wave in the first place (Step 5 of Figure 9.2)!

PARENT: What is Tommy Thunderbolt doing now? Is he louder or quieter than before we ran?

CHILD: He's a lot quieter.

PARENT: Come sit down next to me. Let's go through a worksheet together and figure out what we just learned about Tommy Thunderbolt. Let's also try to figure out where he came from in the first place.

CHILD: Do I have to?

PARENT: You don't have to, but I think it would be a really good idea to learn something new about Tommy the Thunderbolt.

CHILD: Fine.

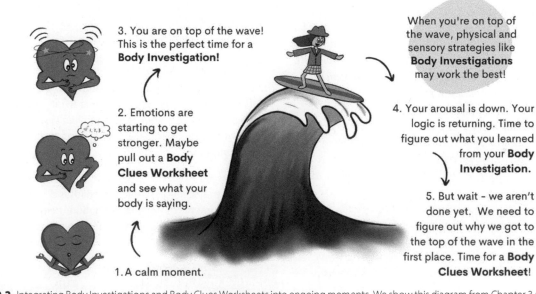

Figure 9.2 Integrating Body Investigations and Body Clues Worksheets into ongoing moments. We show this diagram from Chapter 3 again to remind us about the integration of FBI strategies with intense moments. We can think about in-the-moment Body Investigations as perfect opportunities to turn a high-intensity, top-of-the-wave moment into a fun investigation in which we learn something more about the body. As sensations are starting to get stronger (2), it might be a good time to explore what is going on. After a Body Investigation or an intense moment has happened is another good time to pull out a Body Clues Worksheet to see what happened (4) or what put you on top of the Wave in the first place (5).

Noticing Arousal Increasing

As you will notice, there are two steps in our emotional wave (Steps 1 and 2, Figure 9.2) that we have not yet discussed. Step 1 is when our arousal is low and we may be feeling calm and peaceful. The final sessions of the FBI program focus on increasing our awareness of these relaxing sensations so we can be sure to notice and revel in them when they are happening. But for now, let's travel up the wave. As you go up the left side of the wave in Figure 9.2, arousal is just beginning to increase – emotions or other body states are just starting to get stronger. Alert and savvy detectives can notice this increasing arousal before we get to the top of the wave. Logical strategies work here, so it is a good time to pull out a Body Clues Worksheet and figure out what might be going on. Table 9.2 summarizes the strategies for helping parents implement Body Clues Worksheets and In-the-Moment Body Investigations.

Table 9.2 Tips for parents for practicing Body Clues Worksheets and Body Investigations

1. If you are having a calm and peaceful moment, revel in it (Step 1 on Figure 9.2).
2. If you are noticing that your child is starting to get distressed or aroused by something, it may be a good time to pull out a Body Clues Worksheet and figure out what is going on (Step 2 on Figure 9.2).
3. If a child is having a high-intensity, Top-of-the-Wave moment, try a Body Investigation right then and there (Step 3 on Figure 9.2).
4. If you have just completed a Body Investigation, take a moment to figure out what you learned from your investigation. Maybe use a Body Clues Worksheet to help you. You could add what you learned to your Body Map (Step 4 on Figure 9.2).
5. After an intense moment, it may be a good time to pull out a Body Clues Worksheet to figure out what happened and what to try next time (Step 5 on Figure 9.2).

Dialogue to Introduce the Emotional Wave to Parents

THERAPIST: *It has been a pleasure working with you and your child. We have learned a great deal over the past four weeks. I want to take a minute with you alone over the next several weeks to make sure that I have time to answer any of your questions but also to give you some tools to help you implement what we learned at home. Do you have any questions about things we talked about so far?*

Therapist should plan enough time in the event that the parent has many questions.

THERAPIST: (A diagram of the emotional wave is included in the workbook pages for this session). *I wanted to talk to you a bit more about how to use the Body Clues Worksheets at home and about how to use Body Investigations during intense moments.*

This figure of a wave is designed to represent how strong our emotions can feel at a given moment.

Let's walk through this diagram together. As you notice, as we go up the left side of this wave, our arousal starts to get a bit stronger. Advanced FBI agents are really good at noticing when their arousal is starting to increase. This is a great time to pull out a Body Clues Worksheet and try to figure out what might be going on.

However, as we are just learning how to be FBI agents, we may not be very good at noticing the slight increase in arousal just yet. Instead, it may happen that our arousal – our emotions – get so strong that we go right to the top of the wave. As you can see, there is one important thing that happens as we ascend to the top of the wave: we cross the logic line. When our emotions are very strong, it can be hard to reason things through and think rationally. At the top of the wave, we often just have strong urges to act. Sometimes these actions are not the most effective. For example, if you are on top of the wave and feeling Tommy Thunderbolt, you might have the urge to say something mean or throw something. The strategies that work best at the top of the wave are physical – activities that use up some of our energy. Thus, being on top of the wave is the perfect time for you and your child to design a Body Investigation to see what happens to that arousal. For example, if your child was feeling Tommy Thunderbolt on top of the wave, perhaps you both could go run around the block and see what happens to Tommy Thunderbolt by the time you get back to the house.

Do you have any questions so far? When you think about your child and what your child is like when having strong emotions, can you imagine using a strategy like Body Investigations in that moment?

PARENT: I would really like to try. It certainly seems like a fun way of dealing with the intense arousal and feelings.

THERAPIST: *Terrific! All of this takes practice but you will learn so much as you practice! Let's keep walking through this worksheet together. Once you have performed a Body Investigation from on top of the wave there are two important things you can do afterwards. The first is to figure out what you just learned from the Body Investigation, exactly like we do in session. This can help us learn more about ourselves and generate ideas for the next time your child rides the wave. The second thing you may wish to do is to use a Body Clues Worksheet to explore what sent your child to the top of the wave in the first place.*

The whole purpose of this discussion is to give you some ideas about ways to implement at home what you have learned in sessions. However, you know your child best and you will figure out what works best for you and your family. Do you have any other questions about this?

Framing the strategies that the child and parent try during intense moments as Body Investigations helps to create a context of curiosity around high-arousal emotions.

Joining the Child in a Top-of-the-Wave Body Investigation

Here is one insider tip about helping a child who is experiencing intense emotions. It is really important that parents take ownership of their own emotions in that moment and engage in the activity with their children. Even if the parent is not feeling intense emotions, the child can experience it as patronizing and demoralizing if they are instructed to engage in an activity because of their intense feelings.

"You are on top of the wave. Why don't you go take a walk" does not sound very supportive. Instead, "Boy we are both having some really strong feelings. How about we both do an investigation and try … " – joins you and your child in the situation together, and puts you on the same team.

Back to Parent and Child Activities: Adding to the Body Map

After we are done talking with the parents, we bring everybody back together to summarize the session: including a trip to the Body Map! Ideally, every investigation is followed by a trip to the Body Map to summarize what was learned.

Body Brainstorms

Questions on our Body Brainstorms Worksheet this week include the following:

What are some situations that bring out Betty the Butterfly?

What are the three things that would make Tommy Thunderbolt come out the strongest?

Is there a time of day in which Mind-Racing Mikella is the fastest? What about in the morning before school or when you are lying in bed?

Have you ever gotten Julie Jitters in school? When you were in a performance? When you were playing sports?

Has there ever been a time when you had too many things to do at once? Did you feel Stressed-Out Stella?

Your Fourth Body Investigation Assignment (Home-based Practice)

The family fills out Body Clues Worksheets as a summary of the day and/or after a tough moment. Now that the parent understands the Emotional Wave, when to use Body Clues Worksheets may make more sense. This week we add in the design of Body Investigations if parent and child experience any top-of-the-wave moments.

Body Investigation Journal

In the child's body investigation journal this week, they can draw some pictures of situations that gather butterflies.

Materials Families Take Home from Session 4

Here is a summary of what families get from Session 4.

1. A worksheet that summarizes the characters that they have learned so far.
2. Body Clues Worksheets for practice
3. Coloring pages
4. The workbook pages for their binder, including an ideas page of some home-based body investigations
5. The Body Brainstorms worksheet they completed
6. Optional: Prizes! A stress ball and a compass with a flashlight and a Betty Butterfly Button

Information on getting prizes and buttons can be found at https://fbikids.org

Body Investigations to Practice at Home

Body Investigations to practice at home are always optional. It is important that parents do not feel overwhelmed with what we are asking them to do. However, when these investigations are done at home, they help get the whole family in the spirit of marveling at something cool that the body did.

1. See what happens to Betty the Butterfly when the child is going to do something hard. Is she there to help? How many butterflies came out?
2. What happens if we plan a strategy to try with Tommy Thunderbolt in advance, just like you do a fire drill. If there are situations that Tommy Thunderbolt usually comes out, see what happens if you have a plan. Does he still come? Is he not as strong? Does somebody different show up?

Then you schedule the next session! Congratulations, you've just finished session 4!

Therapist Reminders for Session 4

The families have learned a ton of stuff. Cheerlead, cheerlead, cheerlead.

A Final Reflection for Session 4

Professionals in the health field work with many individuals whose intense emotions seem to have interfered with their functioning. The link between intense emotions and impaired functioning is actually quite complicated. Is it the intensity of the emotional experience, the individual's reactions to that emotional experience, how they channel that emotional experience, or others' reaction to the individual when the person is at the top of the wave? It may be all those things. To really embrace what we are trying to do here – to teach children that emotions are guides and helpers – requires that we believe it ourselves. It may be enlightening to consider what shows up for you personally after doing this session. Hopefully you are feeling a bit kinder towards your emotions.

Questions and Answers for Session 4

Q: Emotions can be scary for kids. What happens if they just refuse to do any of the activities and the parents do too?

A: **In these circumstances, we practice our own wave surfing and proceed to be a phenomenal role model for investigations. If you can, try to get the child involved in a peripheral way. For example, the therapist could perform the Betty the Butterfly exercise and go sit in the dark. You can ask the child to be the timekeeper and to knock on the door when two minutes are up. You can have them do the drawing of what happened to you on your own Body Map.**

Q: What about positive high-arousal emotions, like extreme joy? Why aren't these feelings addressed in this session?

A: Because we have a whole separate section devoted to positive, high-arousal emotions: the Zoomies and Shakies, Part 2! That said, psychological treatments generally target maladaptive tendencies that contribute to distress or impairment (or in this case, tummy pain), so our initial material on emotions focuses on negative, high-arousal states. If a child or parent asks about this quadrant of the arousal-valence emotions framework now, go with it for a bit, while reassuring them that positive emotions will be addressed a few sessions down the road. You can even be genuinely impressed that they are paying close attention to what they are learning and anticipating future FBI strategies! Remember too that FBI sessions are flexible, and that encouraging, reinforcing, and honoring curiosity is a core tenet of the intervention that takes priority over immediate manual content delivery.

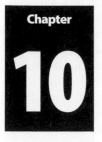

Chapter

10

Session 5: The Blahs

Well I tried to make it Sunday, but I got so damn depressed, that I set my sights on
Monday and I got myself undressed.
Sister Golden Hair by America

Overview of Session 5

We are approaching the Blahs: those sensations that comprise low-arousal, negative emotions. Sadness. Despair. Guilt. Loneliness. We explore the wisdom of these sensations, sensations such as Ricky the Rock, that pit of dread that you may feel in your gut when you have done something wrong, and Blah Bertha, that feeling of heaviness that you may experience when you are feeling quite sad. In Session 6, we are going to dive head-first into pain, so we also use Session 5 to check in with parents and make sure they have the tools to implement the FBI strategies at home so far. We want them going confidently into the session about pain – feeling like they have come a long way and made great progress.

In Session 5, we again spend some time alone with the parents. We started off Session 1 meeting with the parents only. The purpose of this original meeting was to orient parents to the treatment. We also wanted to provide space to make sure that the parent could tell their own story, including their experiences trying to understand and manage their child's pain and perhaps, recounting their own history of pain. We have been trying to emphasize throughout that participating in this treatment is a chance for parents to help create a sense of body trust in their children. Notwithstanding, participating in this treatment with their children could be a new beginning for them – strengthening or building a sense of trust in themselves and their own bodies. Tuning in and responding to our body's needs is something we can all work on. Thus, this treatment offers parents a chance to model this for their children while improving their own emotional capacities. The science behind this conversation with the parents is discussed more thoroughly in Chapter 3. Given that Session 5 marks the halfway point through treatment, it is a good time to check in with the parents and to learn more about the challenges of parenting a child with sensory superpowers. This session follows the same format as the last one.

Session Outline

1. Perform a warm-up Henry Heartbeat exercise
2. Review homework and add new things to the body map
3. Check in with everyone's energy and fuel up with a snack

4. Learn new characters related to low arousal and negatively valenced emotions: Blah Bertha, Nauseous Ned, Empty Eliza, and Ricky the Rock, by going over the workbook pages
5. Perform some Body Investigations
6. Complete a Body Brainstorms Worksheet
7. Spend time with caregivers/parents: Parenting children with sensory superpowers
8. Review the plan for the week
9. Give out coloring pages
10. Optional: Give out prizes

Session Materials

1. Workbook, worksheets, and coloring pages for Session 5 are available for download at www.cambridge.org/fbi-clinical-guide.
2. A snack the child brings or that you have on hand that is in small pieces for sensing our energy and fueling up
3. Optional: Create your own super-hero comic book and Nauseous Ned Button for Session Prizes, see updated links for suggested prizes at https://fbikids.org

Background Information for Session 5

Chapter 3 discusses attachment theory and the importance of safety. The framework of FBI – Pain Division is intended to create safety: a child feeling safe in their body, a parent feeling safe in their body, a child feeling safe with their parent. For some parents, this treatment may offer a fresh start – both in how they parent their children and in how they self-parent. However, the fact that parents are learning some tweaks to their strategies is in no way meant to imply that they have been deficient in their parenting or are to blame for their child's pain. Learning from the past is very different from using decisions made in the past as sources of rumination and regret. Thus, as we discuss parenting styles, it is crucial to emphasize that all of us are students: constantly learning more about ourselves so that we can be our most attuned and effective parents and self-parents. Of course, if a parent starts noticing Ricky the Rock, that is a great opportunity for an investigation.

Parenting "styles" provide a (simplified) framework that is used to classify the way in which parents interact with their children. In fact, parents may have different styles with different children. They may also have different styles with the same child in different contexts. Despite this, it can be really helpful to discuss these frameworks with parents. It encourages them to reflect on how they interact with their children. This can help them be more intentional about how they are building and maintaining a safe context for their child. For ease of this classification, we stick with two dimensions of parenting styles: the degree of warmth a parent displays and the degree of firmness. These dimensions arise from a body of research that we discuss in Chapter 3. In brief, a warm and firm parenting style, also referred to as authoritative style, has been found to be associated with and predictive of positive mental health in children. However, the story is more complicated than that. An adaptive parenting style in one context may not be the same as in another context. For example, one study found that among parents who were raising their children in high-crime neighborhoods, an authoritarian parenting style (higher in firmness, lower in warmth) provided the most benefit. This raises an interesting point. An authoritarian parenting style is often associated with lower warmth. But what does warmth mean?

Warmth is caring and parents express this in their own ways, and differently across contexts. Let's think about the physical sensation of warmth. Imagine you are outside on a sunny and cloudy day. Around you are spots of shade and spots of sunlight. Think of the sun as a parent. To feel warmth, you step into the sunlight and you absorb the sun's rays. Metaphorically and physically, there is a connection between you and the sun. The sun has "seen" you and shares with you some of its energy. If we break this down, we have the essential elements of warm parenting. A child has to feel seen. A child feels that the parent has energy to share. This energy is positive and the experience of receiving it is like you are filled up from head to toe with warmth.

You may notice that parents only control a part of this equation. They cannot control whether their children are willing receivers of this warmth. Part of the trial and error of self-parenting and other-parenting is learning this back and forth of responding to children in a manner that can be received. Some children are much harder to read.

You may also notice that this example of warmth does not include a measure of how mushy-gushy or kissy a parent is. This turns out to be a very important discussion to have with parents. Our experience is that many parents feel guilty about their degree of warmth and their degree of firmness. They may have a vision of what an ideal warm and affectionate parent looks like and feel like their style does not match that. Our job is to validate the wisdom inherent in the parenting styles they have adopted and to explore what warmth and firmness look like for them.

> For a child to experience warmth, it is important that they feel seen. Imagine a child absorbing the rays of the sun.

In FBI, we try to define some principles that may constitute a warm and firm parenting style. First, a child feels seen. Feeling seen means acknowledging a child's experience. Deeply listening. Trying to understand the wisdom of what a child is experiencing in that moment. This is referred to as validation. One aspect of validation that is often confused is that validation is different from empathy and it is different from agreement. With validation, it does not matter that you would not respond to that same situation in that way. Validation is not about your experience at all. That is an essential difference from empathy. When one is empathizing, one is really tuning in and sometimes trying to embody the experience of another. Validation is acknowledging the wisdom of another person's experience for that person at that time. One may have to dig really deep to get into the right space to understand why that experience makes sense for that person, particularly if it is very triggering for you. However, to be effective, validation has to be authentic.

That is the warm part of the equation. The second part involves firmness.

We define firmness as clarifying expectations. It is not about how strict a parent is, it is about how clear a parent is. Here is the challenge: in a state of high negative emotional arousal, our hard-wired responses are to fight, flee, or freeze. Think about the level of arousal present when a parent is issuing a demand. If we think back to the emotional wave of last session, a request might be equated with the level of arousal of climbing the wave, and a demand is nearing the top of the wave. Thus, for children with sensory superpowers, a demand may be experienced as a high-arousal situation. In response, they might fight, flee, or freeze. This can make them look oppositional, when, in fact, they are just overwhelmed. Enter the body mission!

Thus, when a child is faced with a challenging situation that they need to approach, we turn this into a Body Investigation! This solves this dilemma and provides the "firm" of our parenting equation. First, it clarifies expectations. Second, the emotional context is fun and not threatening. The child is part of the planning and thus feels seen and heard. If we put these steps together, a warm and firm parenting style à la FBI –Pain Division has these elements, outlined in Table 10.1 (and sutmmarized in the parent workbook).

Step-by-Step Guide to Session 5
Warm-Up Henry Heartbeat Activity

By this point, it would be great if the child (and sibling if available) designed the Henry Heartbeat activity.

Table 10.1 The components of warm and firm parenting FBI style

1. Listen to your child.
2. Be curious about what your child's (and your own) body is telling you. Explore what those sensations may mean.
3. Authentically validate their experience.
   This means acknowledging that those feelings make sense for them in that moment. It has nothing to do with whether these experiences are adaptive or whether you would feel that way in that situation.
4. If there is a need to gently nudge them to approach a situation, design an investigation together. This allows the child to approach that situation and learn something new about how smart their body is.

Review Homework and Add New Things to Their Body Map

Try to keep up the routine of completing a Body Clues worksheet in that moment if the family has not been able to complete in-home practice sheets. This provides them with some practice and gets the parents more comfortable in seeing how to implement these worksheets with their children.

Assessing Your Energy and Fueling Up

Complete the energy ritual.

Session 5 Workbook: The Blahs

This week's investigative questions ask families to think about the following body mysteries.

Session 5: Body Mystery Questions

What are some things that make people feel sad?
When you feel sad, do you have high energy or low energy?
Have you ever done something that you felt bad about? Like maybe you accidentally broke or spilled something? Or said something mean? What did you do?
When you were feeling bad about what you did, was your body feeling high energy or low energy?

Try to have every family member answer these questions if possible.

Table 10.2 summarizes the characters that are learned or reviewed in this session.

Table 10.2 Summary of body sensation characters

Ricky the Rock

When you feel a pit or knot in your stomach

Have you ever felt a pit or a knot in your stomach, like "Ugh! I can't believe I did that!" It is almost like someone punched you in the stomach! What happened?`

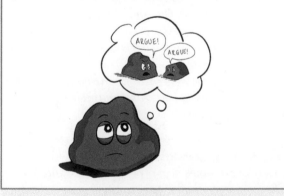

Nauseous Ned

The feeling of nausea or queasiness in your stomach

Have you ever felt like you were going to throw-up but then you didn't? Have you ever seen something that was so gross that you thought you might be sick?

Blah Bertha

The feeling of heaviness, like your body is filled from head to toe with sand

When was the last time you felt really heavy? What did you feel like doing? Did you want to run around and play?

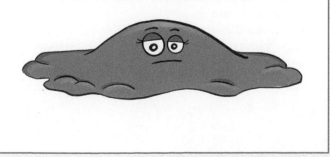

Empty Eliza

You feel like there is nothing inside you: like you cannot think of any ideas, you do not feel any body sensations – it is like your body decided to go on vacation.

Do you ever feel bored? What does that feel like?

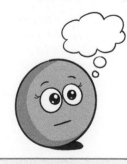

For all sessions, the Body Investigations that we describe are just ideas to help you and your FBI agent-in-training brainstorm your own investigations. Of course, you can try these as written, you can tweak them – whatever works for you. We keep giving you examples so you can understand the basic principles: we are exploring what the body does in different circumstances so we can appreciate different aspects of the body's wisdom. From a logistical perspective, you will probably only have time to do one or two investigations in a 45-minute session.

The Blahs Body Investigations

Ricky the Rock Body Investigation: Revealing a "Dark" Secret

We were first introduced to Ricky the Rock in Session 1. In Session 5 we get to really understand what Ricky the Rock is all about by doing some investigations.

THERAPIST: Let's see if we can design a Ricky the Rock investigation. First let's think about what Ricky the Rock feels like. Ricky the Rock may come around if you did something that you feel bad about.

(Therapist suddenly clutches their stomach). *Urgh! I feel so bad about the argument that I had with my friend. I did not mean to hurt her feelings, but I did by accident. Ricky the Rock can also come up if there's something that's going to happen in the future that you really don't want to do.*

(Therapist puts their hands on their stomach). *Oh! Do I have to go to the doctor? One situation that can really bring up the Ricky the Rock is if you've ever said something that wasn't true or if you did something that you didn't tell anybody about that you feel bad about. Keeping secrets can definitely bring on Ricky the Rock. For our investigation, let's have a private team huddle and see what we can come up with.*

The therapist and children can go and talk privately in a corner and see if there's anything that the children want to bring up that they want to address. There could be two parts to this investigation: the first part is telling the therapist what happened and seeing what happens to Ricky the Rock after they describe what happens. The second part is "confessing" to their parent what happened and seeing what happens to Ricky the Rock after they let their parents know about what they had been hiding.

If no one can come up with any examples, another idea is to come up with a bunch of ideas of things that might make people feel Ricky the Rock. You could write each of these on a slip of paper. Then, one person picks one out and play-acts confessing that mistake to someone else.

Body Investigation: Getting Queasy

Nauseous Ned is one of the new characters that we meet in Session 5. Nausea is actually a bit tricky in terms of whether to put it with the high arousal or low arousal chapters. Some people are nauseated when they feel really anxious and some people are nauseated when they feel really disgusted about something. From a physiological standpoint, nausea is usually associated with activation of the vagus nerve which is associated with your parasympathetic nervous system, the branch of your nervous system known for restoration and repair. Aside from this technical reason, we put Nauseous Ned in this session (the negative low-arousal emotions) because of the action urges that one experiences when nauseated. Rather than feeling like running or fighting, you probably just want to be still and lay down – some very low-arousal activities – and a different kind of protective, defensive response. We learned in Session 3 that disgust is an emotion that protects us from contaminating pathogens. Well, we can think of Nauseous Ned as the messenger or warning bell. Pretty clever system.

THERAPIST: *OK. Who has an idea of an investigation that we could do with Nauseous Ned?*

CHILD: We could watch videos of people throwing up.

THERAPIST: *Wow! That is a great idea! Is that something that you have done before or did you just think of that?*

CHILD: I just thought of that!

THERAPIST: *Very clever. OK. Let's find some. How do you think we should design this investigation?*

CHILD: Well, we could rate how nauseous we feel before the video and then after the video.

THERAPIST: *I really like that. Do we need to make a plan in case we get really, really nauseous? Like have a trash can nearby?*

CHILD: Yeah, that's a good idea.

> A prepared FBI therapist always has a stash of child-friendly videos ready for exposures: clips of people throwing up, sad movie clips, and scary movie clips.

THERAPIST: *Wow. That was really interesting. We all got really nauseated after seeing someone throw-up. Why do you think your body does that?*

CHILD: Well maybe everybody ate something that was really spoiled and dangerous and so everyone should throw it up because it is dangerous. Getting nauseous when someone throws up helps to make sure you get rid of something dangerous, just in case.

THERAPIST: *Whoa! Did you just think of that? That makes a lot of sense to me. You may have something there. That definitely should go on our body map!*

Ideas to Bring on Nauseous Ned

1. Guess how many times you can run in a circle. See who lasts the longest. Guess how long it will take for Nauseous Ned to get weaker.
2. Spin in a chair. See what makes you more nauseous: doing this with your eyes open or closed. Does the nausea get better or worse if you then spin in the opposite direction?
3. Watch disgusting but child-friendly film clips.
4. Make a really gross food mixture.

The fact that, for many people, seeing someone throw-up or smelling vomit increases feelings of nausea and may even cause vomiting is actually quite interesting. As noted, one proposed function of disgust is to protect one from contamination from pathogens. As germs spread, protection from pathogens does not only involve what you do, it also involves how other people behave. Everyone in a group may need to engage in germ-preventing behaviors for the group to remain healthy from contagious diseases. People also often eat in groups. Thus, if a food is contaminated and causes vomiting, it would be advantageous for the group if vomiting (and pathogen removal) was expedited. So, yes, that child was pretty smart. Which is not surprising. They are an FBI agent!

Body Investigation: Getting Up When You Are Weighted Down

Blah Bertha is another character that we meet this chapter. Blah Bertha is the sensation of heaviness you may have when you are feeling extremely sad, or to a more intense extreme, depressed. What might be the function of sadness? In the Body Clues Worksheet, some suggestions of what to do when one is sad is get a hug from someone, snuggle, hold someone's hand, write about or draw what is going on in a journal (and maybe share it with someone), pet or spend time with an animal, or try to find something really beautiful to smell, look at, or listen to. One way to think about the message of sadness is that it communicates that we need more support: from ourselves and from other people. Thus, the activities that are suggested are about connection: connecting with ourselves by thinking about what is going on; seeking out support from others; and/or connecting with the beauty of the world. How can this be the message of sadness when our urge when we are sad is often to withdraw? Well, we can think of that urge to withdraw as a period of restoration (if the person frames it as such and gives themselves permission to withdraw and restore rather than beating themselves up and feeling guilty about withdrawing). After that restoration, we have renewed energy to seek out the support and connection that we need. This can be challenging to do. The investigation that we designed demonstrates that.

THERAPIST: *So Blah Bertha says she feels really, really heavy. Like she is weighted down from head to toe with sand. Has that ever happened to you? It sounds like she could really use a hug. Let's see if we can figure out some investigations of different ways to get a hug when we are feeling really heavy. What do you think of this idea? First, tell me who you want to get a hug from when you are feeling very heavy.*

CHILD: My stuffed bunny.

THERAPIST: *OK. So, we are going to put your stuffed bunny at the other end of the room here. Now we are going to have you lie on the couch. We are going to try to make it as hard as possible for you to get off the couch (of course, we keep things safe). Maybe we can cover you with these blankets – not your head though! Now maybe we can pile on some pillows. Maybe your little brother can climb on top of this heap. (As you may surmise, this is supposed to be very silly, but the point is – it is hard to get up when you are weighted down). OK, now we are going to pretend you are feeling Blah Bertha. You are feeling really heavy – like you really are because of all these blankets and stuff. When you fill out your Body Clues worksheet, you say you are actually feeling really sad. Now, what you need to make you feel happier is a big hug with your bunny that is across the room. What are some things we can investigate that might give you the energy to get up off the couch and go get a hug?*

CHILD: I could roar like a lion and then knock all the stuff off.

THERAPIST: *Well, that makes a lot of sense. Let's try that.*

Child roars like a lion, throws off the blanket, and walks on four legs over to the bunny and gives it a big hug.

THERAPIST: *Well that sure worked well. What should we add to our Body Map about what we just learned about Blah Bertha.*

CHILD: How about, when you need extra strength, you can use your imagination.

THERAPIST: *Great! Let's add it!*

Possible Body Lessons from the Blahs

Ricky the Rock helps me take a good look at my situation and fix things as needed.

Blah Bertha helps me to get the support I need.

Nauseous Ned protects me from germs and other stuff that might make me sick.

Empty Eliza reminds me to use my imagination to come up with new ideas.

Ideas to Bring on Blah Bertha

1. Watch a sad movie clip.
2. Read a sad story.
3. Talk about something sad that happened to you.
4. Make up a sad story and write it as a comic strip.
5. Try things to make one physically heavy as in the example.

Body Investigation: Feeling Nothing

Empty Eliza is a sensation certainly familiar to many parents: when their children complain of feeling bored and cannot seem to generate any content whatsoever about what they are feeling or what they feel like doing. We thought we may as well add this to our list of sensations and see what we can do with it.

THERAPIST: *Have you ever felt bored?*

CHILD: YES!

THERAPIST: *What kinds of things do you do or say when you are bored and your parent asks you, what do you want to do?*

CHILD: I DON'T KNOW! NOTHING!

THERAPIST: *Exactly, that is that Empty Eliza feeling – when you feel like your mind is blank and you just cannot come up with any ideas. So, we are going to play a little game. There are four of us here: me, you, your brother, and your dad. We are all going to take turns and come up with something you can do when you feel Empty Eliza. We have to keep going until we get to 50 things we can do (though it may seem like a lot, we have never had a family not come up with 50). These do not all have to be fun things – chores, etc. count on this list too! Then, after we have this list, we can do an investigation and try out different ways to use it!*

For example, the children can compare what happens when they are feeling Empty Eliza and they just close their eyes and point to something on the list and then they have to do that. Or, they can write the 50 things on different index cards and when they feel Empty Eliza they pick a card, any card. Or, they do not try to do anything with Empty Eliza. They can just sit on the couch and keep Eliza company. For all of these activities, they can explore what happens to Empty Eliza before and after the trial.

Adding to the Body Map

Ideally, every investigation is followed by a trip to the body map to summarize what was learned.

Time with Parents/Caregivers: Parenting Styles

The purpose of this conversation is to validate the challenge of parenting a child with sensory superpowers. It is hard to know when to nudge children who feel things so deeply. When do you encourage them to perform activities? Does pushing too hard have the possibility of creating harm? This can be an underlying concern for parents, one that paralyzes their decision-making. We attempt to ease this dilemma for parents via our framework of body investigations – by infusing every challenge with curiosity, fun, and levity. Thus, this conversation with parents reinforces the "how to" of body investigations and underscores the importance of reflection and validation. The therapist discusses various parenting styles and the wisdom inherent in each. Below and in the parent workbook, we have a diagram that illustrates four basic parenting styles (see Chapter 3, Figures 3.3–3.6). These four styles result from crossing two dimensions: warmth and firmness. The resulting parenting styles are called: permissive (high warmth and low firmness), neglectful (low warmth and low firmness), authoritarian (high firmness

and low warmth), and authoritative (high firmness and high warmth). The therapist will ask the parent to reflect on how they describe their own parenting style and how that has worked and not worked. Together, parent and therapist will arrive at any necessary tweaks to parent behaviors that may help the child more easily approach activities that have been avoided due to the fear of pain.

THERAPIST: *Today we will talk a bit about parenting and the particular challenges of parenting a child who has recurrent abdominal pain. It can be really hard to know when to nudge your child to do something when they are complaining of pain or whether they are better off avoiding the activity. Is that something that you struggle with?*

Therapist allows the parent to discuss their own personal challenges with limit setting and pain management and their children.

THERAPIST: *What we will do next is to take a look at some different parenting styles. We will think about how you would describe your parenting style (and perhaps the parenting style of the child's other parent). We will reflect about what is working well for you in your parenting. We will then consider if there's anything you think would be worth trying differently, in general or in certain situations. I'm going to walk you through four very oversimplified descriptions of parenting styles. They are oversimplified for many reasons. First parents do not neatly fit into one category. We can be different types of parents depending on the situation. We can also be different types of parents for different children. If you have multiple children, you may notice that in yourself.*

Each of these parenting styles is organized around two dimensions. The first dimension is warmth. This does not mean how warm and fuzzy you are. What it does mean is the degree of caring you communicate to your children. Parents communicate their caring in different ways. Some parents are very touchy-feely and give lots of hugs and kisses. Some parents are very attentive and communicative. Some parents are very good at deciphering their child's needs and know when to give their child attentive interaction or when they need a silent physical presence. There are innumerable ways to enact caring. However, we will say that the core dimension of caring, no matter how you express it, is that the child feels seen and heard.

The second dimension is firmness. This dimension refers to the communication of clear expectations and the enforcement of those expectations. After we talk about the different parenting styles, we will share some thoughts about ways that warm and firm parenting can look for children who have sensory superpowers. What is important to understand about this conversation is that you are the expert on your child and you have probably been using different parenting approaches, with trial and error, throughout your child's life to forge your expertise. Therefore, we are reviewing these parenting styles to generate ideas if, in fact, you are ever feeling stuck.

The first type of parent style we will talk about is called the low-resource parent. This parent is low in both warmth and firmness. Usually when we see this type of parenting style, our first thought is that the parent needs help. They do not have the emotional or physical resources to be an involved parent and thus increasing the support of the parent is essential. Do you have any experience with that type of parenting in your own life?

> In the first session, we opened the door for parents to talk about their own history of pain. In Chapter 3, we discuss parenting – including the parent's own history of self-parenting. If a parent has experienced trauma or neglect in their childhood, feelings about this can surge up – sometimes unexpectedly – as waves of grief when parenting their own children. Always be on the lookout for opportunities to address this with parents. In this session, when we describe that a key element of warmth is helping the child to feel seen; a powerful way to demonstrate that is to ensure that the parents experience what it feels like to be seen themselves – by you, the therapist.

THERAPIST CONTINUES: *This next type of parenting style is what is referred to as authoritarian. Authoritarian parents are high in firmness and low in warmth. This type of parenting style has the advantage in that children know very clearly what the expectations are. This may help to decrease their fears of uncertainty. However, this parenting style has the disadvantage of having the child feel invisible. If the rules are the rules no matter what the circumstance or situation, the child can feel faded in the scene.*

Next, we have permissive parenting. This type of parent is high in warmth and low in firmness. We see this type of parenting style often in parents who have a child with pain. When you see a child in distress, it can feel really challenging to set and implement limits. So, the advantage of this type of parenting is that the child feels seen and cared for. The disadvantage is the child's sense of safety can be compromised. Believe it or not, children actually feel safe when they know the rules and they know the rules are going to be enforced in a fair way. Rules provide structure. Just like the structure of a house can make you feel safe from the elements, so goes the structure provided by fair rules.

Finally, we have an authoritative parenting style. This type of parent is high in warmth and high in firmness.

How would you describe your own parenting style? What parts of that style are working well? Are there any aspects that you are trying to work on or would like to work on?

What we have been doing in FBI – Pain Division is an attempt to give you and your child some tools so it is easier for them to try things when they are feeling uncomfortable. A lot of what we have been teaching you aligns with the combination of warm and firm parenting. By respecting and being curious about your child's body sensations and emotional experiences, they feel seen. By being clear and predictable, they feel safe. You are essentially saying to your child, "When you're in pain, you can expect that I will hear you and take that seriously. We will dive into your experience with a body investigation and look for

clues as to what might be going on. We will be curious and I will be open to your ideas. When your experiences become particularly intense, we will team up to discharge some of that energy and figure things out together."

By helping your child be curious about their bodies, you are helping them become more confident that their body is strong and can handle things and be less afraid that something bad will happen to them. Because it is hard to try to nudge a child in distress, we try to make these situations less threatening and more interesting. You and your child can design an investigation whenever they are trying to approach something hard. Then you see what happens. This makes you better prepared for the next time a situation like that arises. Everyone has different ways of parenting. Here in your workbook, we describe some of the core principles that may support a warm and firm parenting style (see "Warm and Firm Parenting Suggestions"). You decide what these elements may look like for you.

> *Warmth*
> Think of the experience of warmth as your child feeling seen, heard, and cared about.
> Imagine that your child is absorbing the rays of the sun.
>
> *Firmness*
> We think of firmness as the communication of reasonable expectations. By reasonable,
> we mean that we set up conditions whereby your child has the capacity to attempt to
> reach those expectations. Designing an investigation is one example of that!

Body Brainstorms

We will end today' session with our Body Brainstorms of the Week.

Questions on our Body Brainstorms worksheet this week include the following:

Can you remember a time when you felt Blah Bertha? What happened? What might you try the next time you feel Blah Bertha?

What you do you want to try the next time you feel Empty Eliza?

What are some things that bring on Nauseous Ned?

Your Fifth Body Investigation Assignment (Home-based Practice)

Home-based assignments are the same as last week. The family fills out Body Clues Worksheets as a summary of the day and/or after a tough moment.

Body Investigation Journal

In the child's body investigation journal this week, since they are becoming expert FBI agents, they can add to their journal when they feel something that they find important to note down.

Materials Families Take Home from Session 5

Here is a summary of what families get from session 5.

1. A worksheet that summarizes the characters that they have learned so far.
2. Coloring pages
3. The workbook pages for their binder with some ideas for home-based body investigations
4. The Body Brainstorms worksheet they completed
5. Body Clues Worksheets
6. Optional: Prizes! A comic book to design your own superhero
7. Optional: A Blah Bertha and Empty Eliza button
8. Information on getting prizes and buttons can be found at https://fbikids.org

Body Investigations to Practice at Home

Body Investigations to practice at home are always optional. It is important that parents do not feel overwhelmed with what we are asking them to do. They are intended to get the whole family in the spirit of marveling at something cool that the body did.

1. Can you find a spot to twirl around? See who feels Nauseous Ned first. Is there someone in your family that does not feel Nauseous Ned no matter how much they spin?
2. See if Empty Eliza shows up this week. Empty Eliza may not show up when they are expected!
3. When Blah Bertha comes around, have a snuggle party!

Then you schedule the next session! Congratulations, you've just finished session 5!

Therapist Reminders for Session 5

Congratulate families on making it halfway through the program.

A Final Reflection for Session 5

Parenting is personal. In this session, we tried to strike a balance between providing information and guidelines but also communicating that parents are the best judges for knowing what this would look like in their own home. As you think about this conversation with your client, how do you think it went? Are there things you would do differently next time to strike a better balance? If you are a parent, how would you have felt participating in this conversation?

Questions and Answers for Session 5

Q: What if I struck the wrong note and the parent gets really defensive when we have this conversation about parenting?

A: One strategy you might try is naming that right then and there. "I worry that I might have said something that came out the wrong way. Is there anything bothering you that we can talk about? I am always trying to strike a balance of giving parents information and also trusting their judgement that they know what is best for their children, but I sometimes may err more on one side than the other." Or something like that …

Q: What if a parent states they are already doing a warm and firm parenting style and they know all of that.

A: Fabulous. Reinforce the heck out of them and ask them for tips that you can pass on to other parents. What are some strategies they have found to be helpful?

Session 6: The Ouchies

Overview of Session 6

We have arrived at pain – The Ouchies. We took a while to get here quite intentionally. We wanted to ensure that children and parents have a solid framework and foundation for body sensations as helpful messengers. With our routines and strategies set, the Ouchies are just another group of sensations that can be very helpful in communicating what we need in a given moment. We have already touched on some body sensation characters related to pain. We met Polly the Pain, our generic pain character, and Patricia the Poop Pain in Session 1. We met Harold the Hunger Pain in Session 2. We will revisit some of these characters and also get into some more nuanced pain sensations: Ella the Emotial Pain, Sore Muscle Stan, Harriet Headache.

In this session, we continue to practice in-the-moment body investigations for when a child is faced with an intense sensation. We do this to ensure that parents are armed with strategies, and the confidence to implement them, when their child is experiencing pain. We spend a few minutes with parents at the end of the session to reinforce how to balance three important components in responding to a child's pain: validating the experience of pain or other body sensations, role-modeling curiosity about what those sensations may be communicating, and working with the child to design investigations to learn more about these sensations and their bodies. The purpose of this balance is to ensure that the child feels seen and heard while we create a playful and curious context to help them approach something that may be hard or scary. Finally, we want to collect data so that we know when pain is something that needs to be explored further.

Now let's investigate some pain!

Session Outline

1. Perform a warm-up Henry Heartbeat exercise
2. Review homework and add new things to the Body Map
3. Check in with everyone's energy using our energy meter and fuel up with a snack
4. Read the Session 6 workbook together to learn new characters related to pain: Ella the Emotional Pain, Sore Muscle Stan, Harriet the Headache
5. Perform some Body Investigations
6. Complete a Body Brainstorms worksheet
7. Time with caregivers/parents: Designing Body Investigations around pain, and learning to balance three essential components when responding to their child's pain
8. Review the plan for the week

9. Give out workbook and coloring pages
10. Optional: Give out prizes

Session Materials

1. Workbook, worksheets, and coloring pages for Session 6
2. A snack the child brings or that you have on hand that is in small pieces, for sensing our energy and fueling up
3. Optional: A disguise mask and an Ella the Emotional Pain button for session prizes. See https://fbikids.org for updated prize lists and links.

Background Information for Session 6

Pain is an important warning signal. If we think of the metaphor of streetlights, there are warning signals such as a flashing yellow light that caution a driver to slow down and pay more attention and there are red lights that signal that the time for action – stopping – is now. A challenge for children with sensory superpowers is that they can experience everything as a red light; with practice, however, they can learn to better distinguish the nuances of different sensations and discriminate the yellow light from the red light. Similarly to how we have handled each body sensation throughout the program, we learn nuanced experiences of pain via different characters, and conduct body investigations, with upbeat curiosity, to observe what happens to the intensity of pain with different maneuvers (did it go from a full circle to a half-circle? Did it stay the same? Go from a half-circle to a full circle?).

An important aspect of pain-related body investigations is, just like with all body investigations, we keep them acceptance focused. To remind you, by that we mean that we conduct an investigation to learn something about the body and to be curious about what happens – but not for the purpose of reducing pain. Thus, an investigation does not succeed or fail, it just is. We can take the information that we learn from it and use that to design and tweak the next investigation. As with any attempt to approach something hard, parents praise the gumption that is required to be an elite Feeling and Body Investigator. A mission never fails, especially when the goal is appreciating the profound wisdom of our bodies.

Step-by-Step Guide to Session 6

- Warm-Up Henry Heartbeat Activity
- Review Homework and Add New Things to Their Body Map
- Assess Energy and Fuel Up

Read the Session 6 Workbook Together to Meet the Ouchies

As everyone reads the workbook out loud together, this week's investigative questions ask families to think about the following body mysteries.

Session 6: Body Mystery Questions

Why do you think people have pain?
What do you think would happen if there was no pain?

As in every session, there are no wrong answers, we are just trying to get the family thinking about pain a bit differently. We encourage consideration of the value of pain. It protects us. It provides a contrast to situations without pain. It signals that something important may be happening. It allows us to have the experience of relief and learn what the body is communicating when it turns off pain signals. It allows us to feel and be more powerful and tough. Because each type of pain in this session has a different message, we discuss each individually below (Table 11.1).

Workbook pages this session provide some playful information about pain. We introduce Brenda the Brain. Brenda

Table 11.1 Summary of body sensation characters

Harold the Hunger Pain

When you feel intense discomfort in your gut because you need nourishment.

Harold is an old friend. We know them well by now. We just need to go grab a snack or meal when he comes around.

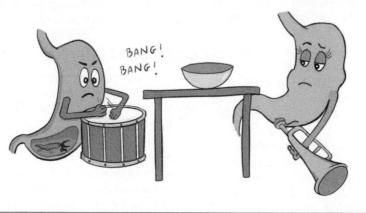

Ella the Emotional Pain

The throbbing pain in your chest that you may feel when you love something so much that it hurts.

What are some of the people or things that you love with all your heart?

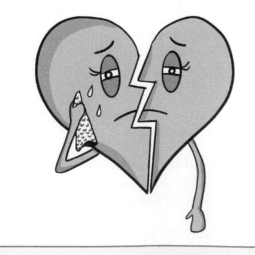

Sore Muscle Stan

The soreness and achiness you feel in your muscles when you have been exercising a muscle that is not used to moving much.

(This is very different than the jolt of pain that signals you should stop what you are doing).

When was the last time your muscles felt really sore? What were you doing?

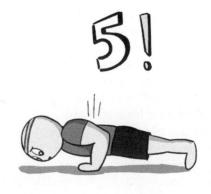

Harriet the Headache

A pounding or feeling of pressure in your head.

Have you ever had a headache? What are some ideas of some investigations you can do if you do have a headache?

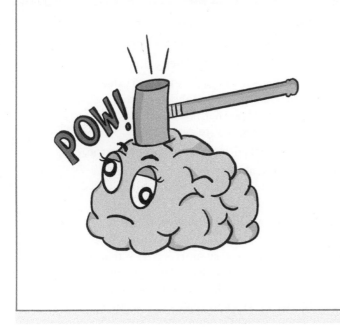

Patricia the Poop Pain

Sometimes when we go to the bathroom, our poops are very hard and rub against our skin. All that rubbing can make us sore sometimes.

Do you know any ways to make your poops squishy?

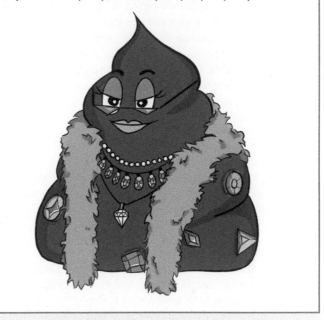

the Brain is a useful character to have around, but does not make it to many of our worksheets, because the brain is not a sensation per se – rather Harriet the Headache or Mind-Racing Mikella are some examples of sensations related to thinking. However, Brenda the Brain helps explain a core concept that we wish to illustrate in Session 6: that while the body and brain work together to manage pain, often the body is smart enough and tough enough to take care of pain on its own (Figure 11.1).

The Ouchies Body Investigations
Oh, the THINGS You Can Do with an Achy Tummy: Polly the Pain in Action

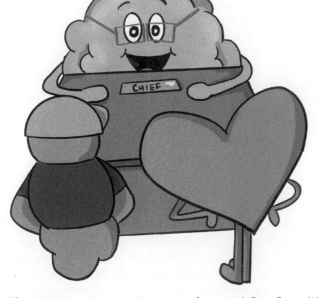

Figure 11.1 Brenda the Brain having a conference with Gassy Gus and Henry Heartbeat to discuss the division of labor for the day.

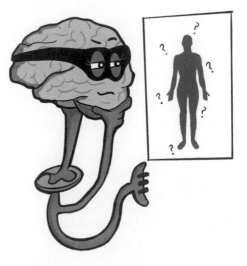

Polly the Pain is our generic pain character. They wear a mask and look stealthy because they can be a bit sneaky sometimes. Though they try to be sneaky, Polly the Pain is no match for a well-trained elite FBI agent. The activities that we describe for Polly the Pain are designed to demonstrate that pain will not get in our way. In this type of activity, we try to make the child a little bit uncomfortable and then see what they are able to do despite that. The way that we have found works well is to have a variety of belts of various sizes in the office, and then to ask the child to wrap a belt around their stomach so that it's just a bit tight. Then, we go about doing lots of crazy body things. For example, we try running really fast, balancing on one leg, solving a math problem – the options are endless. The goal: seeing we can still do things (and even improve at doing things) while being uncomfortable.

> For Polly the Pain investigations, a helpful strategy is to think of different ways to make the child feel a little bit uncomfortable and then show them what they are able to do even when they feel a little uncomfortable.

THERAPIST: *Let's design a Polly the Pain investigation. I want to see how fast you can run, even when we make things a little bit challenging for you. Go ahead and pick out a belt from that stack over there. (We have found it helpful to have a bunch of cheap and colorful belts on hand). Now when someone has a stomach ache, they may think that they cannot do a lot of things. We are going to investigate that! I want to see how fast you can run if we put this belt around your stomach and we tighten it a little bit so it's just a wee bit uncomfortable. Parents do you want to try this too?*

The therapist, parent, and child (and any other family members at the session) all grab belts and tighten them around their stomachs.

THERAPIST: *Okay! Is everybody a little bit uncomfortable?*

CHILD AND PARENT: YES

THERAPIST: *That is terrific. OK, now begin to see how fast you can run from point A here* (therapist marks the spot) *to point B. Serena you go ahead to the starting line and I will count you down.*

Child walks to the starting line at Point A wearing the belt that makes them a little bit uncomfortable.

THERAPIST: *On your marks, get set, go!*

The therapist has a stopwatch going and announces the time.

THERAPIST: *Amazing! You ran that lap in XX seconds while wearing a tight belt around your stomach. Now, let's try and see if you can go even faster?*

The therapist and child repeat that exercise as much as the child wants to.

THERAPIST: *Wow! You keep getting faster and faster! What should we add to our Body Map about this?*

CHILD: That I can run really fast even when I'm a little uncomfortable?

THERAPIST: *That sounds great. Your body sure is tough and can get through lots of stuff – that's for sure.*

CHILD: Yeah, I want to add that to.

THERAPIST: *Let's see what else we can do. What about seeing if we can balance on one foot when we are feeling Polly the Pain?*

> ### Things you can try when the child is uncomfortable
>
> Test their speed and how their speed improves with practice
>
> Test their balance and how their balance improves with practice
>
> Test their problem-solving abilities
>
> For example, you can play the hot cold game where you hide something and you indicate how close the person is getting to the object by saying hot, hotter, etc., or how far away they are getting by saying cold, colder etc.
>
> You can have them solve math problems or read.
>
> Test their artistic abilities.

Body Investigation: Ella the Emotional Pain

Throughout Part 1 of this handbook, we described how one of the gifts of having sensory superpowers is that children live life out loud – they have intense, vital experiences that can really make them feel alive. When we think of positive affiliative emotions like love, this means that these children can love things with tremendous depth. As anyone who has loved things deeply has probably experienced, fear, sadness, and emotional pain are often at the heels of love. When we are feeling a moment of intense love, you may sometimes be surprised that that moment is followed by a moment of intense sadness. The anticipation of losing what we love someday can sneak right underneath that profound feeling of safety and closeness that comes with loving someone (a person, a pet) intensely. In the words of Ella the Emotional Pain:

> Why hello. I'm Ella the Emotional Pain. Believe it or not, sometimes you can have such strong loving and caring feelings that your body may actually ache. While this may seem scary, it is actually a beautiful thing. It means that you care about something so deeply, that you love that thing with your whole body. It is wonderful to care about something that deeply. It is worth it to hurt sometimes if it means you get to love things that much.

Investigations that can evoke Ella the Emotional Pain include telling stories about or watching pictures or movies of animals or people that the family loves – including those individuals who have passed away. Children with sensory superpowers may actually feel emotional pain when they say goodbye to their parents in the morning for school or when they give their pet a hug goodbye for the afternoon. Thus, Ella the Emotional Pain can be a great source of material for in-the-moment body investigations that the parent and child design on-the-fly.

The Power of Sensory Superpowers and Ella the Emotional Pain

What does one do with this challenging universal situation? It is inevitable that we someday lose those people and things that we love most dearly. Is it worth it to feel that intense level of pain? Wouldn't you avoid that pain if you just kept yourself from loving something that deeply? The answer is that once we have experienced that kind of deep love or joy, we keep that precious feeling with us and it makes our lives more meaningful. Life is about moments and we hold these moments in our bodies and minds. We can summon up a memory and allow the joy from that moment and the love from that moment to wash over us again and again and again. Here is where children with sensory superpowers have a special advantage. Because they feel things so intensely, their memories of these experiences are richer. They get the benefit of reliving these moments of joy at a level of intensity that may make reminiscing about these memories even more exhilarating.

Body Investigation: The Power of Sore Muscles

Sore Muscle Stan is that harmless but uncomfortable feeling that you get in your muscles when they have been stretched and are working really hard. We can think of that soreness as a sign that your muscles are getting stronger. Doing investigations regarding muscles soreness and strength is a particularly powerful demonstration of how the body gets stronger with practice. Through these investigations, we typically have children do a hard exercise. Then rest. Then try again to see if they quickly get better with practice. Sore Muscle Stan is also a good source for body investigations that are practiced at home. The child can repeatedly practice an exercise and watch themselves getting better at it. Practicing with exercise can also be a really great frustration tolerance activity, especially when learning a new physical movement that requires coordination. It requires patience to keep approaching it and practicing it so you get

better and overcome the initial struggle. Sore Muscle Stan is our symbol that we are tough enough to stick with it. Sore Muscle Stan is a really powerful and unique kind of discomfort. It is the sign that your body is getting stronger and tougher (see Figure 11.2 and Table 11.2).

> Charts and graphs of the body getting stronger with Body Investigations are great things to add to the Body Map.

Table 11.2 Ideas for Pain Sensation Investigations

Ideas for getting to know Sore Muscle Stan

1. Have the children do a wall squat – where they sit against the wall pretending they are sitting on a chair with their legs at a 90-degree angle. Time how long they can hold it. Have the children rest for a few minutes. Then, do it again. See if they can get even one second longer than the first time.
2. The children can do any exercise that involves repeated movements (jumping jacks, push-ups etc.). Try the same strategy. Do a set. Rest. Then do a second set to see if you get any better (e.g., one more repetition of the exercise).
3. The therapist can keep a record of what the child did and repeat these exercises as treatment progresses so that the child can see improvement in their power and strength over time.
4. For all these investigations, the child can give a rating of how much of Sore Muscle Stan they feel using the FBI circle the character metric (half-circle, three-quarter-circle, etc.) or whatever scale they invent (e.g., 0 to 5 with 0 being no soreness).

Ideas to Bring on Ella the Emotional Pain

1. Look at pictures, videos, or tell stories about an animal the child has lost.
2. Look at pictures, videos, or tell stories about a person the child has lost.
3. See whether Ella the Emotional Pain comes to visit when the child says goodbye to their parents. Maybe an interesting investigation would be to see what happens to Ella the Emotional Pain once the child sees their friends at school. Is Ella the Emotional Pain at recess?
4. For all these investigations, the child can give a rating of how much their heart hurts using the FBI circle the character metric or whatever scale they invent (e.g., 0 to 5 with 0 being no hurt at all).
5. They can then investigate what they would like to try with these different feelings. What happens to Ella the Emotional Pain when everybody snuggles? Or writes down a memory? Learning strategies to sit with Ella the Emotional Pain in the company of loved one can be a very powerful experience.

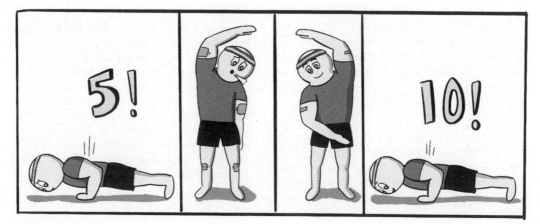

Figure 11.2 Sore Muscle Stan getting stronger with practice.

Body Investigation: Harriet the Headache

Harriet the Headache gives us lots of useful information. When our head is hurting, is it a sign that we are a little dehydrated and need to drink some water? Is it an indication that we have got a lot of on our mind and our muscles are very tense? Only a well-designed body investigation can reveal the answers!

THERAPIST: *Let's see what Harriet the Headache has to say.* (From the workbook:)

Who may come to visit if you are worrying a lot about something, and thinking very hard about it, which then causes your head muscles to get very, very tight?

You guessed it! Harriet the Headache!!!

"Why hello! I am Harriet. I am good friends with Polly the Pain and Harold the Hunger Pain – and all our other muscle, worry, and emotional pain buddies. We all went to school together and learned many of the same tricks. However, I have a specialty degree. My specialty is causing pain in your head, from worrying a lot, being hungry or dehydrated, or other reasons. When I come around, it is usually a good time to take some deep breaths, do some stretches, and maybe make a plan."

THERAPIST: *Let's see if we can figure out an interesting Harriet the Headache investigation. You know about our energy meter, how we use our hands to indicate our increasing energy as we eat food or do different things. Another example of a scale that people sometimes find helpful is a pain thermometer. Let's look at this pain thermometer in your workbook. You see, as someone's pain is getting stronger, the color red is getting darker, that is what is called the mercury in a thermometer. It rises as someone's temperature is going up. So, at the top of the thermometer is the most pain you can possibly imagine and at the bottom of the thermometer is the least amount of pain you can possibly imagine. What if we say that zero is no pain and 10 is the most pain you could possibly have? Now let's listen to our bodies and see what we are feeling like right now. What is your rating?*

CHILD: 2

Measuring Pain

In the clinical trial of Feeling and Body Investigators, we used the Iowa Pain Thermometer[1] as our way to measure pain throughout the treatment. This thermometer has the advantage of using verbal descriptions, numbers, and colors to indicate the intensity of pain, so it gives children lots of options to try to quantify their pain – which was important for the study. For FBI agents, knowing the intensity of pain can be a useful part of an investigation, so that we can track changes during a body investigation. What we learn from these investigations can also help us to make decisions about pain management. For example, a parent and child may learn that at a level of pain at or below a certain threshold, they can still perform certain activities, etc. Because FBI agents are elite investigators, making graphs and charts of changes in ratings can be a really useful image to add to our Body Maps. It can also be a powerful demonstration of the strength of the body, that the body can do many things, even when uncomfortable. In our online materials, we include a copy of the pain diary that we used in our FBI clinical trial.

THERAPIST: *Do you remember when we investigated Mind-Racing Mikella and we listed all of our worries to see how fast they could go? This time, we are going to do something a little bit differently. Now, what if I set a timer and we all think about as many worries as we can. First, you will give me a rating of how much your head hurts before we start this. Then, we will think of all the worries that we can. We will just think of them to ourselves or you can draw a picture of them. Next, I will get another rating of how much your head hurts and we will see if it changes. After that, we can repeat this investigation again but with one important difference. Rather than keeping your worries to yourself, this time everyone will share their worries with each other and see what happens. We will do the same thing: give a rating of Harriet the Headache before, then share as many worries as you can, and then rate Harriet the Headache again and see what happens. We can learn something really interesting from these investigations. We can see whether sharing worries with someone makes Harrier the Headache stronger or weaker than if you keep them to yourself.*

The therapist proceeds to keep track of the time and sees what happens when you keep worries to yourself versus when you share them.

Body Investigations About Harriet the Headache to Try at Home

When a child has a headache at home, parents and children might want to design one of the following investigations.

1. Make a pain rating. Drink some water right then, and take a pain rating every ten minutes for the next 40 minutes. You can also design a longer experiment in which the child increases their water every day for the next week and makes pain ratings as a summary of the day.
2. Trying writing or drawing about worries and then share what you drew or wrote with someone who is a good listener. See what happens to Harriet the Headache before and afterwards.

Body Investigation: Patricia the Poop Pain

We learn a bit more about Patricia the Poop Pain in this session. As Patricia likes to explain it (from the workbook):

"Remember me? Patricia the Poop Pain? The glamourous and fancy piece of poo? It's time for you to learn a few more things about me so you can be the MASTER of POO! As you know, I can feel very differently from one bathroom trip to the next. Sometimes I may be very squishy and come right out, and sometimes I may be very hard and it may hurt your butt a little bit when you poop. That feeling is probably my jewels rubbing against the side of your intestine. Either way, it is a fun ride for me! But do you know how to make your poop nice and squishy? The secret is to eat foods that are full of fiber! Check out our list and see which ones you eat!"

Of course, given the lack of control we have over the timing of a bowel movement, conducting a Patricia the Poop Pain investigation in session would be very challenging to design (however, if

What is the perfect fiber/poop squishiness combination?

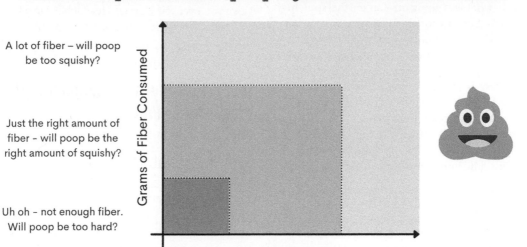

Figure 11.3 An example graph of fiber:poop squishiness.

you come up with a fun one, please share it via our web-based community, https://fbikids.org). Instead, Patricia the Poop Pain is ideal for body investigations to conduct at home. In the workbook, we list some high-fiber foods that it may be fun for the child to try to eat more of to see if it impacts their poop consistency – a very fun thing for children to plot. Of course, there can be too much of a good thing, so it can be interesting to find the optimal amount of fiber for the optimal poop squishiness (Figure 11.3).

Body Investigations About Patricia the Poop Pain to Try at Home

When a child is having trouble with poop pain, the family may want to design an investigation that looks something like one of these:

1. Gradually add fiber to the child's diet over a two-week period and plot the poop squishiness. Make sure the children design their own "poop squishiness" scale.
2. Try different entertaining activities while sitting on the toilet. Find out which one is the most entertaining. See what happens to Patricia the Poop Pain when you do something entertaining.
3. Investigate the relationship between the firmness of poop and the smelliness of farts. Make sure you generate *a priori* hypotheses about this important question.
4. Improve water intake and see what happens to the squishiness of poop. Consider a graph as in #1.

Body Investigation: Gas Pain

So many types of pain! You may have some clients who are very good at passing gas on command, in which case, you can have a lot of fun with the before and after effects of passing gas. We focus more on these types of pain in our Body Brainstorms worksheet and in our home-based body investigations (see below).

Possible Body Lessons from the Ouchies

Ella the Emotional Pain helps me to remember how wonderful it is to love things.

Polly the Pain makes sure I pay attention to things in my body that may need attention.

Sore Muscle Stan is my signal that I am getting stronger and tougher.

Patricia the Poop Pain helps me remember to drink water and eat things that help my poops stay squishy.

Harriet the Headache reminds me to share my worries with someone who is a good listener.

Adding to the Body Map

Do not forget to summarize these lessons on the child's (and parents') Body Map!

Time with Parents/Caregivers: Designing Home-based Body Investigations

Parents have learned several ways to use their Body Clues Worksheets. For example, parent and child can pull out a worksheet following an intense moment to figure out what just happened and to plan for what to do next time. Parent and child can use a Body Clues Worksheet as a way to review the highs and lows of the day, the best and the lowest moments. These examples use our Body Clues Worksheets to learn about the body by being an investigator for things that have already happened. As this treatment has progressed, we have given parents ideas for body investigations that they can perform at home. In Session 4, the Zoomies and Shakies, we got even more sophisticated. We introduced parents to the emotional wave and began discussing how to use Body Investigations to help master high-intensity moments – in the moment. This involved designing an investigation in reaction to what was going on – an on-the-spot, high-tech investigation suitable only for elite FBI agents.

In this session and throughout the rest of the treatment, we continue to practice in-the-moment investigations, including when the child is having different types of pain sensations. If it is helpful to write these down for your child, we introduce Step 5 to our Body Clues Worksheet: Plan your next investigation so the parents and child can jot down their plan.

For example, it might be a good idea to design an investigation when a child complains of pain in the morning on a school day. Rather than keeping a child home from school, the parent can say:

> "Thanks for telling me that your stomach is hurting. I definitely want to help you with that. I have an idea. How about we do an investigation and see what happens to your pain at different times of the school day without us doing anything else. How do you think we should track that? Should we make our own pain scale or use the pain thermometer in your workbook? Should we track this in your journal throughout the day?"

As another example, if the child is about to start something new, like playing on a new sports team, a parent could help the child design an investigation like this.

> "I'm so glad that you told me that you are feeling uncomfortable. Let's see if we can design an investigation about this. You know, I wonder if running around makes you fart more? Should we investigate it? Should we track the number of times you pass gas at the basketball game?"

Table 11.3 lists some ideas to help with in-the-moment investigations

Body Brainstorms

We will end today's session with our Body Brainstorms of the Week.

Questions on our Body Brainstorms Worksheet this week include the following:

What is something that you did that gave you Sore Muscle Stan?

Table 11.3 Investigations to help children (and parents) deal with difficult moments

1. Investigate what happens to pain throughout the school day. Make a hypothesis about which part of the day the pain will be the lowest.
2. Investigate what happens if you do a Henry Heartbeat activity (ones in which you slow down your heartbeat) during different parts of the investigation. How does your body feel then?
3. Get a friend involved. Perhaps a close friend could be doing the same investigation. This is particularly nice if both children have a journal that they can record their observations and share what they have learned. The other child does not have to have pain. They can each design their own investigation about something important to each of them.
4. Rather than monitoring pain, another strategy is to investigate what happens when you actively provoke another sensation. For example, parent and child could see how many times they can bring on Lulu the Laughing Pain during the day (you will meet them in Session 8).

What is a time when you felt Ella the Emotional Pain?

Have you ever felt Harriet Headache? Do you remember what you were doing or what you did?

What is something that you do on the toilet if you are having Patricia the Poop Pain?

Your Sixth Body Investigation Assignment (Home-based Practice)

Keep practicing in-the-moment investigations.

Body Investigation Journal

The body investigation journal will be used this week to record any investigations that parent and child design.

Materials Families Take Home from Session 6

Here is a summary of what families may receive from Session 6.

1. A worksheet that summarizes the characters that they have learned so far
2. Coloring pages
3. The workbook pages for their binder with ideas of some home-based body investigations
4. The Body Brainstorms sheet they completed
5. Optional: Prizes! A disguise!
6. Optional: An Ella the Emotional Pain button
7. Information on getting prizes and buttons can be found at: https://fbikids.org

Body Investigations to Practice at Home

Remind parents to be on the alert for times when they can design a body investigation to learn something about the body while approaching something challenging. Then you schedule the next session! Congratulations, you've just finished Session 6!

Therapist Reminders for Session 6

Congratulate families on making it through the hardest part of the program. It is all fun from here on out!

A Final Reflection for Session 6

Avoiding positive feelings due to fear of loss is something we all experience. FBI is not a mindfulness-based intervention, in that we did not deliberately instruct skills in mindfulness (focusing on the present moment, focusing on one experience at a time, and doing so non-judgmentally). Yet, as you may recognize, we have been working throughout this program on increasing moment-to-moment awareness. By becoming more aware of what we are feeling, we increase the vitality and richness of each moment. Life is about moments, and memories capture these moments. If we are becoming more aware of, and fully experiencing moments as they unfold, we may just be making life a bit more meaningful. Something definitely worth reflecting on.

Questions and Answers for Session 6

Q: Some of these sound like really challenging investigations. What if the parent starts to get nervous that we are doing something that could be harmful to their child?

A: This would be a great opportunity to role model exactly what we want the parents to do when their child is distressed about approaching a situation. You could name that directly if you think that would be helpful. "The situation we are in right now is very similar to a situation you might experience with your child when they are having doubts about approaching a situation. Let's do now what we are trying to do then. Let's design an investigation and let's just see what happens. We have a massive toolbox to help us manage whatever happens from our investigation. We are an elite group of special forces. We are ready for this."

Q: Do you really believe that Ella the Emotional Pain is worth it?

A: We really do.

References

1. Herr, K., Spratt, K.F., Garand, L., et al. (2007). Evaluation of the Iowa pain thermometer and other selected pain intensity scales in younger and older adult cohorts using controlled clinical pain: a preliminary study. *Pain Med*, 8(7), 585–600. https://doi.org/10.1111/j.1526-4637.2007.00316.x

Chapter 12

Session 7: The Drowsies

There never seems to be enough time to do the
things you want to do once you find them.
Time in a Bottle, by Jim Croce

Overview of Session 7

Congratulations! You have made it to Session 7. We are fully into
our session routine. We have learned all the basic techniques.
If you were at a cocktail party, and you overheard someone
mentioning "energy meter," "body brainstorm," "body clues,"
or "body investigation" you would know exactly what they are
talking about and would know that this is going to be a great
party. You have helped parents to further develop a parenting
style that they feel comfortable with when parenting a child
with sensory superpowers and we have given them a toolbox of
strategies to help their children manage intense situations. We
have accomplished a great deal. From here on out, we are just
practicing. Our next set of practices is with sensations that are
pleasant and calming.

In this session, we focus on the sensations around sleeping.
There are entire interventions devoted to improving sleep in
children. This session benefits from the expert consultation of
Allison Harvey at the University of California at Berkeley and
Lauren Asarnow at the University of California, San Francisco.
Dr. Harvey and Dr. Asarnow are both experts on the development and testing of interventions to promote sleep across the
lifespan.[1-7] We learn our sleeping tools in a single session; however, we do have an advantage in that the children are already
experts in body sensations, some of which may interfere with
sleeping. They also already regard these sensations with curiosity rather than fear, meaning that these sensations may be less
likely to interfere with sleeping. We have another advantage in
that families are now well-versed in body investigations. There
are lots of fun investigations that can be done when one is trying
to get better at noticing when they are truly tired, and what happens to the body and one's energy level when they start to adopt
a more regular sleep schedule.

Dr. Asarnow and Dr. Harvey have helped us to distinguish
some essential sensations associated with sleep – such as the
important difference of feeling tired or fatigued versus feeling
sleepy. We will get some visits from some old friends in this
session, namely Mind-Racing Mikella, Sore Muscle Stan, and
Empty Eliza and, of course, meet some new friends. Let's get
cozy.

A well-rested body is best equipped to manage pain. That is
why we devote a session entirely to improving the enjoyment
of bedtimes and the restfulness of sleep.

Session Outline

1. Perform a warm-up Henry Heartbeat exercise.
2. Review homework and add new things to the Body Map.
3. Check in with everyone's energy and fuel up with a snack.
4. Learn new characters related to sleep: Sleepy Steven, Tired
   Tina, Cozy Celeste, Cool Cyrus, Comfortable Cayla, Stuck
   Stephanie, Dark Debra
5. Perform some Body Investigations.
6. Complete a Body Brainstorms worksheet.
7. Review the plan for the week.
8. Give out coloring pages.
9. Optional: Give out prizes.

Session Materials

1. Workbook, worksheets, and coloring pages for Session
   7 are available for download at www.cambridge.org/fbi-
   clinical-guide.
2. A snack the child brings or that you have on hand that is in
   small pieces, for sensing our energy and fueling up.
3. Optional: A mini-stuffed animal and a Cozy Celeste Button
   for session prizes. See updated prize lists at https://fbikids.org.

Background Information for Session 7

Ideally, going to sleep, falling asleep, and staying asleep is something that is easy and pleasurable for both parent and child.
We all know from our own experiences the value of effort-
less, refreshing sleep, and we may have personal experiences
with the profound distress and potential impairment that can
occur when sleep becomes disrupted. In the context of children with sensory superpowers and recurrent pain, the benefits and costs of refreshing sleep become magnified. Poor sleep
impacts immune system function and more acutely, influences

regulatory functions like focusing attention and managing distress. Thus, on days when children sleep poorly, everything can seem harder. The good news is that much like hunger, sleep is one of those body functions that can be trained. Training regular sleep habits and investigating the factors that get in the way of easy and refreshing sleep are perfect challenges for elite FBI forces.

Our bodies can learn to associate going to bed and being in bed with arousal (e.g., Julie Jitters, Mind-Racing Mikella, Henry Heartbeat). Through processes referred to as classical conditioning (see chapter 4 for more information), we form associations between things that commonly co-occur. Let's picture the following two scenarios.

Scenario Number One: The Child Who Has Not Been Through the FBI – Pain Division Intervention

A child has had a very busy day. During the day, some things did not go quite as well as the child would have liked. The child is rushing around until bedtime. They get into bed and immediately their thoughts start racing. They cannot fall asleep. They feel very lonely in the dark in their bed. After a while, they go to wake up their parents so they do not have to be alone in the night. After a few nights of this, the parents have a harder time getting the child to go to bed because the child is dreading facing the racing thoughts and being alone. Whenever the child gets into bed, their thoughts start racing. Meanwhile the parents have decreased capacities to cope because they have had poor-quality sleep over the past several nights.

This scenario is an example of conditioning: the bed has become a cue for thoughts to race.

Scenario Number Two: The Child Is Trained as an Elite Agent on the FBI – Pain Division Special Forces Task Force

The child has had a very busy day. Some things did not go quite as well as the child would have liked. The child is rushing around until bedtime. The child and parent have had days like this before and they remember that the child had trouble sleeping when that happened – they were visited by Mind-Racing Mikella all night, felt lonely, and then went to visit their parents in their bed. They decide to conduct an investigation. They are going to try doing a Sore Muscle Stan stretching routine to see what happens when they do that before sleep. Does Mind-Racing Mikella come to visit or does she keep her racing car in the garage? Because these are elite agents, they decide to make this a sophisticated, two-part investigation. If Mind-Racing Mikella comes to visit, the child's is going to explore what happens if they write or draw the images or words racing through their mind on a notepad by their bed. Then they will imagine tucking Mind-Racing Mikella in bed next to them as Mikella runs out of gas. The next morning, parent and child will review what they learned on their Body Clues Worksheet and tweak the plan as necessary.

These are pretty shrewd investigations. We are making sure that bed is associated with relaxing sensations by trying a stretching routine beforehand to slow us down and then seeing what happens to Mind-Racing Mikella. We also employ the recontextualizing strategies that we discussed in Chapter 4. That is, rather than changing the objective features of a thing, such as the experience of racing thoughts, we change the way that it is experienced. Rather than worries racing through our mind, it is just Mind-Racing Mikella speeding by in their racing car. As always, we frame everything as investigations in which we cannot fail. We just learn new things.

There are multitudes of factors to know about sleep. We only touch on some very basic, over-simplified principles – things that may be helpful for an FBI agent to know. Our focus, of course, is what being sleepy feels like and the investigations we design help us to notice, feel, and act on sleepiness. Sleepy Steven is our sleep character. Sleepy Steven is the signal that sleep is going to come soon. In ideal circumstances, there is a rhythm that develops with Sleepy Steven (that is why Sleepy Steven has music notes on their pajamas – they are a very rhythmic character).[8] Just as one can learn to dance better with practice and have better rhythm, it is the same with the rhythm of sleep.[9] Thus, it is important to have routines – routines give the day a rhythm. As we noted in Chapter 3 when we discussed the importance of a child's experience of safety, routines are predictable, and predictability helps children feel safe. Predictability can include things like the time the child goes to bed and the activities that they perform before bed. Because getting a child to be willing to go to bed can be challenging, a focus of Session 7 is on investigations that explore how children feel before bed. To do so, we investigate some different bedtime routines and examine how these different routines make our bodies feel. These routines may not only make bedtime feel predictable and safe, but they may have the additional benefit of making the bedtime routine playful. Perhaps, this will make it easier for children to be more willing to start getting ready for bed.

It is also important to have comfortable conditions. To demonstrate the importance of this, it may be interesting to try this investigation with yourself. The next time you have a troubling dream, notice whether you were physically uncomfortable while you were sleeping. While not all troubling dreams can be attributed to the physical state of our bodies, you may be surprised at how often they are. To help parents and children remember features of the sleeping environment that we can manipulate, of course, we have some characters that can help. Cool Cyrus reminds us about being aware of our experience of temperature (having a cool room but not feeling too cold ourselves can help with sleep). Cozy Celeste and Comfortable Cayla remind us that part of the joy of sleeping is feeling snug and relaxed. Finally, once we are cool, comfortable, and cozy, we focus on our experience of the light in the room. It is important to make things as dark as possible or reasonable. To help create a context in which the dark is associated with restful snuggles, Dark Debra is the sensation of not being able to see things, but feeling surrounded by a peaceful calm, like a soft, dark blanket covering the world (which is what Dark Debra is).

Because we are not with the children during bedtime, our investigations for this session focus on doing some before and after explorations of various bedtime routines to see how we feel after each and when they might come in handy. We also do some pretending that we are in bed and have different experiences that we investigate. For example, we try to conjure up Mind-Racing Mikella and explore what happens to their racing car with different strategies. We can go back to some investigations in Session 4 to remind ourselves that Betty Butterfly and their friends may come dancing in the dark and we can see what happens when Dark Debra joins the party. Finally, we get to meet Stuck Stephanie. Stuck Stephanie is the feeling we have when we are having so much fun doing what we are doing that we just feel stuck because we don't want to stop. We investigate some different ways to help her get unstuck.

Finally, there is the important difference between Sleepy Steven and Tina Tired. While Sleepy Steven is our trigger for sleep, Tina Tired is more related to our feeling of energy.[8] Tina Tired comes around when we are having trouble maintaining a high enough level of energy to get things done. Tina Tired is a signal that we need to take care of ourselves. Because of the overlap in some of the feelings of Tina Tired and Blah Bertha (the feeling of heaviness we may feel when we are sad or down), we suggest some home-based investigations in which we try some of our Blah Bertha strategies and see what happens to Tired Tina. All in all, this session is about making a habit of getting comfy and cozy. Have a relaxing session!

they will learn. We provide a summary worksheet every week that summarizes all the characters they have learned to date (see Table 12.1). The length of this worksheet is a great experience of mastery for the children as they marvel at all the different characters they have learned.

So, do we expect them to learn all these? We do not expect anything really. We just want these children to have all these sensations at their disposal so they could take advantage of what is helpful to them. And, we think they will love them.

Step-by-Step Guide to Session 7
- Warm-Up Henry Heartbeat Activity
- Review Homework and Add New Things to Their Body Map
- Assessing Your Energy and Fueling Up

Read the Session 7 Workbook: The Drowsies
As in every session, the next step of treatment is that everyone goes through the workbook pages together to learn the new characters and to explore what they mean. This week's investigative questions in the workbook ask families to think about the following body mysteries.

Session 7: Body Mystery Questions
Why does your body get sleepy? What are some body sensations you notice as you start to get sleepy?

The Drowsies Body Investigations
Sleep Match: Sore Muscle Stan Stretching Routine Versus Gassy Gus Exercise Routine Versus Henry Heartbeat Exercise Routine
What is the most effective and most fun way to get your body ready for bed? The answer to this important question requires some sophisticated body investigations.

There are so many sensations! Do we really expect children to learn all these?
Our experience is that one of the most exciting moments of each session is learning the new characters. I (NZ) had to "endure" sessions of deflation when a child saw that there were only a few new characters (or none at all!). That is one reason we ended up creating coloring pages and character buttons – so children could hold onto the characters and use them as reminders of all that they have learned. Some children will indeed learn every single sensation. Other children will adopt a few favorites that

Table 12.1 Summary of body sensation characters from the workbook and questions to discuss

Sleepy Steven	
This is the feeling you have when your body is telling you are about ready to fall asleep. Your eyes are getting droopy, your body may start to feel heavy – so heavy, in fact, that you may feel a strong urge to lay down your head. Sleepy Steven is very good with rhythms and routines. Sleepy Steven is smooth: every night Steven goes to bed with style. Sleepy Steven's body gets more to the beat of sleeping when they start doing the same things at the same time before bed and becomes even more stylish. What are some things that you notice when you are sleepy? What are some things your mom or dad notices when you are sleepy?	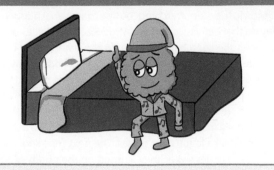

Table 12.1 (cont.)

Tired Tina

Tired Tina is actually a little bit tricky. Tina is good friends with Empty Eliza, that feeling when your mind feels blank and you don't have any urges to do anything in particular. Tired Tina can also feel like she's related to Blah Bertha, that feeling of heaviness we may have when we are sad. Tired Tina comes around when you have had enough of something and you are having a hard time keeping your energy up – like you have been practicing your spelling words for too long. She is sneaky because even though when someone feels Tired Tina they are low in energy, they are not feeling Sleepy Steven. Tired Tina is a signal that you need rest and comfort – not sleep.

What are some things one could try when they feel Tired Tina? Well, since Tired Tina has some similarities to Blah Bertha and Empty Eliza, it could be an interesting investigation to try some of our strategies for Blah Bertha and Empty Eliza and see what happens then to Tired Tina. It might also be interesting to check out some of the routines that we learn in this lesson and see what happens to Tired Tina. However, perhaps the most interesting investigations to try when you are feeling Tired Tina is to see what you can do to bring on Cozy Celeste! You will see what we mean soon …

What are some things that after you've been doing them for a little bit of time you start to feel Tired Tina? Is there anything that you could do for hours and hours and you would never feel Tired Tina? If you were feeling Tired Tina and Blah Bertha at the same time, what could you try?

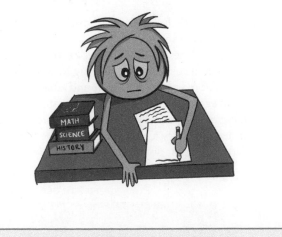

Cozy Celeste

How does one describe what cozy feels like? When we feel cozy, it almost feels like it activates our rooting reflex as an infant: we just want to nuzzle up next to someone warm, like your mom. So, we define cozy as the feeling that you want to nuzzle up to something.

Can you describe what would make you feel the coziest?

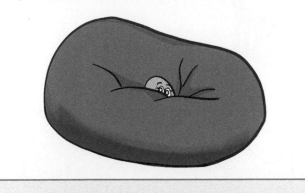

Cool Cyrus

Cool Cyrus is there when you feel like your body temperature is a little bit lower than just right. It is just slightly chilly and you feel very comfortable at this temperature with a blanket on.

When you think about your being in your bedroom when it is time to sleep, do you feel Cool Cyrus? If you do not, can we think of ways to help you feel Cool Cyrus?

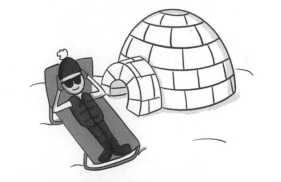

Comfortable Cayla

Comfortable Cayla is when your body feels just right. Your muscles are relaxed after a good stretch and you feel like you are ready to feel Cozy Celeste.

Are there things that you do now to get comfortable for bed? When you are feeling Sore Muscle Stan, what are things you try to bring on Comfortable Cayla?

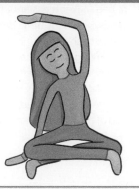

Table 12.1 (cont.)

Dark Debra	Stuck Stephanie
Dark Debra is the sensation you feel when you are looking into the darkness and you cannot see anything or maybe the slight outlines of things. You feel quiet, like there's a dark blanket covering the sky of your room.	Stuck Stephanie is the feeling you have when you are doing something that you really like doing and you're supposed to stop doing it and go do something else – like get ready for bed, but you feel stuck, like you just can't stop doing it.

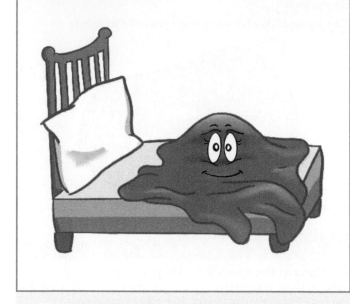 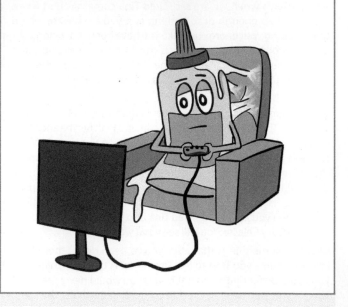

First, choose your outcome measure. Do you want to see which bedtime routine lowers Julie Jitters the most? Which routine is the best at slowing down Mind-Racing Mikella? Which routine brings on the most Comfortable Cayla? Which routine makes you the most Sleepy Steven?

An elite FBI agent knows that there might be a need for different bedtime routines on different days and depending on how we are feeling. That is why it is good to have several routines handy. We give you the example of three different bedtime routines. There are endless creative possibilities for children and parents to invent their own.

As with any well-designed investigation, once we have chosen our "outcome measure," we are going to want to take that measurement before we do the routine and after we do the routine. We might even want to stick with one routine for one week to see what happens when we practice it over time. For example, if the child decides to try a Henry Heartbeat bedtime routine, does Julie Jitters go up or down after the routine with practice?

Henry the Heartbeat Exercise Routine

Performing a Henry Heartbeat exercise routine before bed can help to answer the fascinating question of whether getting your heart pounding before bed makes it easier or harder to get ready for bed. The premise of this exercise routine is straightforward. We choose a few exercises that each get your heart rate up. If you are working with a very elite FBI agent, you can add further manipulations to this investigation such as those listed in Table 12.2. For example, after three days of doing a Henry Heartbeat exercise routine and seeing how fast you get into bed, you could try adding on an exercise to the end of the routine that slows your heart beat down and see if that makes a difference. Table 12.2 summarizes what an investigation could look like, both at home and in-session.

The details of these investigations are not meant to be overwhelming. We provide them as examples. The spirit of these investigations is quite straightforward: we are trying to figure out which routine gets the child in bed the fastest and/or which routine makes the child most comfortable. The same principle can be applied to any of the sensations that promote sleep: Cool Cyrus or Cozy Celeste. The art and style of how you get there is up to you and your FBI-agent!!

Table 12.2 Conducting a Henry Heartbeat before-bed exercise routine investigation

1. First, you need some baseline measurements to compare your investigation against. For a few evenings, have the parent time how long it takes the child to get into bed from the time the parent says "OK, time to get ready for bed" to the time the child actually climbs into bed.

   The parent can have a lot of fun with just this part of the investigation. Parent and child can write these numbers on a sheet of paper and post them on the refrigerator to see if just doing this makes going to bed a bit faster.

   As noted, we can add other "measurements" such as having the child rate how much Comfortable Cayla or Sleepy Steven they are feeling as they climb into bed. Parents can use a simple scale like: "Not at all," "A little bit", or, "A lot." Thus, when families compare this baseline to the results of the Henry Heartbeat investigation, they can address three questions. They can see whether the Henry Heartbeat exercise routine makes going to bed faster, makes going to bed more comfortable, and/or makes them sleepier.

2. After your baseline measurement, you perform your routine. The child (and any other family members who want to join in) performs an exercise routine they have designed that raises their heart rate. Here is an example.
   a. Twenty jumping jacks.
   b. Two push-ups
   c. Ten sit-ups
   d. Run on the spot until you reach a count of 20
   e. Rest for 60 seconds
   f. Repeat this routine three times

3. Following the routine, collect your outcome measures (e.g., how sleepy, comfortable, and/or quick to get to bed was everybody?).

4. The parent and child perform this Henry Heartbeat exercise routine for as many nights as they did their baseline assessments. Then they see what happens. Did bedtime preparation get shorter, longer, stay the same? Did the Henry Heartbeat exercise routines help the child feel more or less comfortable before bed?

In-session adaptations for conducting a Henry Heartbeat before-bed exercise routine investigation

Here are some ideas about ways to do parts of this investigation in session. Some of this will require some play acting or a "simulation" of what the times at home are like.

1. Therapist and child can make up a pretend bed and if you really want to get serious, you can have parent and child bring their toothbrush and toothpaste to session.

2. You will be doing essentially the same investigation except you will be doing the baseline versus Henry Heartbeat exercise routine right after each other (the child's teeth will be very clean on this day).

3. For the baseline session, have the child play around doing something they really enjoy. Have the parent do what they usually do to get the kids to be ready for bed (e.g., get them to brush their teeth, etc.) and start the timer. Once the child lies down in the pretend bed, have them rate their level of Comfortable Cayla (not at all, a little bit, a lot). That is Part 1 of the experiment.

4. For Part 2, parent and child just add in the Henry Heartbeat exercise routine as above. Once that is finished, the parent calls out time for bed in the same way, the therapist starts the timer, and the child once again gives a Comfortable Cayla rating once they are lying in their imaginary bed.

Sore Muscle Stan Exercise Routine

This investigation can be identical to the Henry Heartbeat exercise routine except of course you are just switching out a set of stretching routines for your heart raising activities. Alternatively, you could put the two routines head-to-head and see whether there are any differences in the level of comfort and bedtime speed preparation between the two. Rather than repeat all the steps above, we just outline an example of what a Sore Muscle Stan exercise routine could look like. We have included a few pictures to help illustrate what these could look like in the workbook for this session.

1. Arm stretch. Put your arms straight up over your head, pointing to the ceiling. Grab onto one of your wrists and gently pull your arm over towards your opposite ear. For example, you would grab your left wrist with your right hand and then gently pull your left arm over your head towards your right ear. This gives your left arm and shoulder a good stretch. Hold the stretch for 20 seconds. Repeat with the opposite arm for 20 seconds.

2. Back stretch. Lie on the floor on your stomach. Put your hands on the floor, on either side of your head. Then push into the floor and raise your head, shoulders, and back off the floor (while your legs and stomach are still flat on the floor). This is sometimes called a cobra stretch. This gives your lower back a nice stretch. Hold this for 20 seconds.

3. Butt stretch. Lie on your back and bend your knees with your feet on the floor. Put your right ankle over your left knee like you're sitting in a chair crossing your legs. Then put your hands on your right knee and see if you can gently push it away from you. You may feel a nice stretch in your right butt cheek. Hold it for 20 seconds. Repeat the same stretch on the other leg.

See what this Sore Muscle Stan exercise routine does to feelings of Comfortable Cayla when the child gets into their imaginary bed during a session or when doing an investigation at home.

Gassy Gus Exercise Routine

While an exercise routine that makes you sweat or a stretching routine that stretches sore muscles may seem obvious, you may be wondering – what in the world is a Gassy Gus exercise routine? Well, these are a series of specially selected exercises that can help to release any gas that you have! Nothing like trying to release as much gas as we can before lying down in bed. You can conduct a Gassy Gus exercise routine investigation with the same steps that we listed above. The parent can compare it to their baseline bedtime routine as we describe in Table 12.2. However, now that the parents and child have learned three different routines that they can test out before bed, they may be interested in comparing them to each other. If you want to try that in session, you could do one routine right after the other. If so, you may wish to stick with a rating that the child could make pretty quickly, such as the Comfortable Cayla rating. You may not have time for them to go through the imaginary bedtime preparation routine three times.

Here are some suggested Gassy Gus exercises. These exercises were chosen for their special abilities to bring on gas-passing. However, this is a huge opportunity for family creativity. Encourage them to note activities that they observe increase their own ability to pass gas so that this becomes a personalized routine.

1. The fart rock. In this exercise, you lie on your back on the floor. Bring your knees to your chest. Wrap your arms around your knees, and then rock back and forth so you feel the floor rubbing up and down your spine. In addition to feeling very nice on your back, this is a great farting exercise.
2. The handstand. This one will require parent support. The child can try to get into a handstand with the parent helping to hold their legs. Holding yourself upside down can be a surefire farting strategy. If this move is too complicated, the child can try just lying upside down on a chair with their legs over the back of the chair.
3. The toe touch. Have a child stand up straight and stretch their arms toward the ceiling. Have them reach down and touch their toes. Sometimes you can get some sneaky farts out of this one.
4. The twist. This is an advanced gas-passing move. Lie down on your back and bend your knees, keeping your feet on the floor. Then, slightly lift your head, shoulders, and upper back off the floor as you twist from side to side. This is also a great gut stretch!

The most interesting investigation with the Gassy Gus exercise routine is whether it increases Comfortable Cayla and whether this improves the child's sleep quality.

Body Investigation: Getting Unstuck from Stuck Stephanie

So far, all of our investigations have focused on the sensations that can help a child get ready for bed and be comfortable when they first lie down. Our investigation with Stuck Stephanie continues this theme. As a reminder, Stuck Stephanie is the feeling you have when you are doing something that you really like to do, and you need to stop and do something else but you are having a really tough time stopping (maybe because part of you does not want to stop, or you have to go do something less fun; or just because switching activities in general is harder for some children than for others). For these investigations, we try a number of different strategies (choose as many as you want or, of course, have the child and parent come up with their own ideas) to get unstuck. A basic outline for a Stuck Stephanie investigation may look something like this (Table 12.3).

Body Investigation: Getting Visits from Betty the Butterfly and Mind-Racing Mikella

Now we are ready for an investigation that we perform in bed! We are already good friends with a few sensations that may arise at bedtime or during a night awakening – Betty the Butterfly and Mind-Racing Mikella. In fact, you may have already performed an investigation in Session 4 that involved sitting in the dark and seeing how many butterflies we can raise up by doing various things (sitting in the dark, telling a scary story, etc.). Thus, if Betty the Butterfly and their buddies come to visit at night, that is cause for celebration (as well as some possible investigations). But nighttime may get even more fun than just having a visit from Betty Butterfly. If the child is lucky, they will receive a visit from Betty Butterfly and

Table 12.3 Investigating different ways to get unstuck

1. Find an activity that the child really enjoys doing.
2. One thing you can investigate is how fast the child stops engaging in this activity by trying the strategies below. In addition, or alternatively, you can decide what will be the first step of the bedtime routine and time how long it takes the child to start the bedtime routine (similar to the investigations above). If you are doing this in-session, this will be the "imaginary" bedtime routine. It could be something as simple as starting to brush their teeth (with a real or pretend toothbrush).
3. Decide what the strategies will be to get the child to stop doing this activity (get unstuck!) and then compare them.
4. Some ideas of strategies include:
   a. Randomly shouting stop and the child has to freeze, just like the game freeze dance.
   b. Giving a five-minute warning and setting a timer that goes off in five minutes. You can investigate different lengths of time and see the amount of time that works best (e.g., a ten-minute warning, a 15-minute warning, etc.).
   c. Figuring out an enjoyable activity to do right after the children are ready for bed and right before bed (e.g., reading a story, listening to music) that the child may be motivated to move towards.
5. See how long it takes for the child to stop the activity they are doing and compare which one is the fastest.

Mind-Racing Mikella! Bedtimes are the best! Table 12.4 lists some investigations to explore if the child gets some visitors during the night.

Investigating Cool Cyrus and/or Dark Debra

Similar to our investigations above, we can manipulate the temperature in the room or the degree of lightness or darkness in the room and investigate the effect of this on Sleepy Steven, Cozy Celeste, and Julie Jitters. Elite FBI agents find the optimal light and temperature to promote restorative sleep.

Table 12.4 Investigations for sensations that may join the child in bed

If Betty the Butterfly comes to visit, count how many friends she brought. See if the child can imagine the swarm of butterflies following Betty as the leader and flying right next to the child under the covers to get cozy.

What if Betty the Butterfly **and** Mind-Racing Mikella come to visit? Well, they may be able to go even faster as a team. Imagine Betty the Butterfly catching a ride in Mind-Racing Mikella's race car and just watch them go around and around the ceiling.

Another investigation to explore if both Betty the Butterfly and Mind-Racing Mikella come together is to keep a notepad of paper next to the bed (or maybe your FBI journal). Then, the child can draw or write what they are experiencing. See what happens to Betty the Butterfly and Mind-Racing Mikella when you try that. Do they finally go to bed? Does it go out of your head because it has landed on the paper? Is it fun just to draw that stuff?

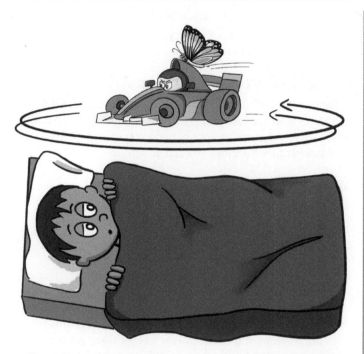

Figure 12.1 Mind-Racing Mikella and Betty the Butterfly having a couple of exciting laps around the mind and stomach.

Sometimes you just find yourself lying in the dark. The dark can be many things, and when Dark Debra is around, the dark is a thick soft blanket covering the sky. When it is just the child and Dark Debra, is it time to do some investigations to get cozy. Read on ….

Body Investigation: Cozy Celeste

Cozy Celeste investigations are some of the best investigations in the whole program. You just try to get as cozy as you possibly can. What could be better than that? Picking out your comfiest pajamas, making a little corner of the bed where you pile up blankets and pillows, having your favorite stuffed animals – those are all great ways to get cozy. See which one makes you the coziest. Here is a fun investigation to try.

1. Take a baseline Cozy Celeste rating. Does the child feel "Not at all cozy?", "A little cozy?", or "A lot cozy?".
2. Now find a pair of potentially cozy pajamas. After getting in pajamas, make another Cozy Celeste rating. Did the child get more cozy?
3. Now build a cozy corner on the bed. Make a running leap into your cozy corner and snuggle in. Take another Cozy Celeste rating. Is it possible that you got even MORE cozy?
4. Now add in a favorite stuffed animal. Is there an upper limit to cozy? Can you get so cozy that you just melt into your bed?
5. For the grand finale, top it all off with a big bear hug. Are you filled up from head to toe with coziness? Only an elite FBI investigator can face this complicated a mission ….

Comfortable Cayla Body Investigation: How Long Does It Take to Feel Stretched?

We are pretty good at getting your muscles to be sore. For example, remember when we did all those investigations to see how strong your muscles got when you practiced over and over again? We then got some practice in making your muscles less sore by designing a Sore Muscle Stan stretching routine to do before bed. With this investigation, we will learn more about Comfortable Cayla. These investigations can help us become master stretchers.

Let's think about some of our favorite stretches. Let's guess how long it takes for a certain muscle to feel stretched out. Then let's see what happens if we hold the stretch for a bit longer. Have everybody pick out: a stretch; an activity that will work their muscles; and at least two different amounts of time for which they're going to hold the stretch. Armed with these decisions, first we will exercise for a certain amount of time, and then stretch for a certain amount of time. We can then rate how relaxed we feel. Then, we repeat with the same amount of exercise, but a different amount of stretch time. These steps are summarized in Table 12.5.

Table 12.5 Comfortable Cayla investigation

1. Perform one of your chosen exercises for a set amount of time (e.g., one minute).
2. Perform one of your chosen stretches for a set amount of time (e.g., 30 seconds).
3. Measure how stretched out you feel. You can use words (a teeny bit, a little, a lot, a whole lot).
4. Write down how you felt so you do not forget.
5. Now repeat that set of steps with the same exercise but with a different length of time that you are stretching.
6. How much time do you need to feel stretched out a "whole lot"?

Adding to the Body Map

Do not forget to write down everything new you learn about the wisdom of the body to the Body Map. Remind parents to fill out Body Investigation Worksheets so you can discuss all these cool investigations that they may repeat at home.

Possible Lessons from the Drowsies
Sleepy Steven lets me know that it is time to start a bedtime routine and get ready to rest.
Comfortable Cayla is my signal that my body is happy and I should just keep doing what I am doing (if I can).
Cool Cyrus reminds me to keep an eye on body temperature to help me get good sleep.
Dark Debra reminds me that I am not alone in the dark: I have a dark comfy blanket surrounding me.
Cozy Celeste helps me to stop and notice wonderful, comfy moments.
Stuck Stephanie helps me realize that everyone has trouble stopping doing things that they like but we can all get better with practice.
Tired Tina is a good signal to add some energy to my current activity and to take good care of myself – by reaching out to someone and/or making myself all cozy.

Body Brainstorms

We will end today's session with our Body Brainstorms of the Week.

Questions on our body brainstorms worksheet this week include the following:

What do you usually do for your bedtime routine?

What are some ways you slow down Henry Heartbeat right before bed?

What do you do to feel Cozy Celeste in your bed?

What are some ways you feel Cool Cyrus in your bed?

Your Seventh Body Investigation Assignment (Home-based Practice)

The investigations we simulate in this session are much more powerful when done at home. If you can, have families decide on some specific sleep routine investigations to try. Remind them to record these investigations on their Body Investigations worksheets so they really keep track of what they have learned.

Body Investigation Journal

This week, the Body Investigation Journal can stay by the bed in case the child needs to draw a picture of Mind-Racing Mikella and Betty the Butterfly.

Materials Families Take Home from Session 7

Here is a summary of what families get from Session 7.

1. A worksheet that summarizes the characters that they have learned so far
2. Coloring pages
3. The workbook pages for their binder with ideas for home-based body investigations
4. The Body Brainstorms sheet they completed

5. Optional: Prizes! A tiny stuffed animal for bedtime
6. Optional: A Cozy Celeste button
7. Information on getting prizes and buttons can be found at: https://fbikids.org

Body Investigations to Practice at Home

Remind parents to be on the alert for times when they can design a Body Investigation to learn to master something challenging or, if needed, to improve bedtimes. Remember to remind parents that this includes investigations of their own bedtime routines.

Then you schedule the next session! Congratulations, you've just finished Session 7!

Therapist Reminders for Session 7

Take a minute to point out how many characters (and by corollary sensations) the family has learned.

A Final Reflection for Session 7

How is your sleep? It may be worth taking a moment and thinking about whether you wake up rested and restored or whether you have to drag yourself out of bed every morning. There are many clever investigations you can design ….

Questions and Answers for Session 7

Q: What if sleep is not a problem for the child? After all, this is an intervention about pain.

A: That is great. Then sleep quality and quantity is one less factor that may be contributing to the child's vulnerability to pain experiences. You can just have a lot of fun making bedtime routines more entertaining, or, if the family already has a bedtime routine that really works for them, you can reinforce the wisdom of that routine by having them act it out in session and exploring the different ways it makes their body feel. Remember that every investigation, even if it doesn't address a problem relevant to a particular child, still reinforces the *process* of turning a problem into a question, and of infusing concerning sensations with curiosity and lightness.

Q: What if families are having a hard time doing investigations at home?

A: Reinforce what they are able to do, to build confidence. Parents often feel awful when they come to a session without having practiced. Help them practice by completing Body Investigations worksheets together at the beginning of every session if they have not been filling them out at home. Brainstorm some ways that you can help the family implement these plans. Who should be in charge of planning and implementing home-based investigations? Children with sensory superpowers may like to be in charge of things. Perhaps they should be in charge of organizing and implementing a home-based investigation!

References

1. Asarnow, L.D., Manber, R. (2019). Cognitive behavioral therapy for insomnia in depression. *Sleep Med Clin 14*(2), 177–184. https://doi.org/10.1016/j.jsmc.2019.01.009

2. Asarnow, L.D., Mirchandaney, R. (2021). Sleep and mood disorders among youth. *Child Adolesc Psychiatr Clin N Am 30*(1), 251–268. https://doi.org/10.1016/j.chc.2020.09.003

3. Asarnow, L.D., Soehner, A.M., Harvey, A.G. (2014). Basic sleep and circadian science as building blocks for behavioral interventions: a translational approach for mood disorders. *Behav Neurosci 128*(3), 360–370. https://doi.org/10.1037/a0035892

4. Dolsen, E.A., Dong, L., Harvey, A.G. (2021). Transdiagnostic sleep and circadian intervention for adolescents plus text messaging: randomized controlled trial 12-month follow-up. *J Clin Child Adolesc Psychol* 1–13. https://doi.org/10.1080/15374416.2021.1978295

5. Faaland, P., Vedaa, Ø. , Langsrud, K., et al. (2022). Digital cognitive behaviour therapy for insomnia (dCBT-I): chronotype moderation on intervention outcomes. *J Sleep Res*, e13572. https://doi.org/10.1111/jsr.13572

6. Harvey, A.G. (2022). Treating sleep and circadian problems to promote mental health: perspectives on comorbidity, implementation science and behavior change. *Sleep 45*(4), 1–13. https://doi.org/10.1093/sleep/zsac026

7. Harvey, A.G., Buysse, D.J. (2017). *Treating Seep Problems: A Transdiagnostic Approach*. New York, NY: Guilford Publications.

8. Neu, D., Mairesse, O., Hoffmann, G., et al. (2010). Do 'sleepy' and 'tired' go together? Rasch analysis of the relationships between sleepiness, fatigue and nonrestorative sleep complaints in a nonclinical population sample. *Neuroepidemiology 35*(1), 1–11. https://doi.org/10.1159/000301714

9. Borbély, A.A., Daan, S., Wirz-Justice, A., et al. (2016). The two-process model of sleep regulation: a reappraisal. *J Sleep Res 25*(2), 131–143. https://doi.org/10.1111/jsr.12371

Session 8: The Zoomies and the Shakies, Part 2

Clap along if you feel like a room without a roof
Clap along if you feel like happiness is the truth
-*Happy* by Pharrell Williams

Overview of Session 8

The Zoomies and the Shakies are back! This time, however, we focus on high arousal, positive sensations. Ernie the Energy Ball, Laughing Pain Lulu, Bursting Bella, Giggling Gina, Tearful Tasha, and Dancing Darren. These are the sensations of happiness and joy. As we noted last session, we are now in a groove. We reinforce what we have learned. We explore new characters and design new investigations. Now is probably a good time to remind you why we start off some chapters with a song lyric. Of course, part of the reason is that we love music. However, it is more intentional that than. Music is a powerful way to bring up or release strong sensations (and emotions). In fact, we will use music as part of one of our investigations this session. Also just for fun, we combined all of the songs we reference into a playlist that you can find on the web-based community associated with this book, at: https://fbikids.org. Music is personal so part of the fun of body investigations in this session is helping the child find some songs that make them want to dance around. Let's go giggle.

Session Outline

1. Perform a warm-up Henry Heartbeat exercise
2. Review homework and add new things to the Body Map
3. Check in with everyone's energy and fuel up with a snack
4. Learn new characters related to high arousal and positively valenced emotions: Ernie the Energy Ball, Laughing Pain Lulu, Bursting Bella, Giggling Gena, Tearful Tasha, and Dancing Darren
5. Perform some Body Investigations
6. Complete a Body Brainstorms worksheet
7. Review the plan for the week
8. Give out coloring pages
9. Optional: Give out prizes

Session Materials

1. Workbook, worksheets, and coloring pages for Session 8, which can be downloaded at www.cambridge.org/fbi-clinical-guide.

2. A snack the child brings or that you have on hand that is in small pieces, for sensing our energy and fueling up
3. Getting some "how to" dance videos bookmarked in case they are needed
4. Optional: A Laughing Pain Lulu button

Background Information for Session 8

> Remember that emotions help us understand how we feel about things, rapidly communicate to us and others what is going on in the world, and help guide us in what to do. So, what is the message of positive emotions? Keep it up.

Take a moment to think about what your body feels like when you experience joyful feelings. Joy feels like an expansion – like your body is filled from head to toe with an energy that feels like it will make your chest burst (Bursting Bella), perhaps make you tear up because you are so moved (Tearful Tasha), and can make you want to reach out and hug somebody. Excitement can feel like you just cannot sit still (Ernie the Energy Ball) and make you want to dance around (Dancing Darren). Feeling silly makes you want to giggle (Giggling Gina). Positive emotions communicate that all is well, or better than well.

Remember that children with sensory superpowers may hold themselves back from experiencing joyous emotions because of the dread of them ending or having to lose what brought on those feelings. There are several tools embedded in our FBI intervention that are aimed to help children lose this fear of joy. First, we have been practicing being fully in a moment. Through our body investigations and by inculcating our observational, investigative mindset, we hope that children have been learning to really stamp in their vivid experiences rather than avoid them. Throughout the program, we have also been trying to enhance our memories of moments – and importantly what we learned about the body in those moments – by systematically adding information to the Body Map. Moreover, the child has been keeping a journal in which they periodically record some body wisdom gained from their home-based practice. We want to stamp positive experiences vividly into our memories, so we can play them over and over again and enjoy them over and over again. To help, we have designed an investigation devoted to this aim.

This is the session about the sensations that accompany joyous and exciting emotions. Why is Tearful Tasha here? Well, becoming tearful about something is wonderful and powerful. We want nothing but positive associations with this incredible form of communication of intense feelings and release from that tension. People often associate tears with sadness, but tearing up can be an index of strong feelings. People tear up when they are furious, when they feel misunderstood, when they are sad, when they are lonely, and when they are so moved by the beauty of something or by the strength of their love. All these examples are powerful. We put Tearful Tasha in this joyous chapter because we want children to be awed by the power of tears – not afraid or apologetic when they feel so strongly about something that their body helps them to get some release by tearing up.

Time for Reflection

To understand what we are trying to do in this session, try to think about the last time you had a joyful moment. Think about a potent way to capture that experience so that you have a vivid way to re-experience it. Think about what happens when you videotape something. It is wonderful to have that video, however, it is detracting from the wonder of your experience in that moment. Perhaps a picture? Perhaps a picture and then writing about what just happened so you can solidify the stamp of that event in your mind? Perhaps just writing about it. The point is, we want to start making deliberate attempts to collect these positive experiences. If we just take a moment right after a wonderful moment has unfolded and allow ourselves to let that moment wash over us again and document it, then we have it for keeps.

Step-by-Step Guide to Session 8
Warm-Up Henry Heartbeat Activity

By now you have been performing at least eight weeks of Henry Heartbeat activities. Perhaps at this point, given all the various exercise routines that we practiced last session, it is time to come up with our optimal (meaning most fun) Henry Heartbeat sequence. The child can reflect on all the different Henry Heartbeat activities we performed that raised or lowered their heart rate, pick out their favorites, organize them in a routine, and then record that routine on their Body Map. In the spirit of the session, we want to make sure that we are holding on to all the strategies that we learned to strengthen our sense of mastery in communicating with our bodies.

Review Homework and Add New Things to Their Body Map

Around this time in the treatment, it is easy to start slacking off on our homework and home-based practice. In part, this could be positive. The hope is that parents and children are getting so

good at checking in with their bodies – during or after intense moments, as a summary of their day, and/or planning body investigations to approach interesting but challenging moments – that they do not need to go through a worksheet every time. The eventual goal would be that children and parents have the skills within them and only need to pull out worksheets if they're particularly stuck. If that is what parents are reporting, strongly reinforce that skill mastery. Notwithstanding, it never hurts to practice a few worksheets at the beginning of a session to just make sure that the family has mastered these skills. Doing so can also give you an indication of the degree to which the skills have indeed been mastered. By now their Body Map should be looking pretty cool.

Assessing Your Energy and Fueling Up
Session 8 Workbook: The Zoomies and the Shakies, Part 2

As you read through the workbook pages this week, here are some investigative questions to think about as a family. This week's investigative questions ask families to think about the following body mysteries.

Session 8: Body Mystery Questions
Why do you think that people tear up sometimes when they are feeling really happy?
Why does it hurt sometimes when you laugh? Remember when we did our exercises to see what happens to Sore Muscle Stan once our muscles got stronger? What do you think would happen with Laughing Pain Lulu if you laughed all the time?

As always, try to get as many family members involved as possible. The more family members that participate, the more that these skills and mindsets become integrated into the way the family, as a whole, relate to their bodies and to each other.

Table 13.1 provides a summary of the characters covered in this session.

The Zoomies and Shakies, Part 2: Body Investigations

In this session, we really play. The investigations in this session are about creating joyous moments and eliminating barriers. It is important to consider the conditions that foster moments of joy or silliness. To fully experience these feelings, a person has to feel free to be able to let themselves go – without worrying that they will be judged or corrected. If you think about what it would be like to let yourself go and perform some expressive dance because you are just having a wonderful time and you are not the greatest dancer from a technical standpoint and you do not have the best rhythm from a precision standpoint and suddenly (!) – someone commented critically about your

Table 13.1 Summary of the characters covered in this session

Ernie the Energy Ball

Ernie is that feeling you have when you so much energy in your body (perhaps because you are really excited about something), that you just cannot sit still.

What are some things that you get excited about? Do you ever get so excited that you feel you are having a hard time waiting for it to happen? Like you have so much energy you feel like you are going to explode? That's Ernie the Energy Ball!

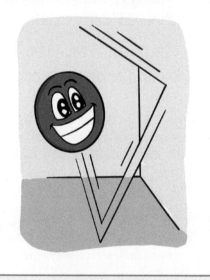

Giggling Gina

Giggling Gina comes around when someone is feeling silly. Giggling Gina is not very cooperative sometimes and comes around when it is not really a good time for a giggle. Maybe that is what it takes to be silly – when you feel like doing something out of the ordinary.

Have you ever had a giggle attack? Have you ever giggled when you were not supposed to?

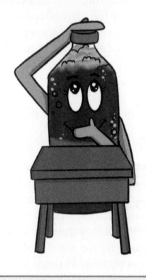

Laughing Pain Lulu

Laughing Pain Lulu comes around when you are laughing soooo hard at something that you might get a cramp in your stomach or even pull a muscle!

Has that ever happened to you? Have you ever laughed so hard that your stomach muscles got so much exercise that they were sore? That sounds like a fun kind of pain, for sure.

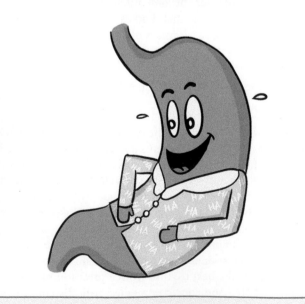

Bursting Bella

Bursting Bella is a very special feeling. Bursting Bella comes around when you are having a moment that is so filled with love, joy, or happiness that you feel that your body is filled from head to toe with a warm energy that feels like it may explode from your chest.

What are your favorite things to hug? What are your very favorite things to do? If you were in charge of planning the perfect day, what would you do? Who would be there? If you were to imagine yourself going through that day, there might be a moment where you are just sooooo happy that you feel Bursting Bella.

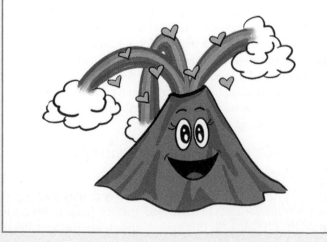

Table 13.1 (cont.)

Tearful Tasha

Tearful Tasha is the sensation when you feel so strongly about something that your body lets the overflow of feelings spill out in the form of tears. Tearful Tasha comes around in all kinds of situations. It might surprise you that when people are bursting with joy (like when they feel Bursting Bella), they often feel Tearful Tasha at the same time. Tearful Tasha lets you know that this might be a moment to cherish.

Have you ever cried when you are really happy? Have you ever seen anyone else do that? Why do you think that happens?

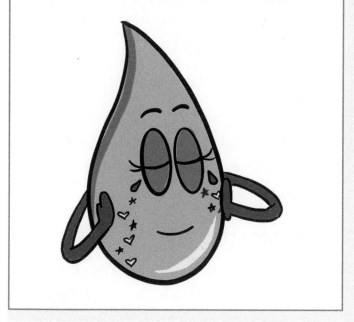

Dancing Darren

Well as you may imagine, Dancing Darren and Ernie the Energy Ball are great friends. It is just that Darren has some moves. Whereas Ernie the Energy Ball just wants to run around in all different directions (perhaps because Ernie is so excited about something), Dancing Darren has a rhythm in their heart and a beat in their feet. Dancing Darren just cannot help tapping their toes, snapping their fingers, and shaking their hips to the beat in their heart. While Dancing Darren does not need music to want to move, that makes it even more fun.

Do you have a favorite song? Do you like to sing? Do you know any dance moves? Is there anything that makes you just want to dance?

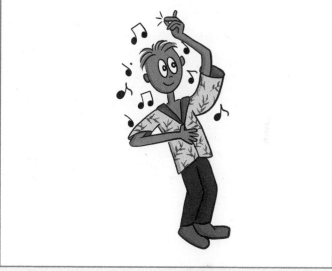

movement skills. It kind of misses the point of the whole thing, doesn't it? By this point in the session, you have had a few conversations with parents about the importance of validation. If you think it would be beneficial, you could have a conversation with parents about just allowing joyous moments to unfold. An example dialogue follows here.

Let joyous moments unfold. If your instinct is to try to tap down intense emotions, pause and assess whether it's a time or place where it would really be inappropriate or dangerous to express joy in whatever way feels right. These situations are fortunately rare, so usually you can let yourself go!

Therapist Dialogue About Letting Go

Therapist and parent meeting alone.

THERAPIST: *I just wanted take a couple minutes to check in and let you know the plan for today's session. From here on out our focus is on more positive and relaxing sensations. Today we focus on high arousal sensations that you might feel when you're having positive emotions such as joy, excitement, or silliness. For a child to really feel those feelings, they have to trust that they can just let themselves go and be who they are without someone judging them or getting in the way. That can be hard to do when you're in someone else's space, like a therapy office. I just want to reassure you that our goal today is to just let your child be silly. Do you have any worries that you have a hard time letting your child do that?*

PARENT: I do worry a little and I really struggle with that myself. When I see my child being silly and acting a bit wild, I worry that they will break something or hurt themselves and I know that puts a damper on things.

THERAPIST: *I agree, it's challenging at times. I wonder if a useful exercise would be that when you have the urge to say something like that, you just pause a minute and ask yourself, do I really need to say something? I'm guessing that the times when there is the potential for real acute danger are quite minimal, relative to our concerns about possibilities.*

PARENT: I think that sounds like a good idea. Now I just have to remember to do that.

Let's Get Dancing and Singing: Dancing Darren and Giggling Gena

As we noted earlier, music can be the secret sauce to get everyone in an uplifted and joyous mood. Incorporating music has gotten so much easier since it is not hard to pull up a child's favorite song on our phones. Creating a playlist of songs to which everyone contributes a few ideas can be the first step in a number of Dancing Darren investigations (Table 13.2).

THERAPIST: *OK. Let's do some investigations that let us feel Dancing Darren. Can everybody tell me one of their favorite songs? Don't worry if you do not have a favorite song. We can all think of ideas together.*

The group chooses a few songs. The therapist pulls up the songs on their phone or computer. If technology is a barrier, the group can choose the person who knows one of the songs by heart the best, and is willing to be the singer.

THERAPIST: *OK. Now we are going to decide what we want to do to this music that we picked out. I have some ideas but let me know if you have some better ideas. We could investigate what kind of music makes us feel like dancing the most? We could see what kind of music is hardest to stop dancing to? For example, we could play freeze dance to show off our best dance moves and see if certain songs make it harder to stop our moves? Or we can all try learning or inventing some new dance moves? What do you think?*

For children who are perhaps a bit too self-conscious to dance, there are some other strategies to get them moving in some fun ways. We do think getting them moving is important, particularly in new ways, such as doing things that throw their bodies a bit off balance or that ask them to take on silly poses.

One idea is to play a variation of Simon Says. The person who acts as Simon makes sure to give instructions that encourage everyone to do some silly things. Table 13.3 has some instructions as examples.

Table 13.2 Ideas to bring on Dancing Darren

1. What song is the hardest to stop moving to?
   a. Somebody is put in charge of the music. Ideally, the "DJ" is hidden from view so that you cannot tell when they are about to stop the music.
   b. Somebody is chosen to be the judge. The job of the judge is to see if anybody moves once the music stops abruptly.
   c. The goal of the game is to freeze all movement once the music stops.
   d. The judge can also be playful and get on those people's cases who tried to cheat in the game by only dancing with the tiniest of moves! To win, people have to be really dancing.
   e. The rules of the game are that the DJ will start playing the music and then randomly stop it and shout freeze.
   f. The players are all dancing like crazy and then they have to freeze in their movements the second the music stops.
   g. To truly make this an investigation, the DJ should have a few rounds with different songs. Then you can tally the number of people that moved for each song.
   h. The judge then walks around and inspects everyone and makes sure no one is moving.
   i. If someone moves, they get a point. (We do not have them leave the round like some versions of freeze dance, because we need them to stay in to complete this serious investigation).
   j. Once the judge has checked everybody out, they tell the DJ to start the music again.
   k. At the end, the judge and DJ see which song caused the most movement.
2. How does dancing make you feel?
   a. If you have a roomful of people who already like to dance, the therapist can just ask everybody to show them their moves and experience the joy of moving. They can investigate how they feel before they started to dance and then afterwards. This can help children investigate what a useful and fun strategy dancing can be.
3. What makes you feel like dancing more – learning some new steps or dancing to your own beat?
   a. Some children may really like to dance, but they may be self-conscious that they don't know a lot of different dance moves. The Internet makes this easy as there are lots of free "how to" dance videos out there that everyone can follow along to in session.
   b. Do not underestimate the coolness of five- to nine-year-olds. They can handle advanced dance moves – no kindergarten or preschool stuff (even if they are kindergartners). See what they can do. Little kids can have serious dance moves.
   c. See what brings out the most Dancing Darren – when they are practicing a new step or just moving to their own beat.
4. What things make you just want to dance?
   a. We can invent our own Dancing Darren rating scale (e.g., 0 you feel like a rock that cannot move a muscle to 10, you have such a strong urge to dance that you just cannot stop).
   b. Then, we can investigate how different things affect our urge to dance. Does getting ready for school make us want to dance? Listening to a favorite singer? Eating a yummy breakfast?

Table 13.3 Exploring Ernie the Energy Ball and Giggling Gena

1. Exploring different ways to feel Ernie the Energy Ball the fastest
   a. Create your energy rating scale.
   b. Decide on a time interval (like two minutes).
   c. Pick a few activities that you think will get your energy up to its maximum level in two minutes.
   d. Investigations to explore:
      i. Does performing sillier things (e.g., walking on all fours with your butt in the air, running backwards, skipping while blowing bubbles) make your energy higher than just moving around a lot (e.g., running or jumping jacks).
      ii. How long can you sit still before you have the urge to bounce around? What is the best way to discharge that energy so you can sit still again? This might be an interesting investigation to do if you have trouble sitting still in class or at dinnertime, for example.
2. What is the most energizing time of the day?
   a. Conduct a longer-term investigation of Ernie the Energy Ball and see when they are strongest: in the morning? After school? Right before bed?
   b. Once you see what you learn, you can design some investigations depending on what needs to happen. For example, if Ernie the Energy Ball is highest in the morning, is there a way to channel that energy to help get ready for school super-fast?
3. Play Simon Says
   a. In this variation of "Simon Says," "Simon" instructs everybody to do silly things such as moo like a cow, meow like a cat, snort like a pig, stand on one leg, put your butt in the air, twirl, jump up and down, slither on the ground like a snake, etc.
   b. The rules of this game are everyone has to do what Simon says until Simon says "Simon says stop." Simon will try to trick everybody into stopping early by just randomly shouting out "stop." However, in order for a person to stay in the game they can only stop when Simon says stop. If they stop at other times they are out of the game.
   c. Often the winner gets to be Simon the next round.
4. Play freeze tag
   a. Freeze tag gets people moving but doesn't require the dance coordination of freeze dance.
   b. One person is "it." Everyone tries to stay away from the person who is it. If that person tags you, you have to freeze. There is usually a spot that is designated as the safe spot for people to rest.
   c. If someone has been frozen, another person can try to save that person by tagging them. They then become unfrozen.
   d. Ultimately, the game ends when everyone is frozen, but it is easier to just set a time limit (like two to three minutes) and then switch who is it.

Creating the Unexpected: Laughing Pain Lulu

Some of the funniest things are when something unexpected happens. Ideas to bring on Laughing Pain Lulu include watching videos such as those from America's funniest home video, designing a playful and harmless prank (such as hiding a whoopee cushion under a blanket), or playing hide and seek (sometimes the unexpectedness of being found can bring on a good laugh or giggle).

Body Investigation: Bursting Bella

Bursting Bella is that wonderful feeling when you feel so much joy, love, and gratitude it feels like your heart is about to burst out of your chest. For this investigation, children can think of someone in their life they love very much who may be going through a hard time. They can make some cards that are intended to make people smile and let them know that they are cared about. Then, they can always be on the lookout for a chance to hand out a caring card to a family member, friend, or stranger who is looking sad. Trying to spread joy to someone else is the greatest feeling ever – a Bursting Bella feeling.

Body Investigation/Discussion: Saving Joyous Moments

Sensations that accompany joy such as Bursting Bella or Tearful Tasha would be challenging to bring on via an investigation. Rather, an alert FBI agent pays special attention to a joyous moment as it is unfolding and takes special precautions to make sure that the moment is stamped in memory. Imagine that you are a photographer (or perhaps you are a photographer). One gift of being a photographer is that you are constantly alert and on the lookout for beautiful moments to capture. An FBI agent is like a photographer in many ways. Because they feel things so strongly, there are opportunities for many intense and potentially beautiful moments to be experienced. As we learned in the opening chapters of this handbook, however, often the events we are paying attention to are those of threatening sensations like pain. What we are trying to do here is strengthen the joyous moments by thinking about different ways to help us record them so we can replay or experience them over and over.

What is the best way to capture a pleasant experience? The therapist will use the pleasant experiences the child and parent have just had and discuss different ways that they want to record that moment to make it indelible. At home, this could be an ongoing investigation.

THERAPIST: So, we just had a bunch of really fun times. First, let's add what we learned about our body to our Body Map as we usually do. I also want us to think about something else.

> When something fun and wonderful happens to you, that is a gift that you can enjoy over and over again. The reason why is because now it is in your heart and in your memory. Because of that, you can think about it happening and it can fill you up with all the warm feelings that you felt when it was actually happening.

Let's think of some ways that can help us to remember something special that just happened. Like let's think about the fun we just had. What are some ideas you have to help us remember it? (Table 13.4)

THERAPIST: *For body investigations at home this week, try to pay special attention to the new characters we just learned when we did our Body Clues Worksheets. We could also do a body investigation in which we practice different ways to help us remember joyous things and see how these methods work.*

Table 13.4 Strategies to help remember wondrous moments

1. Take a picture after it just happened. Make the picture part of a book of joyful memories. Write a little caption underneath the picture describing what happened to you so you can be sure to remember everything.
2. Add a drawing of what just happened to your Body Map so it can be part of the many wonderful things you have learned about your body.
3. Write a story of what just happened and add it to your Body Investigation Journal or pick a special journal where you record very special moments that you want to hold on to.
4. Connect it to something. For example, many of the investigations we just did might have been tied to music. Whenever you hear that song again, you can say to yourself, "I'm going to think about the time my dad and I had fun doing 'x.'"
5. Make up a song about it.

Lessons from the Zoomies and the Shakies, Part 2

Giggling Gina lets me know that I am in a silly mood.

Lulu the Laughing Pain gives me a jolt to help me really notice something very very funny. She might help me make sure I remember it later so I can enjoy it again. She also reminds me that pain can sometimes be fun.

Ernie the Energy Ball gives me the energy I need so I can do all the fun things I am excited about doing.

Tearful Tasha and Bursting Bella let me know that something truly wonderful is happening. I need to let that moment fill me up so I can replay it again and again.

Dancing Darren is a great way for people to express happiness.

Adding to the Body Map

As noted above, adding something to the Body Map can actually be part of the investigation to figure out what ways help families remember these fun moments.

Body Brainstorms

Questions on our Body Brainstorms worksheet this week include the following:

Do you ever get so excited that you feel you are having a hard time waiting for it to happen? Like you have so much energy you feel like you are going to explode?

Have you ever laughed so hard that your stomach muscles got so much exercise that they got sore?

What are your favorite things to hug? What are your very favorite things to do? If you were in charge of planning the perfect day, what would you do? Who would be there?

Have you ever teared up when you are really happy? Can you remember what happened?

Is there anything that makes you just want to dance?

Have you ever had a giggle attack when you were not supposed to giggle?

Your Eighth Body Investigation Assignment (Home-based Practice)

The parent continues as usual: using the Body Clues Worksheet to summarize a day and/or to figure out an intense moment. Parents are planning Body Investigations as needed to help the child approach something challenging. Parents and children are on the alert for the new body sensations learned to document them in a way that they can remember them easily and enjoy them again and again.

Body Investigation Journal

Catching Bursting Bella, Giggling Gina, and any other body sensation that was learned this week would be an excellent thing to add to the child's body journal.

Materials Families Take Home from Session 8

Here is a summary of what families get from Session 8.

1. A worksheet that summarizes the characters that they have learned so far

2. Coloring pages
3. The workbook pages for their binder
4. The Body Brainstorms worksheet they completed
5. Idea page of some home-based body investigations
6. Optional: Prizes!
7. Optional: A Lulu Laughing Pain button

Information on getting prizes and buttons can be found at https://fbikids.org.

Body Investigations to Practice at Home

Body Investigations to practice at home are always optional. It is important that parents do not feel overwhelmed with what we are asking them to do. The investigations are intended to get the whole family in the spirit of marveling at something cool that the body did.

1. Be on the alert for Bursting Bella, Tearful Tasha, Giggling Gina, Ernie the Energy Ball, Dancing Darren, and Lulu the Laughing Pain. Try different strategies for recording what happens and see which you like best.

2. See what happens when you plan a Giggling Gina event into your day – especially if parents can do it with the children. Parents make Giggling Gina moments even more special.

Then you schedule the next session! Congratulations, you've just finished Session 8!

Therapist Reminders for Session 8

The families have learned over 41 characters. That is a ton of material. Who else knows that many different sensations about their bodies? Elite special forces FBI agents, that is who.

Questions and Answers for Session 8

Q: Some parents may not be comfortable being silly or playful with their kids. What should I do in that situation?

A: Children love it when their parents join in – in whatever capacity. As you may have noticed, there are many roles in the activities presented, some of which just require organization rather than playfulness. For example, a parent can be in charge of the music for freeze dance or be a member of the audience if the child wants to sing their favorite song.

Chapter 14

Session 9: The Soothies

I see skies of blue
And clouds of white
The bright blessed day
The dark sacred night
And I think to myself
What a wonderful world
What a Wonderful World, by George David Weiss and Bob Thiele

Overview of Session 9

We have one more lesson to leave you with – how it feels when you are calm, relaxed, and/or fully immersed in the moment that is happening right now.

Our final session (next session) is a graduation ceremony with some fun games to help the children rejoice in how much they have learned about themselves and to revel in how very tough they are.

As you may have surmised, the sensations we have left are positive, low-arousal sensations: sensations like having a very slow beating heart (Henry Heartbeat); having a lightness in your heart and in your body (Cheery Cathy); feeling day-dreamy in your head (Day-Dreamy David); feeling calm in your head (Slow-Thinking Stewart); feeling that satisfied feeling after quenching a thirst (Ahhhh Annie); feeling really focused and engrossed by something (Focused Freida), and feeling very alert and awake – like you are really taking in everything around you and stamping it in your memory (Alert Arnold).

We already have many tools to relax and thus to bring about these sensations. In our Henry Heartbeat investigations, we often practiced lowering our heart beat. In our session on the Drowsies, we practiced many bedtime routines designed to get our body comfortable and explored ways to slow down our mind. In the Zoomies and the Shakies, Part 2, we started practicing how to capture wonderful moments. Being focused in the moment is one important component of mindfulness skills, a set of tools integrated into many therapeutic orientations (e.g., Dialectical Behavior Therapy, Mindfulness-Based Cognitive Behavioral Therapy[1,2]). Relaxation skills form an important element of many pain management programs. For trained elite FBI agents, we can integrate these skills using the framework and routines we already have – we can learn what the sensations of feeling calm and relaxed are like and perform investigations to bring them on. Let's get going on slowing down!

Session Outline

1. Perform a warm-up Henry Heartbeat exercise
2. Review homework and add new things to the Body Map
3. Check in with everyone's energy and fuel up with a snack
4. Learn new characters related to being still, relaxed, and focused: Cheery Cathy; Day-Dreamy David; Slow-Thinking Stewart; Ahhhh Annie; Focused Frieda; Alert Arnold.
5. Perform some Body Investigations
6. Complete a Body Brainstorms worksheet
7. Review the plan for the week
8. Give out prizes and coloring pages

Session Materials

1. Workbook, worksheets, and coloring pages for Session 9
2. A snack the child brings or that you have on hand that is in small pieces, for sensing our energy and fueling up
3. Optional: A scented candle and a Cheery Cathy button for session prizes (https://fbikids.org).

Background Information for Session 9

Children who experience frequent pain can become hyper-vigilant to any signs of potential threat within their body. The entire FBI – Pain Division program is built on this premise and tries to replace threat hypervigilance with curiosity and wonder about what the body can do. We have also tried throughout the intervention to potentiate what we have learned by actively keeping records: in our body journals, on our Body Maps, on our coloring pages, worksheets, and workbook pages. We are now experts in appreciating and utilizing the wisdom of the body. We have only one advanced skill left in this program to get us ready for a lifetime of openness, growth, and wonder about our partnership with our bodies. That skill is being fully awake and alive in a beautiful moment as it is unfolding – to be on the lookout for sensations that signal relaxing and calm feelings

What would it be like if, just like a photographer, these children are alert for moments of wonder? What if, when these moments occur, our FBI agents pause and let the moment wash over them so they can fully experience it? Of course, we do this in FBI style and have a team of characters to help us. Sensations in this session are about these quiet moments in which we take everything in.

Step-by-Step Guide to Session 9
- Warm-Up Henry Heartbeat Activity
- Review Homework and Add New Things to Their Body Map

Assessing Your Energy and Fueling Up
Given our focus on soothing moments, it is also a good time to check in and see how good the family has become at checking in on their energy on a regular basis and eating slowly to really enjoy the taste of food and notice when they are starting to fill up. Remember Umm-ma Uma, the sensation that we feel when we have a bite of something delicious? Take a minute to check in with the family and hear about some delicious food moments.

Read the Session 9 Workbook: The Soothies
As you all read through the workbook pages this week, perhaps you can use this activity itself as an opportunity to cherish a soothing moment. Sitting and reading something together is a lovely moment, indeed.

Session 9: Body Mystery Questions

Wonderful moments happen to people all the time. Sometimes, they do not pay a lot of attention to these moments until it is too late – the moments are over. What would be some good ways to make sure that you are appreciating a wonderful moment while it is happening? Would this be a good thing – if you noticed more wonderful moments? Why or why not?

What would be a good way to remember that wonderful moment?

Do you know what it means to daydream? Why do you think our mind does that?

Why do you think it feels so good to have a drink when you are really thirsty?

Why is it helpful for you mind to be able to focus really hard on something? What are some ways to get better at doing that?

Table 14.1 presents a summary of the body sensation characters from the workbook and questions to discuss.

Table 14.1 Summary of the body sensation characters from the workbook and questions to discuss

Cheery Cathy

When you feel Cheery Cathy, you have a lightness in your heart and in your body. In the words of Katrina and the Waves, you are "walking on sunshine." You are lighter than air, just moving through a moment like a ray of sunshine with a smile on your face.

What are some things that make you smile? Is there anything that you do that makes other people smile? Does other people smiling ever make you smile?

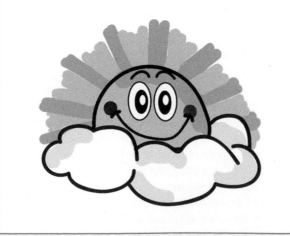

Day-Dreamy David

Day-Dreamy David comes around when you are not focused on what is happening to you in "real life" but instead your mind is drifting off to all sorts of different things. In your mind, you could be on vacation, or playing your favorite game, or with relatives you haven't seen in a long time. Day-Dreamy David can take you anywhere.

Has that ever happened to you? That your mind wanders off and you're thinking about something else even though your body is right here? It's pretty cool, huh?

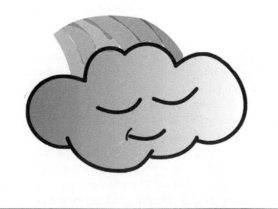

Table 14.1 (cont.)

Slow-Thinking Stewart

Slow-Thinking Stewart is when you feel calm in your head – like your thoughts are moving very slowly and you are seeing things very slowly. Slow-Thinking Stewart feels like you're watching the world in slow motion., like you are on a raft on a lazy river slowly watching the world go by.

Can you do that – move in slow motion? When you move in slow motion, does it feel like everything is slowing down? Even the things in your head?

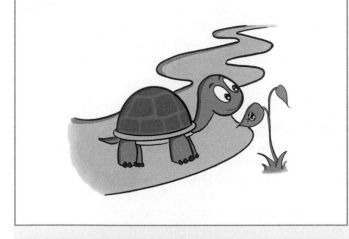

Ahhhh Annie

Ahhhh Annie is a wonderful feeling of relief when you have been feeling really thirsty and you just quenched that thirst. Ahhhh Annie is that gratifying sense of thirst-quenching satisfaction.

Do some drinks make you feel more "Ahhh Annie" than others?

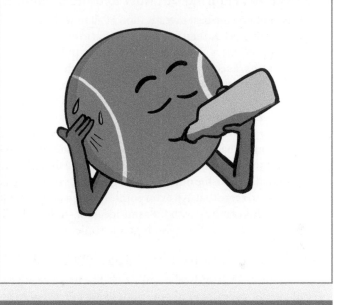

Focused Frieda

Focused Freida is the feeling you have when you are completely focused on something – it takes all your attention and you cannot get your mind off of it. A good test of whether you are feeling Focused Freida is that your parent may need to call your name several times to get your attention because you are so focused you do not even hear it.

Has that ever happened to you? What are some things that you do that really make you feel Focused Freida? Focused Freida and Stuck Stephanie are really good friends. What are some ways they can help each other get unstuck if they need to go do something else for a bit? What are some situations where Focused Freida can really come in handy?

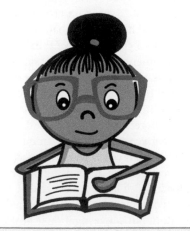

Alert Arnold

Alert Arnold is the feeling you have when you are feeling very alert and awake. It may feel like you are really taking everything around you in and stamping it in your memory. You see everything. You smell everything. You hear everything. You could see that this would be a very useful skill to have when you are an elite special forces FBI agent. You never miss a clue.

Why do you think it would be helpful to feel Alert Arnold? Do you think Alert Arnold would help you to remember things? Why or why not?

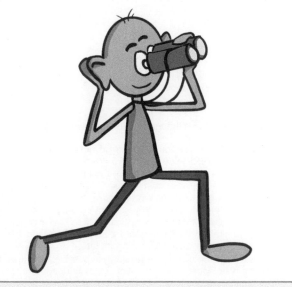

The Soothies: Body Investigations

As with any investigation during any session, these ideas are just that: ideas. It is even better if the children start coming up with their own ideas for investigations. Keep in mind that you will probably only have time for a few investigations in session. Ideas for investigations are also described on the families' workbook pages. Encourage them to try these investigations at home!

Cheery Cathy: Figuring Out How to Bring on Smiles

Well, this might be the best investigation of all time. It is hard to think of anything better than figuring out ways to bring on smiles in ourselves and others. This investigation is the most fun if you break into teams. Each team has to come up with their own plan to make the other team smile (see Table 14.2 for some ideas). Of course, the team that brings on the biggest smiles is the winner. Each team has to go into their own private area to discuss what they are going to do and to plan it out. Then, when time is up, the teams are brought back together and each team takes turns and tries to make the other team smile. What if you take things so far that you actually make the other team laugh? Well, you will need to decide how to score that. An extra point? Losing a point? What happens if teams come up with the same ideas for smiling? Well, then everybody wins and everybody gets to smile.

Slow-Thinking Stewart: Moving as Slow as Possible

We know Mind-Racing Mikella really well. She may like to visit us at night and zoom around our heads as we are trying to go to sleep. Slow-Thinking Stewart is like the opposite of Mind-Racing Mikella. While Mind-Racing Mikella is zooming around the race track, Slow-Thinking Stewart is moving as slow as a turtle. This raises a very interesting question for our investigation. Does moving slowly (or quickly) go together with your thoughts racing or moving slowly? This could be very interesting because it could give us some more ideas about what to do with Mind-Racing Mikella when we are lying in bed. Here is how you might do a Slow-Thinking Stewart investigation (Table 14.3).

Table 14.2 Ideas to bring on Cheery Cathy in someone else

1. Draw them a picture.
2. Sing them a song.
3. Make them a card.
4. Give them a hug.
5. Tell them thank you for something.
6. Write a song or a story about them.

Table 14.3 Getting your thoughts to slow way way down

1. Make a rating of how fast your thoughts are moving. For example, you could rate your speed on a 0 to 10 with 0 = my thoughts could not be moving any more slowly and 10 = my thoughts as going as fast as possible. Alternatively, you could use hand circles to demonstrate how fast your thoughts are circling in your head.
2. Move as quickly as you can. Try this with walking really fast and pumping your arms. (Another interesting investigation to try is whether it works as well with running). Walk really fast for a set period of time and then rate whether your thoughts started moving any faster.
3. Now try the opposite. Try moving as slowly as possible, walking as slow as a turtle. Walk for the same amount of time as you tried walking fast. What happened to the speed of your thoughts?

Body Investigation: Thirst-Quenching Contest

For this investigation, you need some supplies. The goal of this investigation is to figure out what beverage is the most thirst quenching. This may be one of those investigations that the family plans to do at home because ideally this investigation requires data tracking over time. First, you have to figure out some activities that make you thirsty. Ideas include running around in the hot sun, eating a very salty snack, watching a commercial in which someone is drinking a delicious-looking drink, or whatever you can think of. Then have the child rate how thirsty they are. Decide on a set quantity of a beverage (e.g., like a glass), drink it, and then rate your thirst. Record what happens so you can make comparisons on another day. For the second part of the investigation, perform the same activity and drink the same quantity of a beverage (e.g., a glass) but drink a different beverage. Compare the two beverages and see which one is better at quenching your thirst.

Focusing Contest: How Long Can You Feel Focused Freida?

This is a very fun investigation to do. First, you have to decide what being focused looks like. For example, you could decide that a sign of being focused is not lifting up your head or looking around from what you are doing. The next step is to decide on an activity that everyone will be doing at the same time. Good examples include reading a book to oneself, coloring a picture, or playing a game. If you can, try to get everyone to be doing the same activity. Then callout "on your marks, get set, focus!" See who is the first person to look up from what they're doing. The person who can focus the longest is phenomenal Focused Freida. If you want to get even more advanced, you can use a timer to see how long individuals can focus on that chosen activity. Then, everyone can switch to another activity and test the length of their focus. Thus, you can learn that some activities might be easier to focus on than others. You can explore further and see if short attention breaks make it easier to focus for a longer interval overall. The possibilities are endless.

Alert Arnold: Who Notices the Most?

Alert Arnold is the feeling that you have when you are experiencing the full power of all your sensory superpowers. You are a sponge absorbing all that is going on around you. You have the vision of an eagle, the hearing of a bat, the sense of smell of a professionally trained canine. As we think about ways to hold on to beautiful moments, these sensory superpowers help us tremendously. These powers help to make each moment a little more vivid and a little more rich, so that our memories of them can also be a little more vivid and a little more rich. Like any superpower, it gets better with practice. The goal of this investigation is to give everyone a set amount of time and a certain thing to focus on. It could be noticing everything in a room, describing a certain object, focusing on one particular sense, like noticing what you hear, etc. After that set period of time has passed, everyone shares what they noticed. One thing to emphasize when doing this investigation is how much more people notice when they are trying to pay attention and take it all in. This investigation is where we really practice what being a photographer would be like. If you want to make this into a game, you could see who notices the most things, or who finds the most differences between two similar pictures. For this investigation to really be powerful, have families practice this over time – perhaps even repeating the same exercise in session to see if everyone notices more the second time with practice.

> Imagine what it would be like to be a photographer. You're always on the alert for a beautiful moment to capture forever.

Adding to the Body Map

Do not forget to summarize what you learned on the child's (and parent's) Body Map! Here are some possible lessons that you may have learned by performing these investigations.

Possible Body Lessons from the Soothies

Cheery Cathy reminds me to stop and feel this wonderful moment so that I enjoy it while it is happening and perhaps then share this wonderful feeling with others

Day-Dreamy David gives me the power to have new ideas and go to peaceful or exciting places without having to move from the comfortable spot I am now.

Slow-Thinking Stewart helps me to slow down so I can notice everything around me and enjoy the moment for as long as I am able

Ahhh Annie helps to remind me of the importance of drinking enough so that I do not feel thirsty because it feels so good to quench that thirst.

Focused Freida helps me to put exhilarating effort into whatever I am doing because it has all my attention.

Alert Arnold makes sure I do not miss anything that happens. Alert Arnold helps me to make sure I have a very bright, clear picture in my mind of the cool things that happen to me so I will not forget them.

Body Brainstorms

As always, we will try to generalize what we learn in the session to the world around us by completing a Body Brainstorms worksheet.

Questions on our Body Brainstorms worksheet this week include the following:

What kinds of things make you feel thirsty? What do you most like to drink when you are feeling thirsty? Do some drinks make you feel more "Ahhh Annie" than others?

Tell me about something you remember really, really well because Alert Arnold was really strong at the time.

What are some things that are really easy for you to focus on? Focused Freida probably likes those things a lot.

Where are some places you go in your head when you are thinking Day-Dreaming David?

What are some things you do to feel Slow-Thinking Stewart?

What are some things that you do to try to bring on Cheery Cathy in someone else?

Your Ninth Body Investigation Assignment (Home-based Practice)

Families are experts at this point. They know the investigations they may want to try. See what their plans are.

Body Investigation Journal

For the past several sessions, the Body Investigation Journal has been a source to document fun and peaceful moments. Let's keep that up.

Materials Families Take Home from Session 9

Here is a summary of what families get from Session 9.

1. A worksheet that summarizes the characters that they have learned so far included in their Body Clues Worksheet
2. Body Investigation Worksheets
3. Coloring pages
4. The workbook pages for their binder, including an ideas page for some home-based body investigations
5. The Body Brainstorms worksheet they completed
6. Optional: Prizes! A new journal
7. Optional: A Cheery Cathy button
8. Information on getting prizes and buttons can be found at: https://fbikids.org

Body Investigations to Practice at Home

Parents may wish to be on the lookout for calm and relaxing moments so everyone can be focused on those moments and take it all in.

Congratulations, you've just finished Session 9! On to the graduation ceremony!

Therapist Reminders for Session 9

Remind families that the next session is graduation and that you will talk about next steps from there.

A Final Reflection for Session 9

During the second half of this program, we have focused on tuning into pleasant sensations and collecting joyous moments. The song quote that starts off this session is actually a powerful example of doing just that. Consider all that you and this family have been through together. What a wonderful world.

Questions and Answers for Session 9

Q: What if families are getting overwhelmed by the number of characters?

A: Reassure them that it is the principle that is important: not memorizing every character (though the child likely will). The principle is that our body has numerous sensations that communicate different

127

things and that we can learn to listen and get to know and trust ourselves well. The characters are intended to make this self-exploration fun and accessible for young children. What is important is that the family focuses on what works for them. Are there a few characters that they find really useful to talk about? Does everyone in the family have a favorite character? Part of this journey is for the family to integrate these concepts in the way that best helps them continue to learn about themselves and to encourage their children to trust themselves and explore. There is no one way to do this.

Q: Why did you make so many characters?

A: Demand among the children was high. There was always the demand for more characters each session

and I would get pictures of children's bedrooms with row after row of characters that they had colored and hung on the wall. It became habit-forming. Now we cannot stop coming up with new characters. One of the fun aspects of the web-based community associated with this book and program is that children (or parents) can submit their own characters that they have created. It's a character population explosion.

References

1.   Linehan, M. (2014). *DBT Skills Training Manual* (2nd ed.). New York, NY: Guilford Press.

2.   Segal, Z., Williams, M., Teasdale, J. (2018). *Mindfulness-Based Cognitive Therapy for Depression* (2nd ed.). New York, NY: Guilford Press.

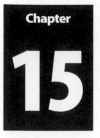

Session 10: The Celebration… and the Next Leg of Our Journey

Overview of Session 10

> We are so tough. We are so strong. We are so very wise.
> We can handle anything.

Children with sensory superpowers are invincible. Even at their young age, they know themselves oh so well now. It is incredible what they have just accomplished with their families. Everyone, including the FBI therapist, made it. This is the last session.

Our final session is a graduation ceremony with some fun games to help the children rejoice in how much they have learned about themselves. To appreciate what you have accomplished, let us take a moment to reflect on all you have done. Your core mission was to help children with frequent pain, who considered themselves vulnerable and weak, to completely change their mindset and their experience of embodiment. They have sensory superpowers. Their bodies are infinitely wise. These children know themselves better than most (almost all?) five- to nine-year-olds. Frankly, they know themselves better than many adults. They have learned that whatever happens – puberty, injury, intense volatile emotions, etc., they can handle it.

We have a lot to celebrate. We have come a long way. And we are on a lifelong journey to keep learning more about ourselves as we develop. At this graduation session, we spend some time considering next steps. These include ways to implement the Feeling and Body Investigator program in your practice, your classroom, and/or your home and ways for your patients to become connected to other families that have participated in the FBI program. To do so, we leave you with information to stay connected to the FBI – Pain Division online communities of providers and patients. This final session is a marker of how far we have traveled as well as the exciting things that lie ahead. A goodbye and a hello.

Session Outline

1. Perform a warm-up Henry Heartbeat exercise
2. Review homework and add new things to the Body Map
3. Check in with everyone's energy and fuel up with a snack

4. Conduct your graduation ceremony
5. Play the character memory game (and/or repeat your favorite Body Investigations)

Session Materials

1. A graduation certificate
2. A snack the child brings or that you have on hand that is in small pieces, for sensing our energy and fueling up
3. Optional: A memory game of all the characters learned

Background Information for Session 10

This session begins with our usual rituals. However, rather than learning new characters and conducting new Body Investigations, we have a graduation ceremony that celebrates the child's official classification as an FBI agent. We conduct this ceremony with the fanfare it deserves – much like a knighting ceremony. We have the child get down on one knee, bow their heads, touch them on both shoulders (with a ruler or something else that represents a scepter) and award them a certificate of completion. We usually give them some symbolic prizes – a fancy journal, a cool pen, a button that has their FBI badge. We also laminate their final Body Clues Worksheet and Body Characters Sheet so that they can use them again and again in the future. After this, we see if the children want to play a memory game – we paste two versions of each of the characters (49 characters total) onto decks of playing cards (there are 52 cards in a deck, so you have cards for any characters that the child may have spontaneously come up with on your journey). You can prepare these in advance using two decks of playing cards. We include some instructions on how to play the memory game as well. We have found that this is a wonderful souvenir for the children, a way for them to practice and show-off what they have learned. We then see if they want to have a booster session in a month, join our online community, and/or join one of our online groups. Saying goodbye to a therapeutic relationship is hard for anyone, but perhaps especially for children, so we try to provide some gentle exits. These options change a farewell to a "till next time." This stage is much easier for those of you integrating FBI into your pediatric primary care practice, as your relationship and contact with the child will be ongoing for the next ten or so years. Otherwise, we prepare ourselves to face all the mixed feelings (Bertha Blah, Bursting Bella, Tearful Tasha, Ella the Emotional Pain) that come with goodbyes.

Step-by-Step Guide to Session 10
- Warm-Up Henry Heartbeat activity
- Review homework and add new things to their Body Map
- Assessing your energy and fueling up

The Graduation Ceremony

THERAPIST: *Today is a special day. You have worked really hard to become an FBI agent and today is your graduation. We get to celebrate that you are now officially an FBI agent. How do you feel about that? Are you proud of yourself?*

CHILD: Yeah.

MOM: Well, I am very, very proud of you. You really worked hard. I can tell that you know your body really well and have gotten really strong.

THERAPIST: *I agree. To honor this, I have a special certificate that I would like to award you. Let's be official. How about you get down on one knee like this (the therapist demonstrates), I will officially dub you an "FBI agent."*

The therapist grabs some type of longish thing (e.g., a ruler) as a substitute for a sword in a knighting ceremony and reads from the certificate (Figure 15.1). After reading the certificate, the therapist touches both shoulders of the "agent" with the ruler and hands the child the certificate.

THERAPIST: *This Feeling and Body Investigator Certificate of Excellence is hereby awarded to CHILD'S NAME.*

*For showing **bravery** in the completion of all body investigations,*

*For showing **curiosity** in learning more about stomach pain, emotions, and all the messages that the body gives you, and for*

*Showing **determination** that went beyond the call of duty in the completion of all ten sessions of the FBI training academy. Congratulations!*

Everybody claps. Do not underestimate what a wonderful moment this is for families. There are usually lots of hugs and pictures.

Following this, the therapist awards any prizes (e.g., a journal and pen and laminated Body Characters and Body Clues worksheets).

The Memory Game

THERAPIST : *As part of our celebration, we can do your favorite Body Investigations or I have this game that I am going to give you that we can play. Have you ever played the game Memory in which you have to remember the location of two pairs of a match? Well, we made a memory game of all FORTY-NINE characters you have learned and the FBI badge you just received. This is a really tough memory game because it has 104 pieces!! Do you want to try it?*

They almost always want to try. If you are worried about the game being too hard and long, you can always divide it in half (just make sure you divide it up so that you have matching cards).

The rules of the memory game are in Table 15.1.

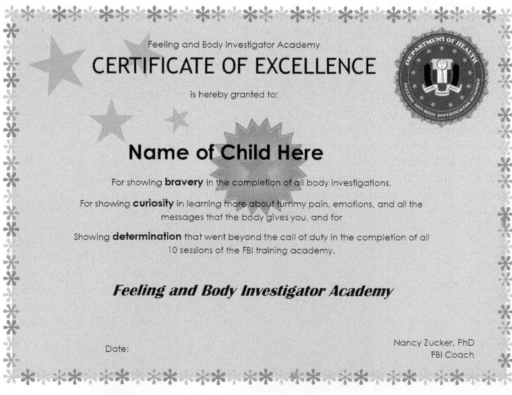

Feeling and Body Investigator Academy

CERTIFICATE OF EXCELLENCE

is hereby granted to:

Name of Child Here

For showing **bravery** in the completion of all body investigations,

For showing **curiosity** in learning more about tummy pain, emotions, and all the messages that the body gives you, and for

Showing **determination** that went beyond the call of duty in the completion of all 10 sessions of the FBI training academy.

Feeling and Body Investigator Academy

Date:

Nancy Zucker, PhD
FBI Coach

Figure 15.1 The "official" Feeling and Body Investigator Graduation Certificate.

Table 15.1 The official FBI memory card game

1. Shuffle the decks of cards well to make sure that pairs of cards are not next to each other in the deck (some inevitably will be, but an unshuffled deck may have all the pairs together which would not make for a very fun game).
2. Lay out the cards face down in a grid. For example, with 104 cards, you could make 13 rows with eight cards each, eight rows with 13 cards each, 26 rows with four cards each, and so on …
3. The first person turns over a card. **Each player must keep the card in exactly the same place where they turned it over.** Then, they turn over a second card.
4. If the cards match (they are the exact same picture), then they keep the pair and get to go again.
5. If the cards do not match, they turn the cards over and it is the next player's turn.
6. The game ends when all the matches have been found. The person with the most matches wins.

Playing on teams is another great way to play this game. At the end of the game, the child gets to keep the game as a souvenir of all that they have learned.

Options for Goodbye

THERAPIST : *You have done such a great job. Now let's talk about what our next steps can be. First, we could be finished here and you can keep practicing your skills and getting stronger and stronger. Or, if you want, we can schedule a booster session for a month from now to check in and see how you are doing. Or, if you want, you can join one of our online groups of other children that have been through this program. You could be part of a group that meets or you can just post things to the community if you feel like it (e.g., characters you invent, drawings that you make).*

Follow-up

In the trial of Feeling and Body Investigator, improvements in abdominal pain were seen at three-month follow-up from the treatment. We did not formally test any booster sessions or online communities. However, with the rapid advances in telehealth opportunities, we saw no reason not to strengthen gains from treatments by building communities. So, they are there if the families would like them and they may be a great source of comfort even if they are not needed.

After the family has made their plans for next steps …

THERAPIST : *I'm really proud of you and I'm going to miss you. I really had fun working with you.*

CHILD : Me too. Goodbye.

MOM : Goodbye. Thank you for everything. Thanks for these options for follow-up. I think we are good but it certainly is a relief to have them!

And that's a wrap.

Materials Families Take Home from Session 10

Here is a summary of what families get from Session 10. See our online community at: https://fbikids.org

1. If possible, a laminated Body Clues worksheet.
2. If possible, a laminated Body Characters worksheet.
3. Optional: Prizes (journal, pen, memory game, a button of the FBI badge).

Body Investigations to Practice at Home

Remind families to continue to practice their skills until they are second nature. Perhaps they can start teaching them to other families!

Therapist Reminders for Session 10

Take some time to celebrate yourself. You also made it through this program.

Questions and Answers for Session 10

Q: Will parents think the program is not enough if we offer options for follow-up and ongoing support?

A: Hopefully not if our messaging has been consistent – that we are always learning about ourselves. You can reassure them that the program has been found to be successful with all the skills they have. These are just options for them to have if they want them. Our experience is that parents are pleased with the offer even though they do not feel that they need them.

The Next Leg of Your Journey

Online Implementation

The Feeling and Body Investigator program was developed a seeming lifetime ago, before the COVID-19 pandemic, when therapy was done in person. Since the transition to telehealth for many providers and families, we have also implemented FBI remotely. Let us say that we were very nervous about the potential challenge of maintaining children's attention and excitement via a video conference. After trying it, we were pleasantly surprised with the positive experiences in delivering FBI via telehealth. Minor adaptations to the protocol for online delivery are listed in Table 15.2.

Group and Classroom Implementation

The Feeling and Body Investigator program is ridiculously fun and relatively seamless to implement in a group format.

Table 15.2 Adaptations for FBI in an online format

1. We have made the workbook available as slides that are easy to share on your screen. These are available via our downloadable materials.
2. We have found it helpful to shorten sessions for telehealth delivery, covering fewer characters and Body Investigations at a time. Thus, sometimes the content for a session will last two sessions rather than one. For younger children, we try to keep sessions to 30 minutes with the child. We can then check in with parents as needed after that.
3. For session materials, we have emailed parents worksheets and workbooks. However, not all parents have printers or like reading things online. A parent and child self-guided workbook will be published that will be particularly helpful when delivering FBI online.[1]
4. We have found that generalization of skills is even better when FBI is delivered online since the children are already practicing the skills in their home.
5. For materials like buttons and prizes, see: https://fbikids.org

Table 15.3 Suggestions for a group format – live or online

Henry Heartbeat Activity

This goes exactly as in individual sessions. It is just a lot more exciting when a group full of children are bouncing up and down and raising and lowering their heartbeats. You can have the children call out the numbers but be careful that any activity is collaborative, not competitive; remember that there are no wrong answers here. You can use all the different values to show how everyone's body is wise in its own way and adapts as it needs to.

Homework Sharing

1. Everyone finds and lays out their Body Maps.

2. The group leader asks everyone to add anything to their Body Map that they learned during the past week. The group leaders get a few volunteers to share what they have learned. Every few sessions the group practices completing a Body Clues Worksheet focused on how everyone is feeling right now. Group members can raise their hands (either live or via the hand raise function via a telehealth platform like Zoom®).

Energy Meter and New Characters

1. Children can check in with their energy and eat their snack while they are hearing about new characters – like a story hour. The group leader needs to remember to stop periodically to have everyone check in on their energy.

2. While reading about new characters, the group leader will ask the group for examples of times they may have felt a given sensation. For an online format, children may want to put their answers in the online chat. You can play interactive games like what is the best emoticon for this sensation? Put it in the chat.

Body Investigations

Body Investigations are conducted just as they are in individual sessions. Everybody does them and the group discusses what they just learned about their bodies. Then everyone adds it to their Body Map.

Body Brainstorms

Completing Body Brainstorms worksheets works well in a group – everyone can chime in responses.

The flow is the same and the learning and potency may even be intensified as children and parents can learn from watching other children or parent–child dyads. We have delivered this both ways – children alone or parent–child dyads. We have also had child-only online groups. Table 15.3 lists some suggestions for a group format – both live or online.

Classroom Activities

Of course, the materials and themes of this program work very well for a monthly classroom theme. One can imagine: posters of characters with themed bulletin boards; Henry Heartbeat activities to start off a class – children practice raising and lowering arousal, which may increase readiness to learn; science experiments around different Henry Heartbeat activities or related to other body sensations; and writing assignments about Bursting Bella moments. There are endless possibilities. In our downloadable materials, we have some posters that can be printed if helpful (https://fbikids.org.)

Integration with a Primary Care Practice

The Feeling and Body Investigator program was designed so that healthcare professionals with different educational training and backgrounds could feel confident in its administration. Thus,

any range of personnel within a primary care practice is able to deliver this intervention. Integration of this program into the short visits and busy flow of a pediatric practice is another challenge, and working through the logistics of this is an ongoing adventure. However, one can imagine a brief nursing check-in of homework, learning one new character, and providing the materials for at-home practice with the workbook and materials. These brief individual check-ins could be coupled with a group practice visit which may follow some of the suggestions above. It is one of our hopes and intentions that, with the online provider community we create, we can learn from each other tips about billing, time management, and other logistical challenges. However, one can imagine a monthly feature at a practice in which there are posters of characters related to a given theme and all children leave their primary care visit with workbook and coloring pages every time they visit the doctor. Ultimately, we hope that the framework of FBI spurs everyone's creativity about body curiosity and connection and makes visiting the doctor a lot more fun.

Goodbye and Hello

As we wrap up our description of the FBI – Pain Division program, take a moment to appreciate just a few specific accomplishments you have facilitated for the family:

1. First and foremost, you have inculcated an attitude of respect and awe towards the body.

2. You have helped families learn to decode the meanings of a wide range of sensations and link them to actions. Through this, and with the help of the Body Clues Worksheets, you have increased families' self-knowledge and trust; everyone has learned to be (or to be a better) self-parent.

3. You have helped families learn more about what their body is capable of and how wise it is via our Body Investigations.

4. You have changed sensations that can be scary (e.g., Polly Pain, Victor Vomit, Patricia the Poop Pain) into playful, informative messengers.

5. You have helped children with sensory superpowers become more confident in, and better at, their skills in raising and lowering their level of arousal. We have done this in many ways, especially with the Henry Heartbeat exercises at the start of every session.

6. You have helped children with sensory superpowers savor food and tune into their hunger and fullness signals.

7. You have helped children notice and relish joyous and soothing sensations as they are unfolding, as well as play them over and over again in their minds and bodies, accessing pathways to self-regulation on demand.

8. You have ensured that children have stamped what they have learned in their memories by recording the wisdom of their bodies on their Body Map.

9. You have given parents language and tools to help guide their children through difficult moments. This includes the Body Investigation worksheets that parents complete with their children.

10. You have helped parents feel seen and heard and perhaps, have given them a chance to learn to listen to and know themselves in a way that they had missed out on previously.

Overall, you helped parents and children attune and be responsive to sensations and emotions from their bodies that they perhaps could not understand before. At the same time, you helped them modify their perception of and reactivity to sensations to which they previously hyper-focused; specifically, you turned fearful, uncomfortable, and confusing body and mind experiences into objects of curiosity, humor, and playfulness. The end result is the creation of a mindset in which we are in awe of the body's wisdom and power. We are all invincible.

We hope that it has been invigorating to help transform a vulnerable child into a being with sensory superpowers. We hope that watching children learn to know and trust themselves has been inspiring, and that this program will make your practice more meaningful and more fun. We look forward to hearing about your journey. Till next time.

References

Zucker, N.L. Gagliano, M.E., & Loeb, K.L. (in preparation). *A Parent's Guide to Treating Functional Abdominal Pain in Children with Feeling and Body Investigators*. Cambridge: Cambridge University Press.

The Feeling and Body Investigator Program
Session 1

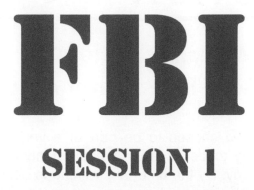

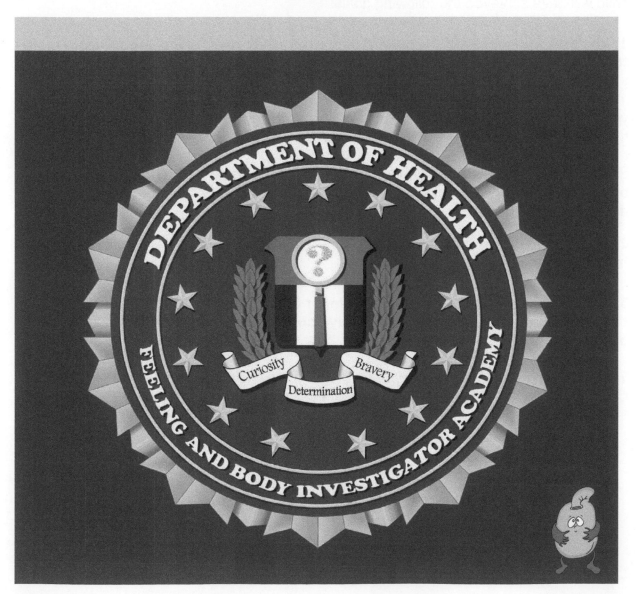

INTRODUCTION

Welcome to the
Feeling and Body Investigator Academy!

You and your child have been chosen to be part of a very special team of investigators. We are training to be experts in understanding the mysteries, power, and wisdom of the body. By the time this training is over, you and your child will have achieved the following goals:

1. You and your child will be able to figure out what your bodies are trying to tell you.

Your child (and you) will be better at knowing what your body is trying to tell you. Pain can have many different messages. Your stomach has many different messages as well. Some common reasons children may notice sensations in their stomach are that they are feeling scared, hungry, guilty, or having other, different feelings. Your child (and you) will also be able to tell the difference between different types of pain (e.g., gas pain, hunger pain, muscle pain, and emotional pain).

2. Your child will not be as worried or afraid of sensations they are feeling in their body.

3. Your child will be less likely to let pain, or other body sensations, keep them from doing their normal day-to-day activities, trying new adventures, or having fun.

The first section of this workbook will introduce you to what you can expect during our journey together through the FBI Academy.

SECTION 1:
BACKGROUND CLUES

In this section, you will learn all sorts of fun things! We'll give you new information to help you and your child learn more about your bodies. You will learn all sorts of things in your live sessions, but you will also have a workbook to help you remember the things you learned. To help you and your child learn new things, we have asked some special friends to assist us. Meet some of them below.

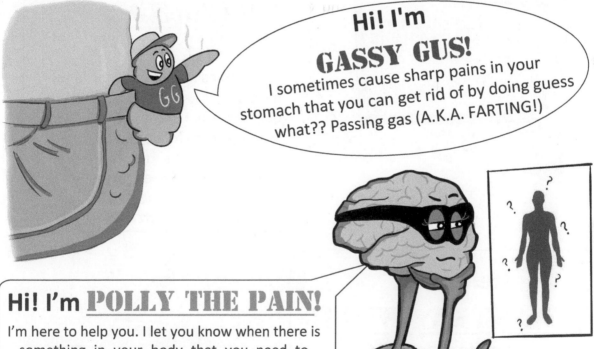

Hi! I'm
GASSY GUS!
I sometimes cause sharp pains in your stomach that you can get rid of by doing guess what?? Passing gas (A.K.A. FARTING!)

Hi! I'm POLLY THE PAIN!

I'm here to help you. I let you know when there is something in your body that you need to pay attention to. Sometimes, in fact, a lot of the time, you may not need to do anything. Your body is really smart and can figure out how to take care of a lot of things on its own. But if you are unsure, we can always do an investigation together to figure out what I am trying to tell you!

Hi! I'm <u>BETTY THE BUTTERFLY!</u>

I cause a fluttering in your stomach when you feel anxious, worried, or maybe even excited about something.

Hi! I'm <u>RICKY THE ROCK!</u>

I sometimes make you feel like you have a tight knot or heavy stone in your stomach. I usually come around when you are feeling guilty or sad about something. I may also come around when there is something coming up that you may not be looking forward to at all.

Hello! I'm <u>SAMANTHA SWEAT!</u>
Sam for short!

I like to come visit you when your body is preparing for a challenge (like when you are going to take a difficult test or run a race). I help keep your body cool so you can face the challenge.

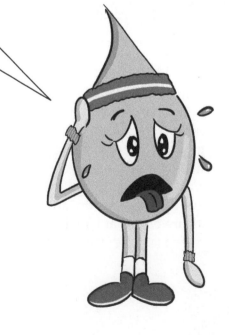

Hello! I'm HENRY THE HEARTBEAT!

I am a very powerful machine that pumps blood to all of the parts of your body. The harder you work, the more I pump. I am like a secret decoder ring. Based on how fast or how slow I am beating, you may be able to tell whether something important or relaxing is going on. My beats are the secret to the code.

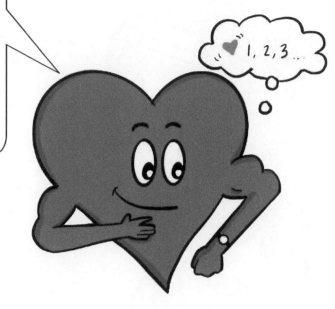

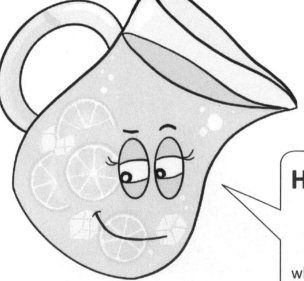

Hi I'm GERDA GOTTA GO!

I am the sensation you feel when you have to pee. However, I can also be a very sneaky gal. Sometimes I make you think you have to pee when you really could wait. Hee! Hee! I'm quite a tease. I hope you don't learn to outsmart me. It will take some investigations to figure me out!

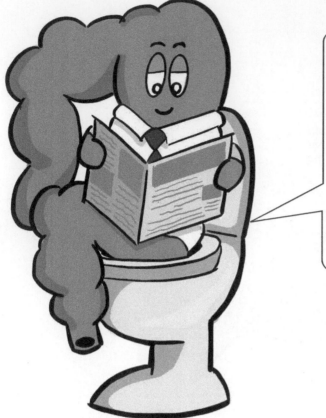

I'm that feeling you get when you have to go poop! Sometimes, it is very easy to know when I am going to come. For example, some poops may happen at about the same time every day. But sometimes, I may try to surprise you... we will learn more about that later!

I'm

GORDON GOTTA GO!

Hello! I'm
PATRICIA THE POOP PAIN!

I know it is not usually glamorous to talk about poop, but I am very important. I take myself very seriously and treat myself very glamorously. I dress up super fancy – complete with all my jewels. If I think it will be a long ride down your intestine, I may as well live it up!

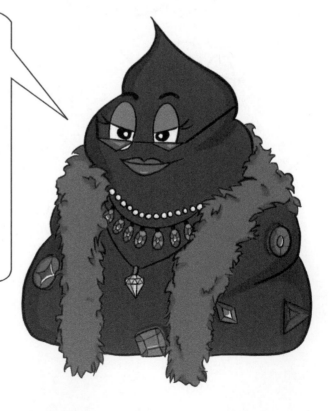

SECTION 2:
BODY INVESTIGATIONS

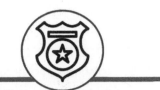

In this section, we will give you ideas about some body investigations that you can try at home. Some of these investigations may sound familiar as you may have already practiced them!

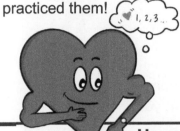

Henry the Heartbeat
I am a very powerful machine that pumps blood to all of the parts of your body. The harder you work, the more I pump.

Henry the Heartbeat Body Investigation #1

1. With your child, choose 2 activities that you think may make your hearts beat faster.
2. With your child, choose 1 activity that you think may make your hearts beat more slowly.
3. Decide on how long you are going to perform each activity. To be more scientific, you should do each activity for the same amount of time.
4. Find your heartbeat! Have your child find their heartbeat. It is important that they sense their heartbeat by taking their own pulse rather than having an adult do it for them or using some kind of gadget. This will help your child practice tuning in and listening to their body. An adult may need to help the child find their heartbeat initially. Sometimes, when a heartbeat seems particularly tricky to find, the child can jump up and down for a few seconds to make the heartbeat easier to detect.

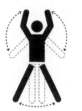

5. If possible, it is ideal that every member of the family (or as many members as possible) try this activity together. So everyone, try to find your heartbeat!
6. Find a stopwatch and assign someone as the time keeper.
7. The timekeeper will say "on your mark, get set, count!" After 10 seconds, the timekeeper will say "stop!".

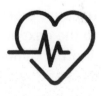

8. The timekeeper will then ask everyone how many heartbeats they counted and record this on a piece of paper. This is their baseline heartbeat.

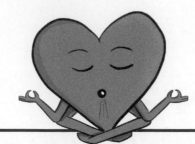

9. Now, everyone should make a guess about which activity (#1 or #2, for example, jumping jacks or running) is going to make their hearts beat faster. If people want to get super-fancy, they can make a guess as to how many beats their heart will go up when they do each activity.

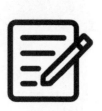

10. Together, decide on how long everyone will perform each activity. The timekeeper will set the timer and might say something like this: "Ok, I'm going to set my timer for XX seconds (whatever was agreed upon) and then you are going to do Activity #1 (for example, doing jumping jacks). When I say stop, you will stop and we will count your heartbeats (and see whose guess is the closest)."

11. The timekeeper will time the activity and all participants will take their heart rate. The timekeeper will write down what everyone's heartbeats were after the activity.

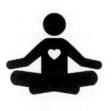

12. The next step is to lower your heartbeat so that it is back to where you started from. The timekeeper can say something like this: "OK, now for the next minute, we are going to do the activity that we picked to bring our heart rate back down. On your mark, get set, slow down your heartbeat!"

13. After the minute is up, the timekeeper will once again direct everyone to count their heartbeats. If it is back to baseline, you can continue on to the next activity. If not, perform the heartbeat reduction activity for another minute.

14. Repeat these steps for the second heartbeat raising activity and then repeat the heart reduction activity.

15. Now look at the data you collected. What did you learn? What activity made everyone's heart beat faster? Was it the same for everyone? Or, did people's hearts adjust to what their body needed? How long did it take to slow your heartbeat down? Did it take shorter, longer, or the same time than it took to raise it back up? At the end of this activity everyone will have learned the following: which activity causes their heart to beat faster; how long (approximately) it takes to bring the heart rate back down to baseline; and who had the best guess! But the main lesson that everyone learned is that your heart is really, really smart and knows how to adapt to different situations.

SECTION 3:
BODY MAP

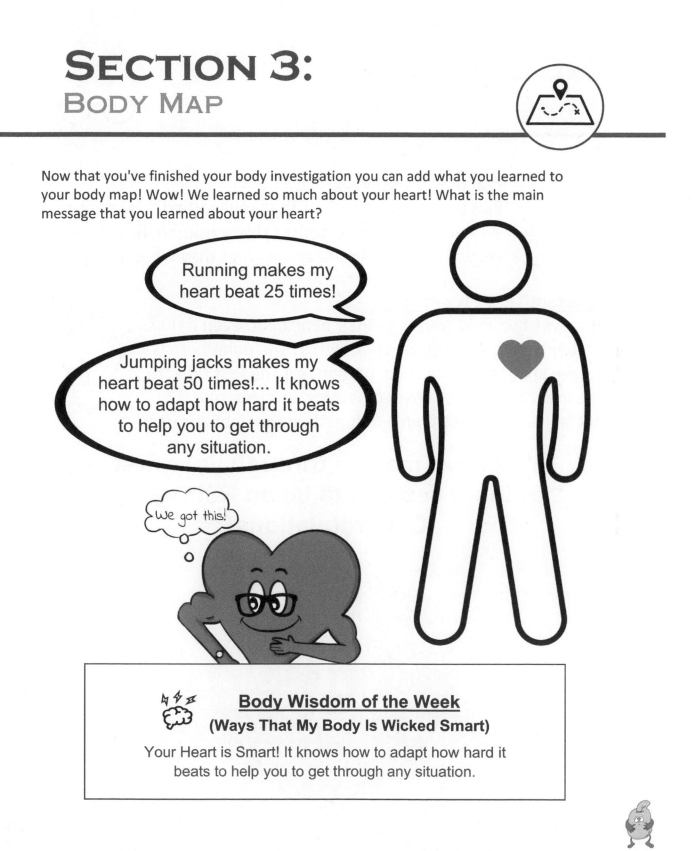

Now that you've finished your body investigation you can add what you learned to your body map! Wow! We learned so much about your heart! What is the main message that you learned about your heart?

Running makes my heart beat 25 times!

Jumping jacks makes my heart beat 50 times!... It knows how to adapt how hard it beats to help you to get through any situation.

We got this!

Body Wisdom of the Week
(Ways That My Body Is Wicked Smart)

Your Heart is Smart! It knows how to adapt how hard it beats to help you to get through any situation.

SECTION 4:
PRACTICES & TIPS

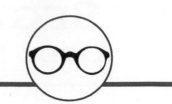

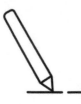

Practice of the Week
Pick two body sensations that you learned this session. Whenever your child notices this sensation, have them write or draw a picture about what they were doing.

Important Tip #1 for Parents
Whatever the child counts as their heartbeat, even if that number seems illogical, we stick with it. The point here is that we are getting the child, perhaps for the first time, to tune into their body, sense something, and describe it. That is the important point – not getting the right answer.

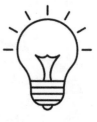

You have made it through your first training session to be an FBI Agent. Congratulations!

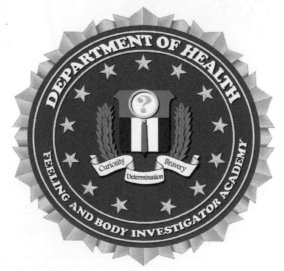

FBI BODY BRAINSTORMS
PRACTICE 1

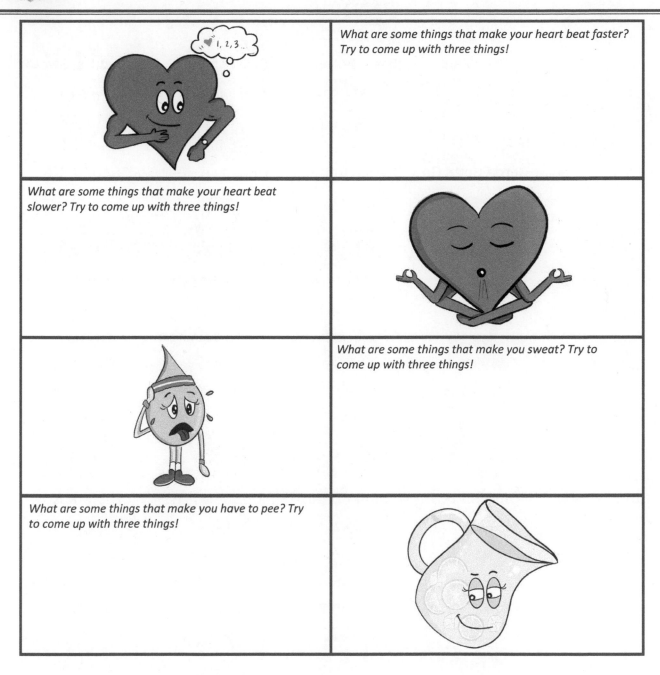

What are some things that make your heart beat faster? Try to come up with three things!

What are some things that make your heart beat slower? Try to come up with three things!

What are some things that make you sweat? Try to come up with three things!

What are some things that make you have to pee? Try to come up with three things!

FBI CHARACTER SHEET

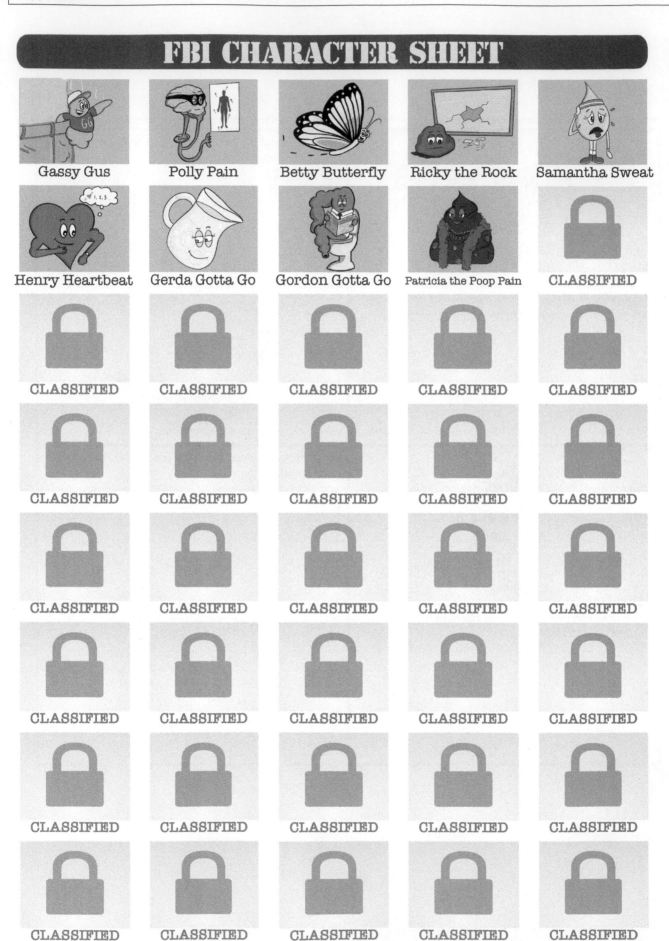

Gassy Gus — Polly Pain — Betty Butterfly — Ricky the Rock — Samantha Sweat

Henry Heartbeat — Gerda Gotta Go — Gordon Gotta Go — Patricia the Poop Pain — CLASSIFIED

CLASSIFIED CLASSIFIED CLASSIFIED CLASSIFIED CLASSIFIED

CLASSIFIED CLASSIFIED CLASSIFIED CLASSIFIED CLASSIFIED

CLASSIFIED CLASSIFIED CLASSIFIED CLASSIFIED CLASSIFIED

CLASSIFIED CLASSIFIED CLASSIFIED CLASSIFIED CLASSIFIED

CLASSIFIED CLASSIFIED CLASSIFIED CLASSIFIED CLASSIFIED

CLASSIFIED CLASSIFIED CLASSIFIED CLASSIFIED CLASSIFIED

The Feeling and Body Investigator Program

FBI

SESSION 2: THE EATS

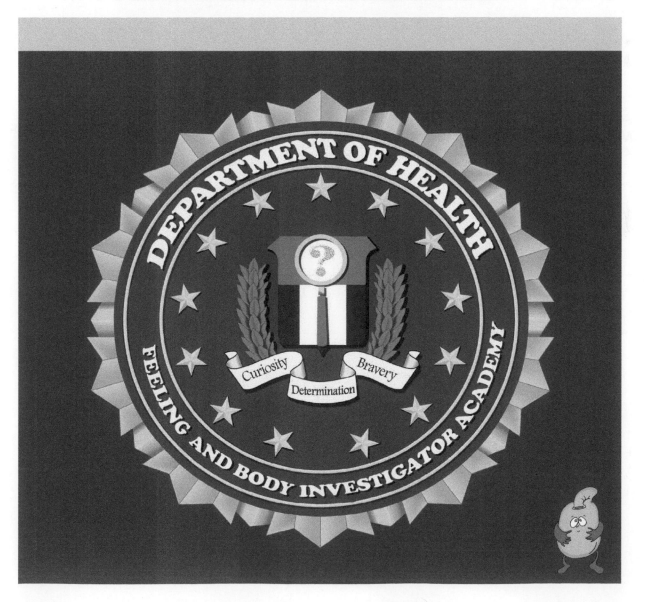

SECTION 1:
BACKGROUND CLUES

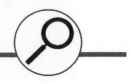

ABOUT HUNGER AND FULLNESS

Let's take a few seconds to come up with some answers to the following investigative questions.

1. Why do you think people have hunger pains?

2. What might happen if you notice a hunger pain and then you ignore it?

3. What happens if you are eating a food that tastes so good that even though you feel full, you keep eating it?

See some interesting clues about hunger on the next page and see how many you and your agent discovered from your investigative interviews!

Important investigative facts about hunger

Hunger pains let you know when your body is low on energy.

What would happen to a car that didn't have any gas in it? It would stop! A car needs gas to run. Your body needs food to work. Food is like the gas for your body. What happens if you don't have enough food for your body to run?

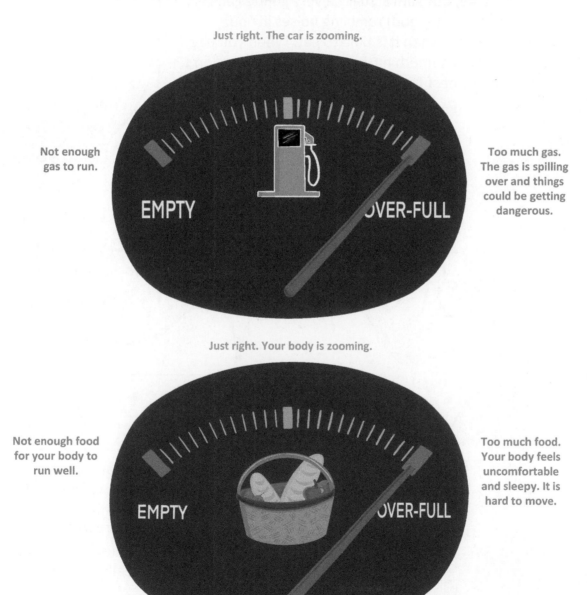

Just right. The car is zooming.

Not enough gas to run.

EMPTY

OVER-FULL

Too much gas. The gas is spilling over and things could be getting dangerous.

Just right. Your body is zooming.

Not enough food for your body to run well.

EMPTY

OVER-FULL

Too much food. Your body feels uncomfortable and sleepy. It is hard to move.

You guessed it! Your body slows down and doesn't work properly. Since giving your body fuel is so important, we need to learn more about hunger and fullness. Now it's time to meet some new friends!

Hi! I'm GEORGIA THE GUT GROWLER!

I may sound very scary, but I am actually a very gentle gal. I like to make soft (or sometimes loud) rumbling noises in your stomach to let you know when it is time to eat. When you pay attention to me and eat something, I get quiet. But if you don't, I may need to call in my best friend HAROLD to help me out...

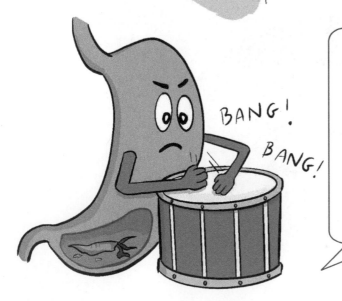

Hi! I am HAROLD THE HUNGER PAIN!

You usually feel me when you have let your body get way too hungry. I am NOT quiet and I can really hurt. That is because I WANT YOU TO PAY ATTENTION TO ME! I need lots of attention because when I give you the signal, it is really time to eat!

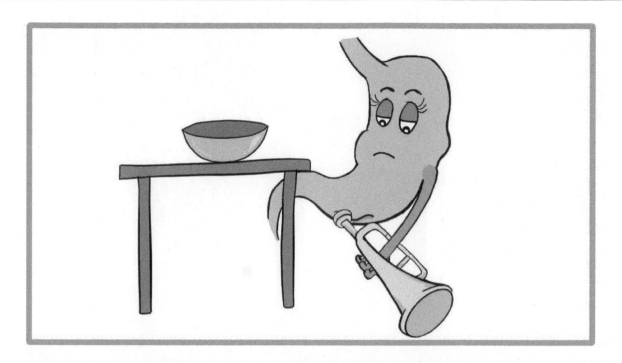

In the beginning, **GEORGIA THE GUT GROWLER**'s person was not very good at hearing her. She would grumble and grumble but nothing happened. Her person was getting hungrier and hungrier but still not noticing until...

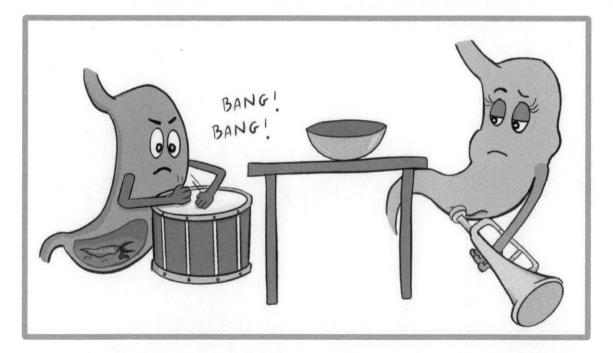

GEORGIA THE GUT GROWLER had to call in her old buddy **HAROLD THE HUNGER PAIN** to help. When **HAROLD** is banging on his drum and causing hunger pains, it can get pretty uncomfortable and his person notices.

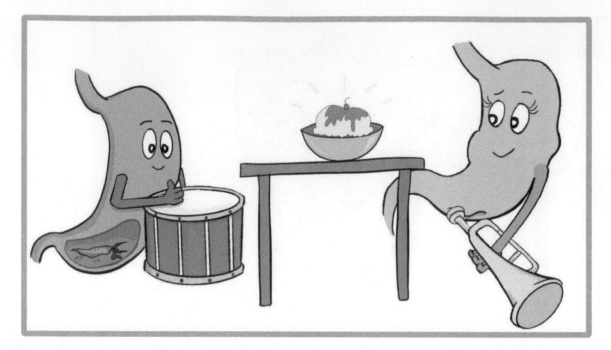

At last! Their person notices their hunger and gives **HAROLD** and **GEORGIA** the food they need. Both **GEORGIA THE GUT GROWLER** and **HAROLD THE HUNGER PAIN** are satisfied. Now, all that needs to happen is practice so that their person gets better at noticing **GEORGIA THE GUT GROWLER**.

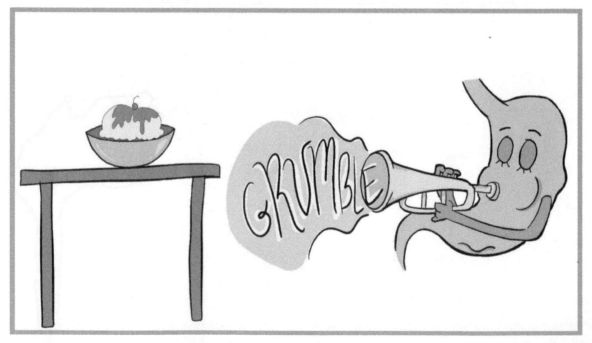

Ah-ha! With practice, **GEORGIA**'s person gets better at noticing their hunger. They notice when they feel **GEORGIA THE GUT GROWLER** and learn that that is a signal they are hungry. No need for **HAROLD THE HUNGER PAIN** this time!

Let's take a minute to do some body investigations.

What are some things that you notice in your body when you have the different feelings of hunger shown below?

Let's fill in the boxes for:

Starving, Hungry, and Getting Energized

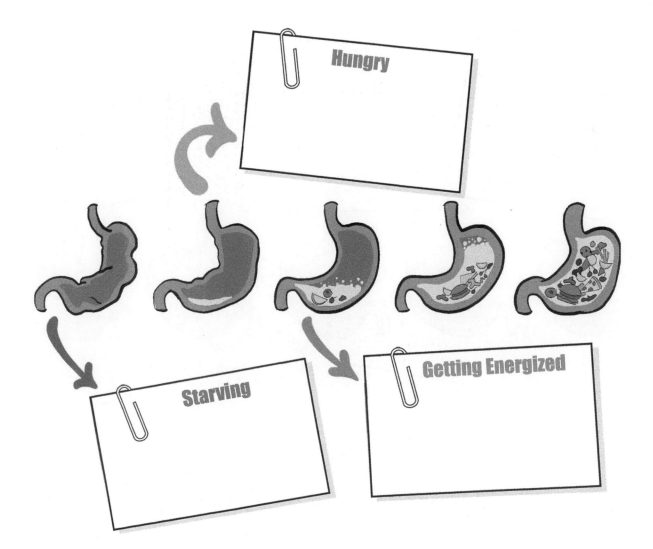

Our stomachs can also get grumpy if they get too much food. Let's go back to our hunger meter and think about what it feels like after a meal when we have given our body a comfortable amount of food and when we have given our body an uncomfortable amount of food.

Now let's fill in the boxes for:

the **Satisfied** and **Stuffed** parts of the hunger meter.

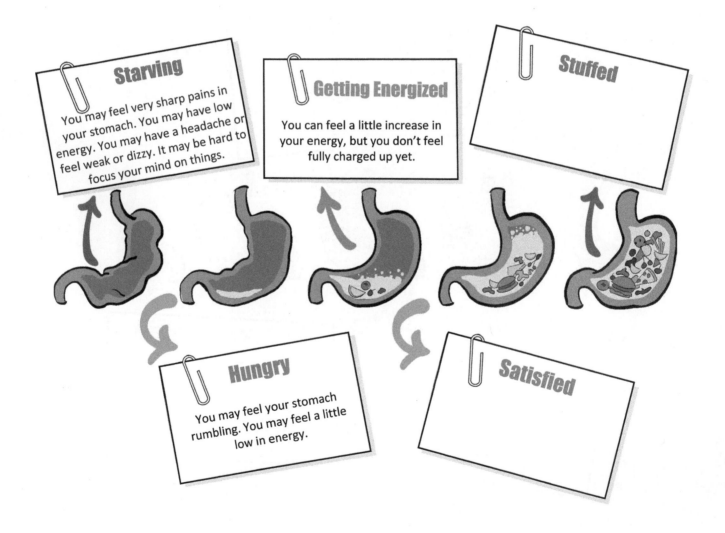

Starving

You may feel very sharp pains in your stomach. You may have low energy. You may have a headache or feel weak or dizzy. It may be hard to focus your mind on things.

Getting Energized

You can feel a little increase in your energy, but you don't feel fully charged up yet.

Stuffed

Hungry

You may feel your stomach rumbling. You may feel a little low in energy.

Satisfied

Of course, this means that it is time to meet some new friends.

Meet **SABRINA STUFFED** and **SOLOMON SATISFIED**

Hello. I am
SABRINA STUFFED!

I have some trouble stopping things that I am doing – especially when it is something that I really like to do – like eat! I really love food so I have a hard stopping myself from eating, until... you guessed it – I AM STUFFED! I guess that is where I got my name from. Everyone gets STUFFED every once in awhile. However, if you find that I am hanging around all the time, it may be time to start listening for **SOLOMON SATISFIED**.

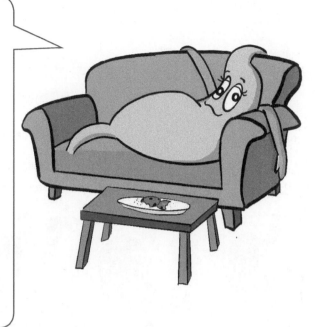

Why, hello. I am Mr. Satisfied,
SOLOMON SATISFIED, that is.

I am always peppy, energized, and ready to go because I always have just the right amount of food that I need to fuel my body. My only problem is that I can be a bit quiet at times (I am rather shy). When the food tastes really good and **SABRINA** is getting excited because she doesn't want you to stop, it can be really hard to hear me. Once we get to know each other better, you will find that I have a lot of interesting things to say and it will be easier to notice me!

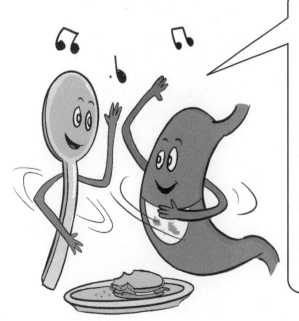

155

A complete hunger and fullness meter may look something like this:

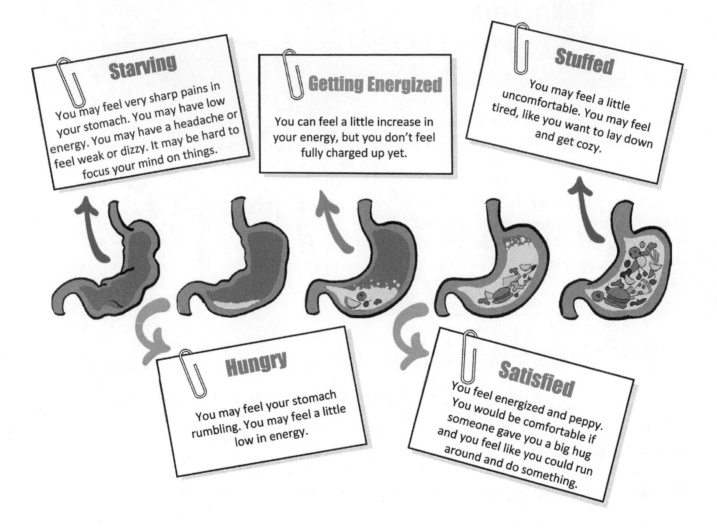

Starving

You may feel very sharp pains in your stomach. You may have low energy. You may have a headache or feel weak or dizzy. It may be hard to focus your mind on things.

Getting Energized

You can feel a little increase in your energy, but you don't feel fully charged up yet.

Stuffed

You may feel a little uncomfortable. You may feel tired, like you want to lay down and get cozy.

Hungry

You may feel your stomach rumbling. You may feel a little low in energy.

Satisfied

You feel energized and peppy. You would be comfortable if someone gave you a big hug and you feel like you could run around and do something.

Now its time to meet two more friends!

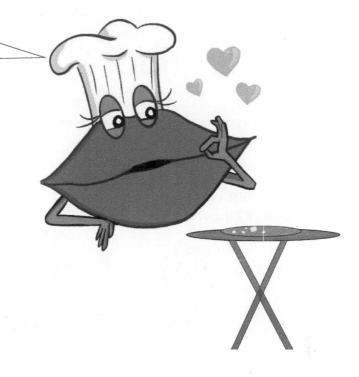

Hello. I am

UMM-MA UMA!

UMMMMMMM!!! I am that feeling of utter deliciousness when you have the most wonderful taste of a scrumptious food. I am the signal that you may want to slow waaaaay down and enjoy every tasty second to make each bite last.

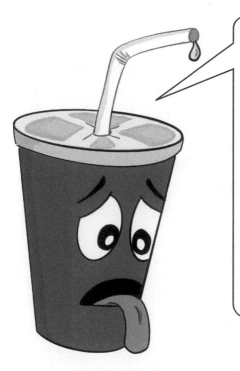

Greetings! I am

THIRSTY THEO!

I'm that feeling that you get in your mouth and throat when you really feel like you need to drink something – like lots of water. Since water makes everything all moist and sloshy, when your mouth feels very dry, it can be a signal you are thirsty. You may be surprised to know that if you get too thirsty you can get a headache or your muscles can ache. Drinking water can be an interesting investigation to try in lots of situations.

SECTION 2:
BODY INVESTIGATIONS

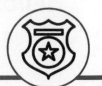

Paying attention to when you are hungry and when you are full can be very tricky. It takes practice. Luckily for us, we have an energy meter that can help us figure out when our bodies are telling us we need more energy. Check out the meter below!

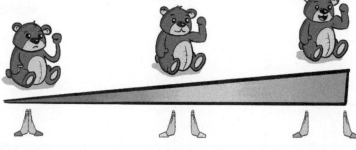

We can use our hands to show how our energy is changing when we do certain things (like run around) or eat different kinds of foods.

If you were very low on energy, like being a gas meter on empty, you would put your hands together just like this picture

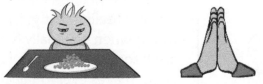

This creature has started to get fueled up! His energy is going up so he moves his hands wider and wider apart!

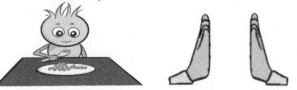

Whammo!! The creature is fully energized! Time to flex those muscles.

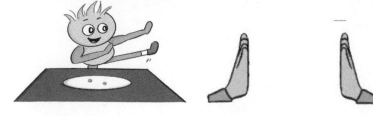

Our Body Clues Worksheets

Time to begin learning one of our secret tools: our Body Clues Worksheet. We will build on the worksheet below throughout your treatment sessions, so this is something we will use quite often!

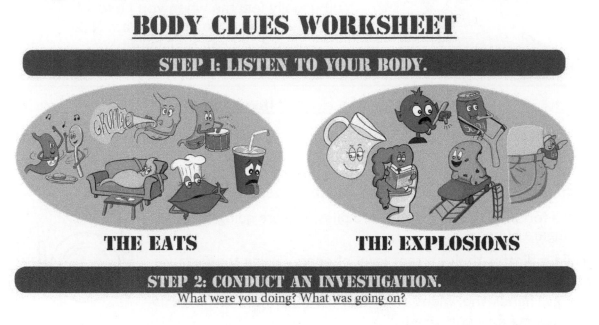

These worksheets can be used by anyone in the family (or even a family friend). The more people who fill out them out, the easier it will be for your child to learn how to fill them out themselves. Children learn a lot by watching others. This can also help the treatment work better for your child!

When someone notices a sensation in their body, and they are not quite sure what the sensation is, pull out a sheet! Then go through the sheet and ask about each of the sensations that we have learned about so far. Another way to practice is to fill out a sheet at the end of every day.

Were you feeling GERDA GOTTA GO? GASSY GUS? THIRSTY THEO? SABRINA STUFFED? HAROLD THE HUNGER PAIN? ... and so on. Think about the biggest, strongest sensations of the day or the high points and low points of the day and use those moments to guide the completion of a worksheet. Each worksheet will have a picture of every character we have learned. Circle all the characters your child notices (or that you notice in your own body).

For **Step 2**, write down or draw what you were doing before and/or during the sensation.

159

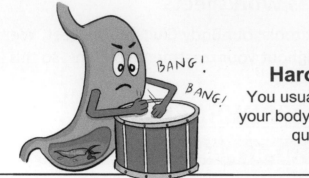

Harold the Hunger Pain
You usually feel me when you have let your body get way too hungry. I am NOT quiet and I can really hurt.

An Example of a Hunger Investigation

This week is all about hunger, thirst, fullness, and deliciousness. Here are some investigations you can try at home.

Note: As with all investigations, these are just suggestions. Children can be encouraged to come up with their own investigations and that may happen increasingly over time.

1. Pick out a food that is easy to split into piles. You are going to use it to investigate hunger.

2. The child indicates their current level of energy using the distance between their hands on their energy meter. Hands closed is equal to no energy, hands the widest they can be with muscles flexed is equal to feeling fully energized.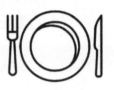

3. The child makes a prediction about how much food it will take to get fully energized. The parent can also make a prediction about how much food they think it will take for the child to become fully energized. In this way it is like a contest to see who is more accurate. Ideally, the parent will also do the investigation and make their own guesses about how much of the snack food it will take to get themselves fully fueled up. Similarly, the child can make a guess about how much it will take for the parent to get fueled up.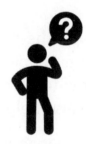

4. Divide the food up into piles. This way it is easy to remember to check in with everybody's energy level after consuming each pile.

5. Have parent and child consume a small pile of food. Then have them pause, check in with how their body is feeling in terms of their energy levels, and indicate their energy levels with their hands.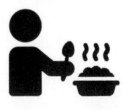

6. Continue this until everyone feels fully energized.

7. See whose guess was the closest.

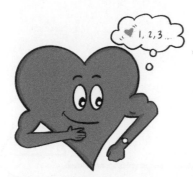

Henry the Heartbeat

I am a very powerful machine that pumps blood to all of the parts of your body. The harder you work, the more I pump.

Ideas for Henry Heartbeat Investigations

Here are some more ideas for some Henry Heartbeat investigations you can try at home!

1. What makes your heart beat faster, watching a scary movie clip (G-rated or child appropriate, of course), or running down the hall? What slows your heart down more, taking slow deep breaths or doing a stretch (like sitting on the floor and bending over to have your hands touch as far away from you on the floor as you can – a great back and shoulder stretch!)?

2. How long does it take to slow your heartbeat down after doing jumping jacks for 10 seconds? How about after you do jumping jacks for 20 seconds?

3. If you practice jumping jacks every day for 7 days, does your heart start beating more slowly than it did when we measured it before?

4. What about if you do it for 14 days? If it does, why do you think this is?

5. Does your heart beat faster when you are excited about something? Let's see!

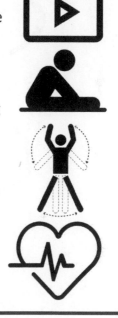

SECTION 3:
BODY MAP

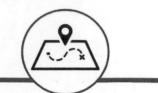

Now that you've finished your body investigation you can add what you learned to your Body Map! Wow! We learned so much about your hunger! What is the main message that you learned about your hunger?

It took me 4 bites to get a little bit energized!...I can get better at listening to my body's energy levels with practice.

It took me 10 bites to get fully energized!...My body can tell me that I need energy and when I'm fully energized.

⚡⚡⚡ Body Wisdoms of the Week
(Ways That My Body is Wicked Smart)

1. My body can tell me that I need energy and when I'm fully energized.
2. I can get better at listening to my body's energy levels with practice.
3. Feeling thirsty is a very unique sensation. It must be an important message.
4. Delicious food tastes even more delicious when you pay close attention to how the food tastes.

SECTION 4:
PRACTICES & TIPS

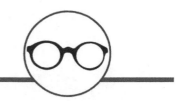

Practice of the Week

Pull out a Body Clues Worksheet after an intense moment and/or at the end of the day to review the high points and low points of the day. It would be great if every family member practiced this. Please bring your sheets to your next session.

Important Tip #1 for Parents

Feel like conducting some hunger, fullness, and deliciousness investigations at home? Here are some ideas.

1. Family members can monitor their energy levels during a meal.
2. Children can try to slow down their eating and see what happens to the deliciousness of the food (they can do ratings of food deliciousness before slowing down eating and afterwards).
3. If they feel extra full after a meal, the child can investigate what happens to Sabrina Stuffed if they go on a walk.
4. They can investigate how long the energy lasts from different meals. For example, if they had a fruit or vegetable with their meal, what is their energy like? How long does their energy last?

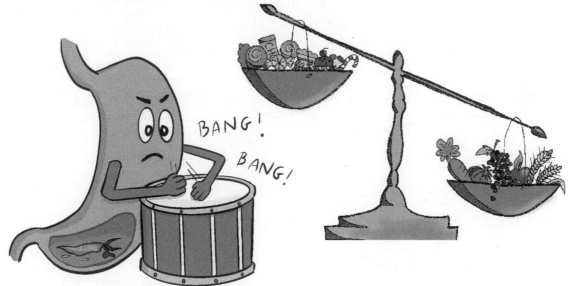

STEP 1: LISTEN TO YOUR BODY.

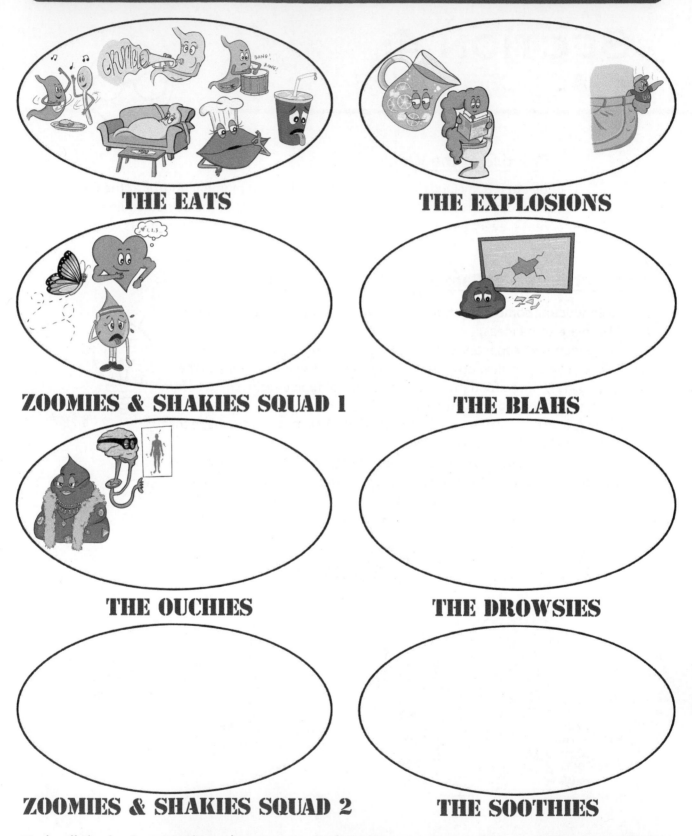

THE EATS

THE EXPLOSIONS

ZOOMIES & SHAKIES SQUAD 1

THE BLAHS

THE OUCHIES

THE DROWSIES

ZOOMIES & SHAKIES SQUAD 2

THE SOOTHIES

Circle all the body sensations that you are feeling. You can draw a few circles if you are feeling the feeling A LOT. Or, you can draw part of a circle if you are feeling the feeling a little bit.

STEP 2: CONDUCT AN INVESTIGATION.

<u>What were you doing? What was going on?</u>

FBI CHARACTER SHEET

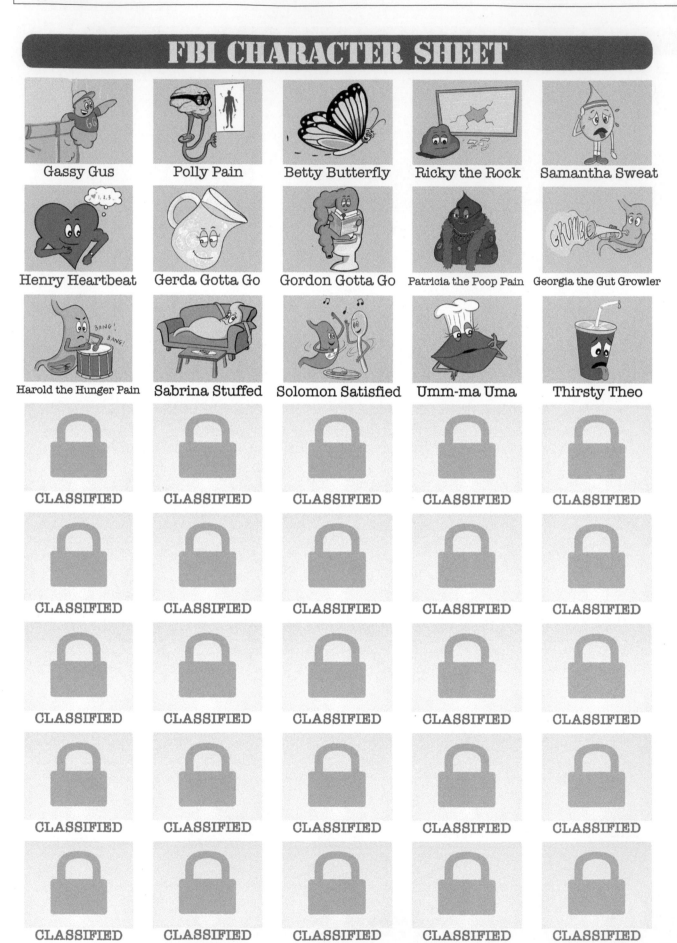

Gassy Gus

Polly Pain

Betty Butterfly

Ricky the Rock

Samantha Sweat

Henry Heartbeat

Gerda Gotta Go

Gordon Gotta Go

Patricia the Poop Pain

Georgia the Gut Growler

Harold the Hunger Pain

Sabrina Stuffed

Solomon Satisfied

Umm-ma Uma

Thirsty Theo

CLASSIFIED CLASSIFIED CLASSIFIED CLASSIFIED CLASSIFIED

CLASSIFIED CLASSIFIED CLASSIFIED CLASSIFIED CLASSIFIED

CLASSIFIED CLASSIFIED CLASSIFIED CLASSIFIED CLASSIFIED

CLASSIFIED CLASSIFIED CLASSIFIED CLASSIFIED CLASSIFIED

CLASSIFIED CLASSIFIED CLASSIFIED CLASSIFIED CLASSIFIED

FBI BODY BRAINSTORMS
PRACTICE 2

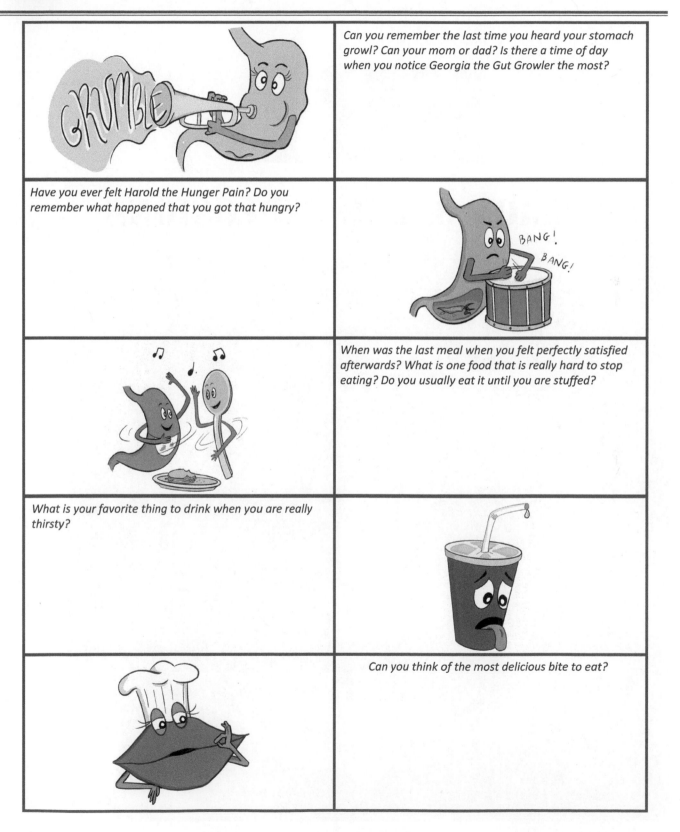

Can you remember the last time you heard your stomach growl? Can your mom or dad? Is there a time of day when you notice Georgia the Gut Growler the most?

Have you ever felt Harold the Hunger Pain? Do you remember what happened that you got that hungry?

When was the last meal when you felt perfectly satisfied afterwards? What is one food that is really hard to stop eating? Do you usually eat it until you are stuffed?

What is your favorite thing to drink when you are really thirsty?

Can you think of the most delicious bite to eat?

FBI

SESSION 3: THE EXPLOSIONS

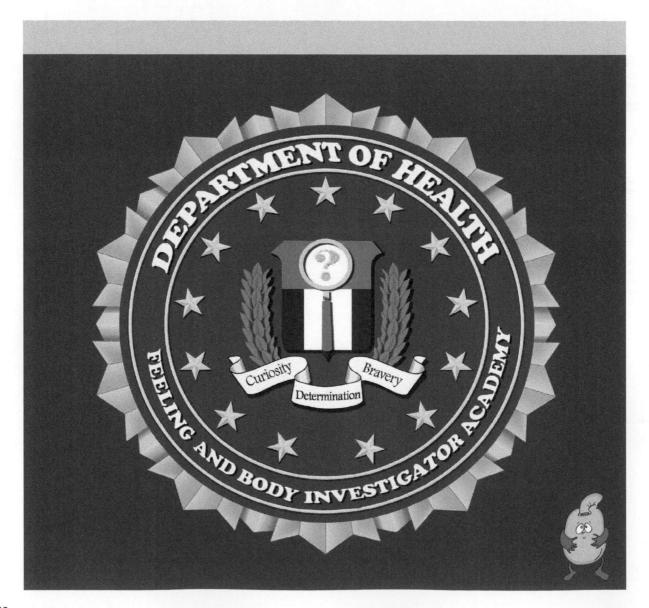

SECTION 1:
BACKGROUND CLUES

ABOUT EATING

Let's take a few seconds to come up with some answers to the following investigative questions.

1. Why do you think that bodies are designed so that they throw up?

2. Why do you think that we pass gas?

This week, we are going to learn about all the different things that can happen to food once you eat it. But first, let's meet a few more friends!

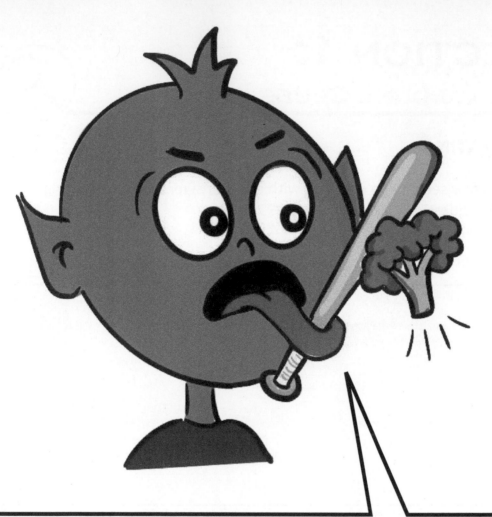

Hello! I'm GAGGY GREG!

I'm a reflex. Did you ever have a doctor hit your knee with a hammer and your foot flies up? That is kind of like me. If I sense something that feels a bit unexpected or unfamiliar, I may get activated and I try to protect you by gagging.

Once I get used to something, I stop. For kids with sensory superpowers, it just may take me a bit longer to get used to stuff, but I can and I will.

SECTION 2:
BODY MYSTERIES

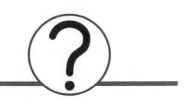

The First Meeting

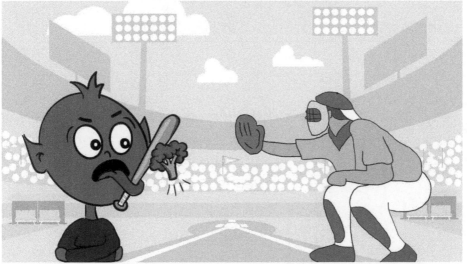

When first approached with a new or different taste, smell, or texture, GAGGY GREG's powerful initial reaction may be to gag - like his mouth is swatting the food away like a baseball batter.

The Tenth Meeting

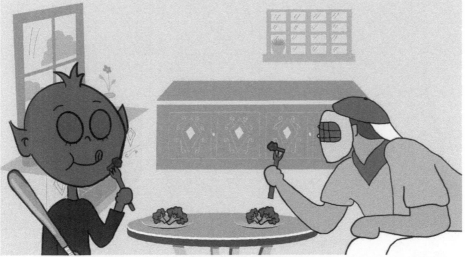

With repeated meetings, GAGGY GREG gets used to the new sensation so he knows what to expect. He may even start to like it. Who knows?

Hi FBI Agents and Chiefs! It's me, VICTOR VOMIT!

I know it might be hard to see me hidden underneath all of this barfed up food! I love action and adventure! For me, every time you throw up, I get to go on a super-speed roller coaster ride!! Whoo-eeee!!

That is what vomiting is. There are sensors throughout your body on the lookout for harmful substances. If the sensors detect something dangerous, the muscles of your stomach use ALL THEIR POWER, and with great FORCE and SPEED, force the bad things out of your stomach, back up your throat, and out of your mouth! Whammo!!! Vomit time!!!

For me, it is a super fun ride – but it may not be as fun for you!

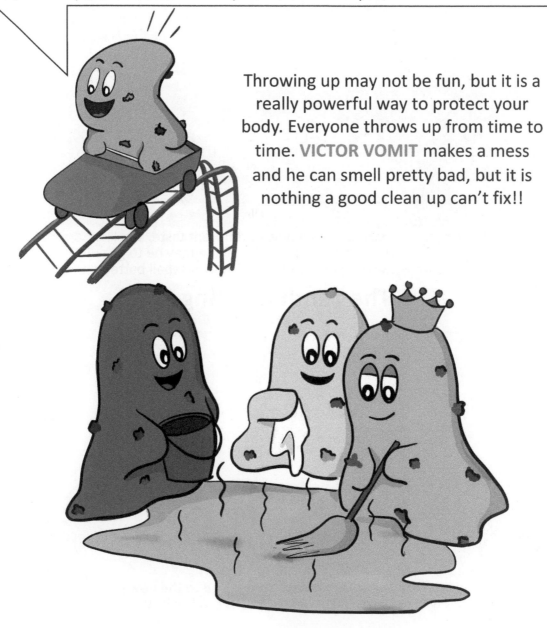

Throwing up may not be fun, but it is a really powerful way to protect your body. Everyone throws up from time to time. VICTOR VOMIT makes a mess and he can smell pretty bad, but it is nothing a good clean up can't fix!!

What Happens to Food Once You Eat It?

Your Digestive System is super cool!

Your **teeth and saliva** get the party started! They help break the food into smaller pieces so you can swallow.

Once you swallow, your food travels down your **esophagus**, or your throat. This is how the food travels from your mouth to your stomach.

After traveling down the esophagus, the food enters your **stomach**. Your stomach contains acid to break down the food even more and destroys the germs.

Other organs like your **liver**, pancreas, and gallbladder also help break down food.

The **small intestine** absorbs nutrients. It passes water and waste to the large intestine.

The **large intestine** absorbs water and makes waste.

Finally, the waste (poop!) exits through the **rectum**.

Digestion works much like a bowl of food being passed around the family dinner table: everyone takes what they need and passes on the rest. The organs of your digestive system take what they need and pass on the rest.

Why Do We Have Gas?

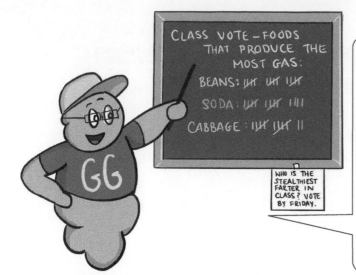

I'm back! It's good ole Gassy Gus! You may be wondering why you pass gas. Well, I'm so glad you asked! Some foods are too hard for your digestive system to break down. These food parts travel to your large intestine. There, the healthy bacteria that lines your intestine turns these food products into – you guessed it –

GASSY GUS!

Certain foods may cause a lot more of me than other foods. What foods give you gas? I love beans! Beans really love good ole Gassy Gus!!

What food gives you the most gas? Who passes the most gas in your family? Do you think it is what they eat or are they just a super gas-passer? I wonder what foods make farts the smelliest.

Have you ever drank a carbonated soda and then afterwards, you could not stop burping? If so, you and I are already old friends! Why I am

BURPY BERNIE!

I am often that noisy explosion that occurs when your body is trying to release some gas pressure that has built up. After burping, people sometimes feel a release of pressure like some air coming out of a balloon.

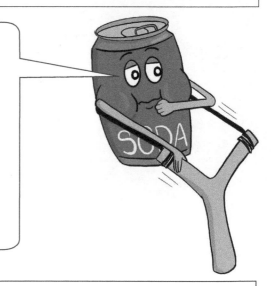

Does eating too quickly give you the burps? What about talking really fast? Do different types of carbonated beverages lead to different degrees of burping? Does being at a fancy dinner where you are expected to be polite and not burp actually make it harder to keep from burping? These are all very important investigations to try.

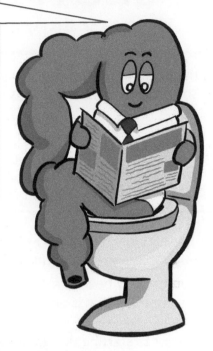

The Routine
GORDON GOTTA GO

Hi! I'm GORDON GOTTA GO!

Remember me? I'm that feeling you get when you have to go poo! I'm a body sensation that is a big fan of routines – but I also love surprises. Usually, there is a certain time of day when I may come visit you. For example, some people have a good poo every night before they go to bed. But, if I feel like I want to create some excitement, I may surprise you and show up when you least expect it! Yippeee!!! There's nothing I love more than a big poo surprise!!

The Surprised GORDON REALLY REALLY REALLY GOTTA GO

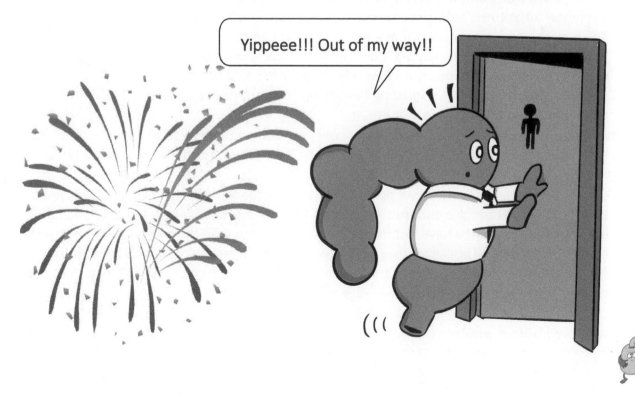

Yippeee!!! Out of my way!!

SECTION 3:
BODY INVESTIGATIONS

In this section, we will give you ideas about some body investigations that you can try at home. Some of these investigations may sound familiar as you may have already practiced them!

Gaggy Greg

I'm a reflex. Did you ever have a doctor hit your knee with a hammer and your foot flies up? That is kind of like me.

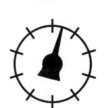

Gaggy Greg Body Investigation #1

Trying something that might be gross or just might be really different

1. In the jelly bean game, children combine both the experience of tasting something that is unexpected with the possibility of tasting something really disgusting.
2. Prior to starting this game, we get ready for the potential that everyone who plays might throw up. We get our garbage cans ready along with some napkins and Kleenex just in case.
3. Everyone takes turns and spins the spinner that comes with this game. The way the game is set up is that each color jellybean can have one of two flavors. One of these flavors is delicious and one is utterly disgusting. The player does not know which they are going to get until they taste it. Examples of disgusting flavors include barf, dog food, and stinky socks etc. You get the picture.

Playing this game is a great example about how your body protects you from things that you are not supposed to ingest. Furthermore, it does so in a funny way so that responses like our gag reflex can be viewed with awe rather than fear.

1. Of course, this investigation can be done with any challenging food – not just gross jelly beans! Have parents and children each pick a food that is manageable but challenging – ideally a food that they have not had before. For children who have sensory superpowers to new tastes or textures, this may be a new food. For those children who try new foods quite easily, family members can try this with a food from a highly unfamiliar cuisine.
2. Decide what your investigative approach is going to be: are you going to go all in and just take a bite or are you going to design baby steps to approach the food gradually? Either way, we observe whether Gaggy Greg shows up.

3. If Gaggy Greg shows up, perhaps design another investigation: come up with a routine that may help to shake it off. Maybe wiggle your body from your head to your toes? Once you have wiggled for a while and Gaggy Greg is off doing other things, approach the food again and see what happens to Gaggy Greg. Does Gaggy Greg get quieter? Louder?

Remember: as an FBI Agent, we are just curious about what happens. An investigation does not succeed or fail. We just learn something new.

Gaggy Greg Body Investigation #2: Embracing the Unexpected

What happens to something unexpected when you expect the unexpected? Does it become expected? We can have a lot of fun with this with Gaggy Greg.

1. Pick a new or challenging food.
2. Make a guess at what it will taste and feel like. Crunchy? Salty? Creamy? Sweet?
3. Make a plan for the unexpected: if you are way off in your predictions, is it time for celebration? Time to wipe off your tongue with a napkin?
4. Take a taste and see how off your predictions were. Then compare your strategies to embrace the unexpected. For example, you could compare shaking it off with rinsing your mouth out with water. Did Gaggy Greg show up with one strategy more than another?

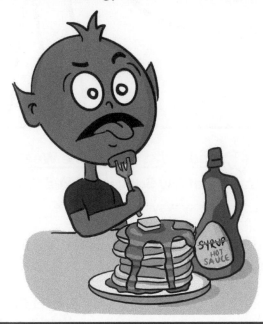

SECTION 4:
BODY MAP

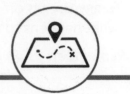

Now that you've finished your body investigation you can add what you learned to your body map! Wow! We learned so much about how your body handles eating and drinking! What are some of the main messages that you learned?

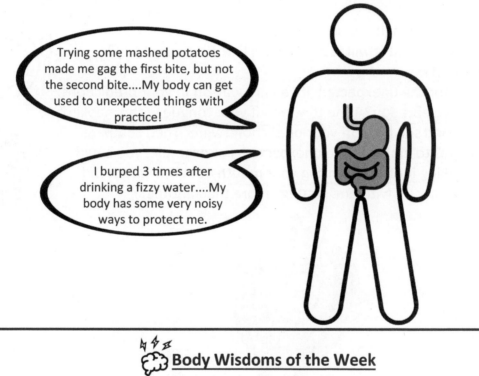

Trying some mashed potatoes made me gag the first bite, but not the second bite....My body can get used to unexpected things with practice!

I burped 3 times after drinking a fizzy water....My body has some very noisy ways to protect me.

Body Wisdoms of the Week
(Ways That My Body is Wicked Smart)

1. My body has some very noisy ways to protect me.
2. My body gives me lots of helpful warning signs.
3. My body can get used to unexpected things with practice!
4. My body has a lot of automatic things that it does that are trying to protect me from harm.
5. Sometimes my body is oversensitive and thinks something is harmful. At those times, I can give it several more tries and see if my body gets used to it and decides it is not harmful after all.
6. Certain foods may make me more gassy than others.
7. Certain foods may make my gas more smelly.
8. Eating things fast may make me burp.

SECTION 5:
PRACTICES & TIPS

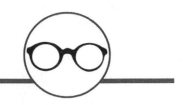

Important Tips for Parents

Sensations in our body communicate many things. Our job is to teach our children to be curious about what their body is telling them, but not afraid of it. Your Body Clues Worksheets are designed to help you and your child figure out what your bodies may be trying to communicate. Let's think of a few examples

- Feeling tired, weighted down, and slow may mean that you are feeling sad. Your sadness may be telling you that you need support and comfort.

- Feeling butterflies in the stomach, sweating, and feelign your heart beating may mean you are feeling anxious. Your anxiety may be telling you that there is potential danger and you should get prepared.

- Grumbling in your stomach may mean that you are hungry. Your hunger is telling you that you need to eat.

Because children are just learning how to read their body messages, they may sometimes confuse the different messages their body is sending them.

This sounds like a job for an FBI agent!

Our Body Clues Worksheet can help with this. Here are some questions to think about as you fill it out.

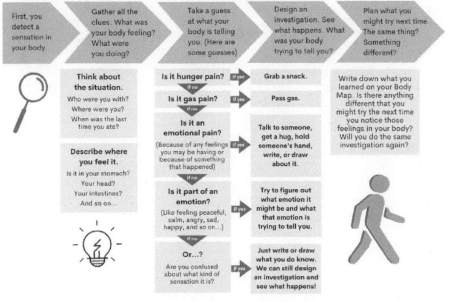

179

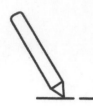

Practice of the Week

Feel like designing some investigations at home this week? Here are some ideas!

1. Come up with your own scale to measure the intensity of passing gas. Family members can post a chart on the refrigerator and everyone can mark their own intensity to determine who is the gas champion.

2. Children can try to add or subtract some foods that are supposed to be gassy and see whether that really effects the frequency, intensity, or smelliness of their farts.

3. If the children have a sensitive gag reflex to new tastes, they could see what happens to the intensity of their gag after they have had that food 1 time, 2 times, 3 times, etc.

4. See which beverage causes the most burping. Decide on at least two things that you are going to compare. Let's say lemonade versus a carbonated lemon drink. On one day, drink a glass of lemonade. Record how many burps you have for the next 60 (or whatever time you choose) minutes. On the next day, pour yourself the same amount of drink #2. Record your burps. See which drink wins!

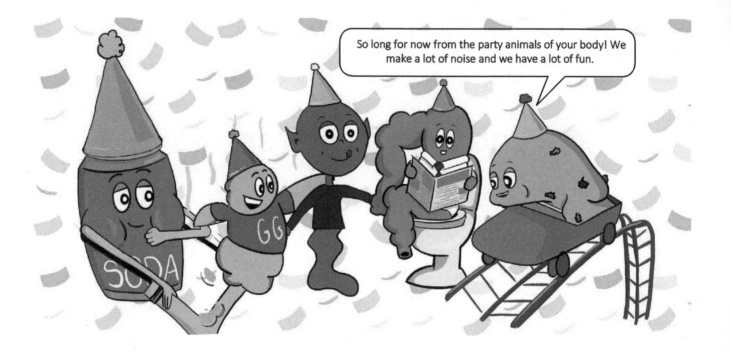

FBI BODY BRAINSTORMS
PRACTICE 3

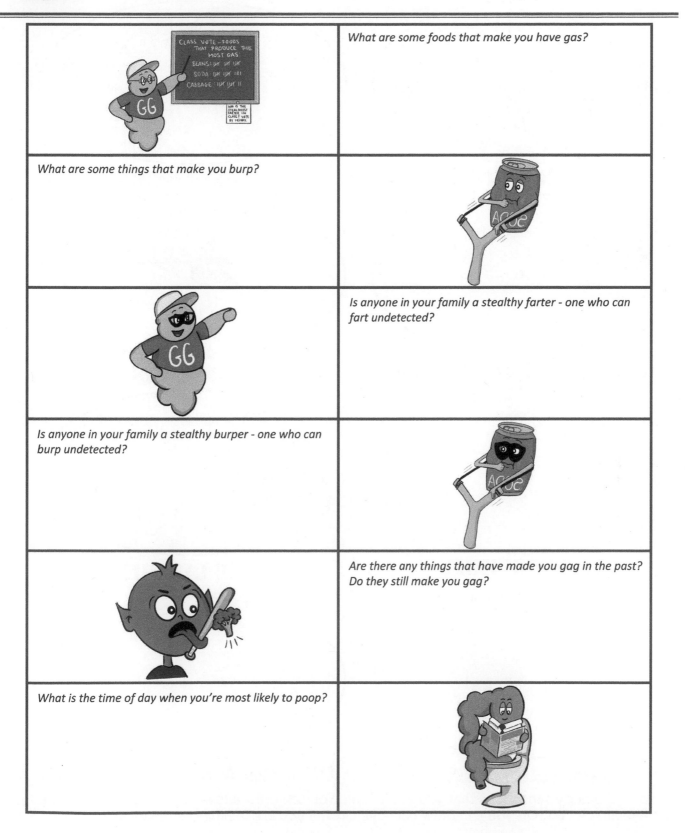

What are some foods that make you have gas?

What are some things that make you burp?

Is anyone in your family a stealthy farter - one who can fart undetected?

Is anyone in your family a stealthy burper - one who can burp undetected?

Are there any things that have made you gag in the past? Do they still make you gag?

What is the time of day when you're most likely to poop?

BODY CLUES WORKSHEET

STEP 1: LISTEN TO YOUR BODY.

THE EATS

THE EXPLOSIONS

ZOOMIES & SHAKIES SQUAD 1

THE BLAHS

THE SOOTHIES

THE OUCHIES

THE DROWSIES

ZOOMIES & SHAKIES SQUAD 2

Circle all the body sensations that you are feeling. You can draw a few circles if you are feeling the feeling A LOT. Or, you can draw part of a circle if you are feeling the feeling a little bit.

STEP 2: CONDUCT AN INVESTIGATION.
What were you doing? What was going on?

STEP 3: TAKE A GUESS AT WHAT THE SENSATION MAY MEAN.

Is it a feeling?

- I'm feeling excited.
- I'm feeling happy.
- I'm feeling scared.
- I'm feeling nervous.
- I'm feeling sad.
- I'm feeling disgusted.
- I'm feeling mad (at my friends, at my parents, at my teacher, at my siblings...).

Something else?

- I'm missing my parents
- I'm feeling lonely.
- I'm feeling tired.
- I'm feeling bored.
- I'm feeling hungry.
- I'm feeling hangry.
- I'm feeling calm.
- I'm feeling relaxed.
- I'm feeling sleepy.
- I'm feeling guilty.
- I'm feeling loving.

Is it a type of pain?

- It is gas pain.
- It is hunger pain.
- It is overstuffed pain.
- It is muscle pain.
- It is emotional pain.
- It is worry pain (from thinking too hard about something).

Or write or draw what you think the sensation means.

STEP 4: DESIGN AN INVESTIGATION AND SEE WHAT HAPPENS.

If you are feeling excited or happy
- Dance around!

If you are feeling scared or nervous
- Talk to someone.
- Take some slow, deep breaths and close your eyes.
- Count your butterflies as you face your fears.
- Do something that makes you laugh.

If you are feeling mad or disgusted
- Get your energy out and then make a plan.
- Do slow deep breathing and walk around.
- Make a firm but polite request about what you need.

If you are feeling sad or have emotional pain
- Get a hug from someone or hold someone's hand.
- Draw a picture or write about it.
- Snuggle with something.
- Make up a song about it.

If you are feeling loving
- Share that feeling with someone or something.

If you are feeling lonely or missing your parents
- Call or talk to someone.
- Write a letter.
- Play with an animal.

If you are feeling hunger pain or feeling hangry
- Eat.

If you are feeling overstuffed pain
- Lay on the couch.
- Go on a slow walk.

If you are feeling gas pain
- Go to the bathroom, or pass gas.

If you are feeling calm or relaxed
- Keep doing what you are doing! Make sure to write about it in your journal so you remember what things help you feel relaxed.

If you are feeling muscle pain
- Get someone to rub your muscles or your ears.
- Lay on a heating pad.
- Take a nice hot bath.

If it is a worry pain
- If you can do something about it, make a plan. If you can't do anything, boss your worry around!

If you are feeling guilty about something
- See if there is a problem that you need to fix.

If you are feeling bored
- Make a list of 50 things you can do (ask for help if you need it). You can use this list again later.

If you are feeling sleepy
- Rest.

Something else?

Write or draw what you tried, how it went, or what you are planning to try!

FBI CHARACTER SHEET

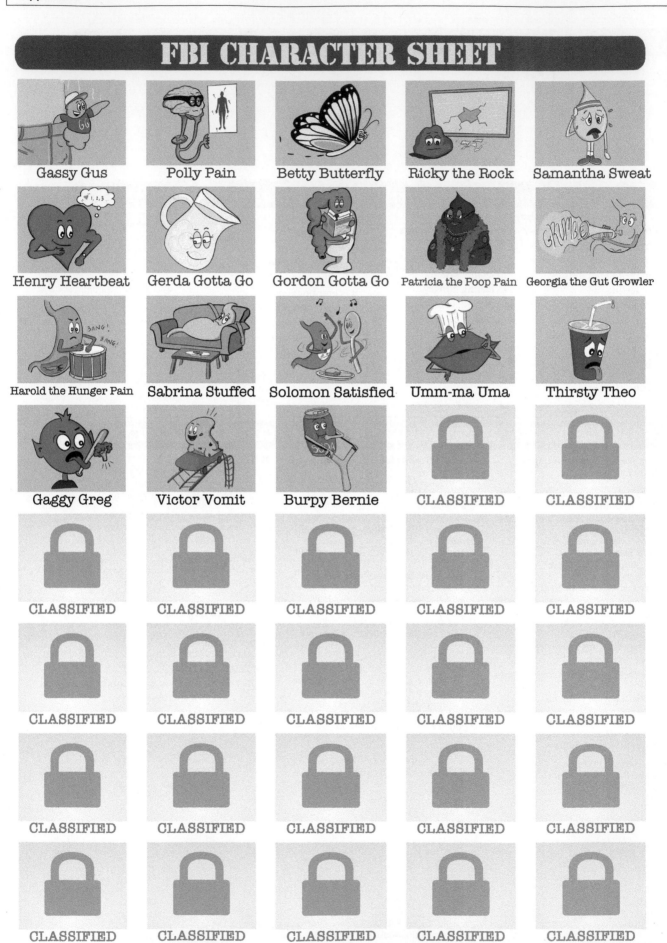

Gassy Gus	Polly Pain	Betty Butterfly	Ricky the Rock	Samantha Sweat
Henry Heartbeat	Gerda Gotta Go	Gordon Gotta Go	Patricia the Poop Pain	Georgia the Gut Growler
Harold the Hunger Pain	Sabrina Stuffed	Solomon Satisfied	Umm-ma Uma	Thirsty Theo
Gaggy Greg	Victor Vomit	Burpy Bernie	CLASSIFIED	CLASSIFIED
CLASSIFIED	CLASSIFIED	CLASSIFIED	CLASSIFIED	CLASSIFIED
CLASSIFIED	CLASSIFIED	CLASSIFIED	CLASSIFIED	CLASSIFIED
CLASSIFIED	CLASSIFIED	CLASSIFIED	CLASSIFIED	CLASSIFIED
CLASSIFIED	CLASSIFIED	CLASSIFIED	CLASSIFIED	CLASSIFIED

Index

abdomen, flat plate of the, 40
abdominal CT scan, 40
abdominal exam, 38
abdominal migraine, 3, 40
abdominal pain, 37
  children with, 2–3
  comprehensive history of, *38*
  diagnostic tests for chronic, 40
  diagnostic work-up and, 40
  differential diagnosis for acute,
    38–39
  differential diagnosis for chronic,
    39–40
  differential diagnosis of, 37
  evaluating, 37
  functional, 40
  history of in diagnosing the child,
    37–38
  physical examination and,
    37–38
  recurrent, 2
abdominal pain episodes, statistics
  for children and adolescents, 2
abdominal ultrasound, 40
absenteeism, chronic, 2
Achy Tummy, 99–100
adventures, seeking, 34–35
age group, selection of, 1–2
Ahhhh Annie, 123, 125, 127
Ainsworth, Mary, 22
  Ainsworth's Strange Situations
    Paradigm, 23
Alert Arnold, 127
Alert Arnold, 123, 125, 126–127
anal fistulae, 37
anxiety disorders, 2, 19, 32, 34
appendicitis, 37, 38
  perforated appendix, 38
arousal, 85
Asarnow, Lauren, 106
assignments
  eighth body investigation, 122
  fifth body investigation, 96
  first body investigation, 52
  fourth body investigation, 87
  home-based, 96
  ninth body investigation, 127
  second body investigation, 64
  seventh body investigation, 114
  sixth body investigation, 104
  third body investigation, 77
asthma, 39

belching. *See* burp
Betty Butterfly, 10, 19, 50, 81, 82,
    108, 114
  and Mind-Racing Mikella, 112

Blah Bertha, 11, 89, 91, 93–94, 96,
    108, 109, 130
  ideas for, 94
Blahs, the, 7, 91
  body lessons from, 94
bloating, IBS and, 39
blood
  gross blood in stool, 39
  in stool, 39
  occult blood in stool, 39
blood count, complete, 40
body
body brainstorms, 7, 62, 72, 87, 96,
    104, 106, 114, 122, 127
Body Brainstorms of the Week, 96,
    104, 114
body brainstorms worksheet, 49, 51,
    61, 87, 103, 104, 122
  first, 52
body characters
  Betty Butterfly, 50
  Gassy Gus, 49
  Henry Heartbeat, 50
  learning about, 49
  Polly the Pain, 50
  Ricky the Rock, 50
  Samantha Sweat, 50
  sheet, 129
body clues, 106
Body Clues worksheets, 14–16, 66,
    79, 87, 96, 122
  as a reviewing tool, 35
  as an activity tool, 36
  completed step 3, *75*
  during FBI intervention, 26
  final, 129
  how to use the, *26*
  introduction to, 62
  parents use of, 103
  reviewing characters on the, 33
  step 1, 19, 62–63, *63*
  step 2, *16*, 63–64
  step 3, *17*, 72–73, *74*
  step 4, 73–77
  steps 4 and 5, *18*
  time with parents and caregivers,
    84
  tips for parents practicing, 85–86
  use of, 7
  using the, 35
body investigation assignment
  eighth, 122
  fifth, 96
  fourth, 87
  ninth, 127
  second, 64
  seventh, 114

sixth, 104
third, 77
body investigation journal, 64, 77, 87,
    96, 104, 114, 122, 127
body investigations, 6, 19, 34–35, 106
  assignment for first, 52
  Betty Butterfly and Mind-Racing
    Mikella visits and, 112
  Blah Bertha, 93–94
  Bursting Bella, 121
  butterflies and, 82–83
  components of, *35*
  Cozy Celeste, 113
  designing, 35
  dramatic enactment of, 82
  eating gross foods, 71
  Ella the Emotional Pain, 100
  Emotional Wave and, 86
  Empty Eliza, 94
  energy meter and, 59–60
  gag reflex, 71
  Gaggy Greg, 72
  gas pain, 103
  getting queasy, 92–93
  Harriet the Headache, 102
  Henry the Heartbeat, 51
  home-based, 103–104
  homemade, 29
  in bed, 112
  integrating with Body Clues
    worksheets, *85*
  in-the-moment, 97
  Julie Jitters, 84
  Mind-Racing Mikella, 83
  Ouchies, the, 99–100
  Patricia the Poop Pain, 102, 103
  power of sore muscles, 101
  practice at home, 64, 77, 114, 122,
    127
  Ricky the Rock, 92
  saving joyous moments, 121
  step 4, *75*
  stretched-out Comfortable Cayla
    Body Investigation, 113
  Stuck Stephanie and, 112
  the Drowsies, 108
  thirst quenching contest and, 126
  tips for parents, 85–86
  to practice at home, 96, 131
  worksheets, 113, 132
body journal, 35, 58, 121, 122, 123
body lessons, 35
  from the Blahs, 94
  from the Eats, 60, 61
  from the Explosions, 72
  from the Ouchies, 103
  from the Soothies, 127

from the Zoomies, 84
session 2, 61
body map, 7, 35
  adding lessons to, 61
  adding to, 117
  adding to the, 8, 52, 56–57, 61,
    67–68, 72, 79, 87, 94, 97, 103,
    108, 113, 122, 124, 127, 130
  adding to their, 91
  creating the, 48–49
  review homework, 124
body mystery questions
  session 4, 80
  session 5, 91
  session 6, 98
  session 7, 108
  session 8, 117
  session 9, 124
body sensation characters, 14, *15*, 59,
    91, 98–99
  session 7, *108–110*
  session 9, 124–125
Body Sensation Characters, 6
body sensations, 6
  investigations for bedtime, *113*
  investigations of, 33–34
  misinterpreting, 32–33
  session 2 and, 54
Body Sensations Characters, *80*
Body Sensations experiences, 68
body trust, 2
Bouncy Bart Butt, 8
bowel movements. *See also* Gordon
  Gotta Go
Brenda the Brain, 98, 99
  and Gassy Gus and Henry
    Heartbeat, *99*
burp, 39, 70, *72*
  lessons from, 72
Burpy Bernie, 70
Bursting Bella, 14, 116, 118, 121,
    122, 130
  body investigations, 121
butterflies. *See also* Betty Butterfly
  ideas for, 83
butterflies, gut indicator of, 10

calm, staying, 27–29
Cannon, Walter, 10
caregivers. *See* parents
Celebration, The, *7*
celiac disease, 39
central nervous system (CNS), 19
Centrality of Events scale, 20
challenging situations, 35–36
characters
  session 8, 117–119

Cheery Cathy, 123, 127
  bringing to others, 126
  smiles and, 126
child/children
  and parent did no homework, 68
  effect of abdominal pain on, 2–3
  Emotional Wave and, 84–85
  introducing FBI-Pain Division
    to, 48
  primary caregiver relationship, 22
  validating experience of, 19, 25–26
chronic absenteeism, 2
classroom activities, online, 132
classroom implementation, 131–132
Comfortable Cayla, 107, 110, 111,
    112
  Body Investigation, 113
  Sore Muscle Stan and, 111
  stretched-out investigation, 113
comorbid psychopathology, 19
complete blood count, 40
conjunctivitis, 39
constipation, 37, 38, 39, 40
  Celiac disease and, 39
  IBS and, 39
Cool Cyrus, 107, 109, 110, 114
  investigating, 112
Cozy Celeste, 107, 109, 110, 112, 114
  body investigations, 113
Craske, Michelle, 34
C-reactive protein (CRP), 40
Crying Cassie, 116

Dancing Darrin, 14, 116, 119, 120
  ideas for, 120
danger, 10
Dark Debra, 107, 108, 110
  investigating, 112
Day-Dreamy David, 123, 124, 127
Diabetes Mellitus, Type I, 39
diarrhea, 37, 38, 39, 40
  appendicitis and, 38
  food poisoning and, 39
  gross or occult blood in, 39
  IBD and, 39
  IBS and, 39
difficult moments, dealing with, 104
digestion, 10
disgust, experience of, 67
disorders
  gut-brain axis, 3–5
  major depressive, 78
distress, undifferentiated, 23–24
diverse mindsets, 11
Drossman, Douglas A., 20
Drowsies, the, 7
  body investigations, 108
  lessons from, 114
  session 7, 108
dysuria, 38, 39

Eats, The, 6, 54
Ella the Emotional Pain, 33, 97, 98,
    100, 103, 104, 130
  sensory superpowers of, 101–103
emotional experience, organization
    framework of, 79
Emotional Wave, 80
  Body Clues worksheet and, 84
  body investigations and, 86
  dialogue for introducing to
    parents, 86
  scenario of, 84–85
emotions, 10–11, 78–79
  awareness of, 15
  intense, 86

Empty Eliza, 92, 94, 96, 106, 109
  body investigations and, 94
Energy Ball, 120
energy meter, 55, 59–60, 59, 65, 80,
    106, See also energy
  and new characters, 132
energy, assessing your, 68, 80, 91, 97,
    108, 117, 124, 130
enteric nervous system (ENS), 19
Ernie the Energy Ball, 116, 118, 120,
    121
eructation. See burp
Explosions, the, 66, 68
  body lessons from, 72

family-level suffering, 2
FBI agents, 1, 11–12, 85, 96
  Body Clues worksheets and, 17
  body sensations and, 15, 16, 32,
    33–34
  challenges for, 12
  children as, 14, 129
  conditioning of, 14
  elite, 11, 32, 104, 112
  exercise and, 110
  importance of understanding
    sleep, 107
  job as, 2
  optimum conditions for sleep, 112
  pain and, 102
  Pain division, 8, 33
  parents as, 23
  Polly the Pain and, 100
  self-reflections and, 20
  Victor Vomit and, 69–70
  vocabulary of pain, 33
FBI characters
  Betty Butterfly, 10
  FBI character sheet, 16
  Henry Heartbeat, 10
  Julie Jitters, 10
  Samantha Sweat, 10
FBI intervention, 26
  beginning of, 1
  parents and, 28
FBI investigator, 113, See also FBI
    agents
  path to being an, 15
FBI via telehealth, 131
FBI-ARFID, 25, 61
FBI-Pain Division program, 2, 10,
    25, 29
  accomplishments for the family,
    132–133
  adaptation for online, 131
  aim of, 13
  as an asset, 9
  body investigations and, 19
  children not going through, 107
  components of, 6–7, 6–8
  disorders of Gut-Brain
    Interactions, 5
  explanation of, 43
  intervention, 107
  introducing children to, 48
  introduction of parent to, 44
  introduction to the framework,
    44–48
  Mind-racing Mikella and, 83
  online communities, 129
  outline for session 1, 43
  parenting styles and, 90
  parents and, 29–31
  special forces task force, 107–108
  take-home message, 44
  threat hypervigilance and, 123

  use of fear in, 32
fear, 10
  gut indicators of, 10
Feeling and Body Investigator
    Academy, 46
Feeling and Body Investigators
    program
  beginning of, 1
  clinical trial of, 102
  FBI agents, 1
  users of the program, 1
fever, 37, 38, 39
firmness, 95
flat plate of the abdomen, 40
Focused Frankie, 123, 127
Focused Frieda, 125, 126
focusing contest, 126
follow-up, 131
food. See also Eats, the
  as fuel, 54–55, 57–58
  digestion, 70
  digestion of, 66–67
  eating gross, 71
  enjoying, 61
food poisoning, 39
freeze tag, 120
fueling up. See energy, assessing your
fullness
  hunger and, 57
  noticing, 59
functional abdominal pain. See also
    abdominal pain
  not otherwise specified, 3
Functional Gastrointestinal
    Disorders, 3

gag, 67, 77, See also Gaggy Greg
  as a protective process, 66–67
  gag reflex, 69, 71, 77
Gaggy Greg, 66, 69, 71
  surprises, 72
gas pain, 103
Gassy Gus, 8, 26, 33, 49, 70
  and Henry Heartbeat and Brenda
    the Brain, 99
  exercise routine, 112
  vs Henry Heartbeat exercise
    routine, 108
gastroenteritis, 39
gastroesophageal reflux disease
    (GERD), 39
gastrointestinal (GI) sensations, 66
gastrointestinal disorders, 3, 20
  nosology for diagnosing, 3
gastrointestinal pain, 26
  over-simplified conceptualizations
    of, 19
gastrointestinal symptom onset, 4
gastrointestinal tract, 10
Georgia the Gut Growler, 58, 62
GERD (Gastroesophageal Reflux
    Disease), 39
Gerda Gotta Go, 51
giardia
  stool for antigen test, 40
Giardia infection, 40
Giggling Gena, 116, 118, 120, 121,
    122
  singing and dancing with, 120
gluten sensitivity, 39
good-bye, options for, 131
Gordon Gotta Go, 51, 70–71
graduation ceremony, the, 130
Groovies and Shakies, the, 6
group implementation, 131–132
growth chart, 37, 40

guessing game, 23
gut. See also gut-brain axis
gut, impact of stress on the, 17–18
gut-brain axis, 3, 19, 20
  communication, 17–18
  conceptualizing disorders of, 3–5
  disorders of, 3, 4, 5, 9
  probe of, 5
  stressful life events and, 17
gut-brain interaction. See gut-brain
    axis

Harold the Hunger Pain, 33, 58, 97,
    98
Harriet the Headache, 33, 97, 99, 102,
    103, 104
  body investigations and, 102
Harvey, Allison, 106
headaches, 40, 102, See also Harriet
    the Headache
hematochezia, 39
hematuria, 39
Henry Heartbeat, 6, 10, 35, 50, 80, 82,
    107, 114, 123
  activity, 36, 68
  activity for a group, 132
  before bed exercise routine
    investigation, 110–111
  exercise routine, 110, 111
  first body investigations, 51
  ideas for investigations, 56, 67
  investigations, 35, 51, 56, 67, 79,
    82, 111, 123
  warm-up activity, 56, 67, 79, 90, 97,
    108, 117, 124, 130
  warm-up exercise, 66
hepatosplenomegaly, 38
home assignment
  first body investigation, 52
  session 2, 64
  session 3, 77
homework, 132
  child and parent did not do, 68
  parent and child and the, 68
  review, 56–57
homework review, 67–68
  session 10, 130
  session 4, 79
  session 5, 91
  session 7, 108
  session 8, 117
hunger, 55
  feelings of, 55–56
  fullness and, 57
  noticing, 58
hunger investigation, example of, 60

IgA serum, 40
Inflammatory Bowel Disease (IBD),
    39
interoceptive exposures, 33–34, 82
  acceptance-based, 34
  body investigation activities, 34
intuitive decisions/decision-making,
    17–19
  as a sensory superpower, 10
Irritable Bowel Syndrome (IBS), 39

Jelly Belly BeanBoozled® game, 71, 71
jitters. See also Julie Jitters
  getting the, 84
Julie Jitters, 10, 11, 80, 87, 107, 112
  bedtime routine and, 110

Keefe, Frank, 20
knee-jerk fear reaction, 13, 14

LaBar, Kevin, 33
lactose intolerance, 39
Laughing Pain Lulu, 116, 118, 121
Lawrence the Laughing Pain, 33
LeDoux, Joseph, 32
liver function tests, 40
logic line, 28
Lulu the Laughing Pain, 121

major depressive disorder, 78
malaise, 39
malrotation, 39
mass/masses
    abdominal, 38
    non-stool, 38
    palpable, 39
Mayer, Emeran, 17
    *Mind-Gut Connection and the
    Gut-Immune Connection*, 19
medical community, 19–20
    self-reflections, 20
memories, 32, 34, 101, 104, 116, 126,
    132
    creating new, 34–36
    joyful, 121
memory game, 130–131
    memory card game, *131*
mesenteric adenitis, 38
metabolic panel, 40
Miller Endowed Chair at the
    University of California, Los
    Angeles, 34
*Mind-Gut Connection and the
    Gut-Immune Connection*
    (Mayer), 19
Mind-Racing Mikella, 2, 81, 83, 87,
    99, 106, 107, 110, 114, 126
    and Betty the Butterfly, 112
    ideas for, 83
    sleep and, 107–108
Muscle Pain Michael, 97
muted sensibilities, 9

National Institutes of Health, United
    States, 1
nausea, 38, 39, 40, 66, 67, 70, 92–93,
    See also Nauseous Ned
    gut indicator of, 10
Nauseous Ned, 91, 92–93, 94, 96
    ideas for, 93
Noisies, The, *7*

obesity, pediatric, 55
obstruction, malrotation with, 39
online implementation, 131
    classroom activities, 132
Oppenheimer Center for
    Neurobiology of Stress at the
    University of California, 17
Ouchies, the, *7*, 97
    body investigations, 99–100
    body lessons from, 103
    meeting, 98–99
ovarian torsion, 39

pain
    as a threatening experience, 32
    diurnal pattern to, 35
    experiences of, 20, 79, 114
    fear avoidance model of, *13*
    maladaptive fear conditioning
    from, *12*
    measuring, 102
    memory of, 32
    parents' journey of, 29–31
    reducing experiences of, 1

session 6 overview, 97
    vocabulary of, 33
Pain Prevention Research Program,
    Duke University, 20
pancreatitis, 39
panic disorder, 32
parenting, 96, *See also* self-parenting
    depiction of challenges of, *23*
    FBI style, 90
    FBI-Pain division and responsive,
    26
    responsive, 22–24, 31
    sensory superpowers and, 26
parenting styles, 29, 90, 106
    authoritarian, 95
    FBI, 90
    permissive, 95
parents
    and child activities, 87
    and child and the homework, 68
    and child confidence and belief
    strategy, 35
    and child did no homework, 68
    and child high intensity moments,
    29
    and child interaction, 22
    as FBI agent, 23
    designing home-based body
    investigations, 103–104
    dialogue for introducing the
    Emotional Wave, 86
    introduction to the framework
    of the FBI-Pain Division to,
    44–48
    parenting styles and,
    reflection and, 44
    responsive, 29
    session 1 and introduction to FBI-
    Pain Division, 44
    time with, 84
    tips for practicing Body Clues
    worksheets, 85–86
Patricia the Poop Pain, 33, 51, 97, 99,
    102, 103, 132
    Ouchies and, 103
pediatric obesity, 55
Peptic Ulcer Disease (PUD), 40
perception, 14, 33
    sensory superpowers, 11–14
    shaping, 13–16
perforated appendix. *See*
    appendicitis:perforated
    appendix
peri-anal fistulae, 39
permissive parenting, 95
Perry, Lisa, 20
pharyngitis, 39
physical exam
    abdominal pain and, 37–38
    features to consider in a, *38*
physical sensations, 1
physician-patient relationships, 20
Pleasantville, 9
    Pleasantville trap, 9
pneumonia, 39
Polly the Pain, 19, 33, 35, 50, 97,
    99–100, 103, 132
polydipsia, 39
polyphagia, 39
polyuria, 39
poop questions. *See also* stool
post-ingestion symptoms, 64
sensory superpowers, 101–103
primary care practice, 132
primary caregiver, child relationship,
    22

prizes, 52, 54, 64, 66, 77, 78, 87, 89,
    96, 97, 104, 106, 122, 127, 130
    for session 1, 52
    session 1, 52
protection, 11
psychoeducation, 33
psychological interventions, 33
puberty, 39, 129
    onslaught of, 2

queasy. *See also* nausea; Nauseous
    Ned
questions and answers
    for session 1, 53
    for session 10, 131
    for session 2, 65
    for session 3, 77
    for session 4, 87–88
    for session 5, 96
    for session 6, 105
    for session 7, 114
    for session 8, 122
    for session 9, 127

rage, 11
rash/rashes, 38, 39
recurrent abdominal pain (RAP), 3
reflections
    for session 1, 52
    for session 2, 64
    for session 3, 77
    for session 4, 87
    for session 5, 96
    for session 6, 104
    for session 7, 114
    for session 8, 117
    for session 9, 127
    moment of, 46
    time for, 22, 59
relaxing sensations, awareness of, 85
Ricky the Rock, 19, 35, 50, 89, 91, 94
    body investigation, 92
Rome Foundation, 3, 20
ROME IV classification system, 3

Sabrina Stuffed, 59
safety
    exploration and, 29
    importance of, 22
    staying calm and, 27–29
    the experience of, 22–24
safety signals, over-reaction to, 32
Samantha Sweat, 10, 50, 82
saving joyous moments, 121
scary sensations, 14, 33
    detoxing, 14
sedimentation rates (ESR), 40
self-attunement, processes of, 19
self-awareness, 15–16
self-parent
    children learning to, *24*, 24
self-parenting
    parent's own, *27*
self-reflections, 20, 31
    FBI agents and, 16
self-trust, building, 16–17
Selyve, Hans, 18
Sensation Wave, *28*
sensations
    high arousal, positive, 116
    of happiness and joy, 116
sensitivity, as an asset, 10
sensory superpowers, 6, 9, 22, 30,
    32–33, 60, 114, 126, 132
    body investigations and, 35
    detecting threats and, 69

eating and, 66, 71
emotional pain and, 100
intuitive decision-making as a, 10
invincible children and, 129
joyous emotions and, 116
learning from fear, *45*
parenting a child with, 26, 29, 89,
    106
perception and, 11–14
recurrent pain and, 106
remembering beautiful moments
    and, 124
self-awareness and, 16
staying calm with, 27
trusting, *46*
session 1
    final reflection, 52
    home assignment, 52
    material for, 43
    outline, 43
    parent introduction to FBI
    framework, 44
    prizes, 52
    questions and answers, 53
    take-home materials from, 52
    therapist and, 43–44
session 10
    adding to their body map, 130
    background information, 129–130
    follow-up, 131
    Henry Heartbeat warm-up activity,
    130
    materials for, 129, 131
    outline, 129
    overview, 129
    questions and answers for, 131
    review homework, 130
    therapist reminders for, 131
session 2
    adding to the body map, 56–57, 61
    background information for,
    54–55
    body brainstorms, 62
    Body Clues worksheet, step 2,
    63–64
    Body Clues worksheets, 62
    Body Clues worksheets, step 1,
    62–63
    body lessons learned, 61
    final reflection for, 64
    guide to, 54–55
    home assignment, 64
    home-based practice, 64
    materials for, 54, 64
    outline, 54
    overview of, 54
    questions and answers for, 65
    reflection on, 59
    review homework, 56–57
    the workbook, 57
    therapist reminders for, 64
session 3
    adding to the body map, 67–68, 72
    body brainstorms, 72
    Body Clues worksheets, step 3,
    72–73
    Body Clues worksheets, step 4,
    73–77
    body investigations to practice at
    home, 77
    body mystery questions, 69–71
    digestion and, 66–67
    home assignment, 77
    materials, 77
    materials for, 66
    outline, 66

session 3 (*cont.*)
  overview of, 66
  questions and answers for, 77
  reflection for, 77
  review homework, 67–68
  therapist reminders for, 77
  warm-up Henry Heartbeat activity, 67
  workbook, 68
session 4
  adding to their body map, 79
  background information for, 78–79
  body brainstorms, 87
  body investigation journal, 87
  body investigations at home, 87
  body mystery questions, 80
  guide to, 79
  Henry Heartbeat warm-up activity, 79
  homework review, 79
  materials for, 78, 87
  outline, 78
  overview, 78
  questions and answers for, 87–88
  reflections for, 87
  therapists reminders for, 87
  workbook, 80–81
session 5
  adding to the body map, 91
  adding to their body map, 94
  assessing your energy, 91
  background information, 89–90
  body investigations to practice at home, 96
  body mystery questions, 91–92
  Henry Heartbeat warm-up activity, 90
  materials for, 89, 96
  outline, 89
  overview, 89
  questions and answers for, 96
  reflection for, 96
  review homework, 91
  workbook, the Blahs, 91
session 6
  adding to their body map, 103
  background information for, 97
  body investigation assignment, 104
  body investigation journal, 104
  body investigations to practice at home, 104
  body mystery questions, 98
  Henry Heartbeat warm-up activity, 97
  materials for, 97, 104
  outline, 97
  overview, 97
  questions and answers for, 105
  reflection for, 104
  therapist reminders for, 104
  workbook, 98
session 7
  adding to their body map, 108, *113*
  assessing your energy, 108
  background information, 106
  body brainstorms, 114
  body investigation assignment, 114
  body investigation Journal, 114

body investigations to Practice at Home, 114
body mystery questions, 108
body sensation characters, *108–110*
Comfortable Cayla investigation, *113*
Drowsies body investigations, 108
guide to, 108
Henry Heartbeat warm-up activity, 108
homework review, 108
materials for, 106, 114
outline, 106
overview, 106
questions and answers for, 114
reflection for, 114
stretched-out Comfortable Cayla Body Investigation, 113
the Drowsies, 114
therapists reminders for, 114
workbook, 108
session 8
  adding to the body map, 122
  background information for, 116–117
  body brainstorms, 122
  Body Clues worksheets, 122
  body investigation assignment, 122
  body investigation journal, 122
  body investigations, 121
  body mystery questions, 117
  guide to, 117–120
  Henry Heartbeat warm-up activity, 117
  materials for, 116, 122
  outline, 116
  overview, 116
  questions and answers for, 122
  reflection, 117
  review homework, 117
  therapist reminders for, 122
  workbook, 117
session 9
  adding to the body map, 127
  Alert Arnold, 126–127
  background information, 123
  body brainstorms, 127
  body investigation assignment, 127
  body investigation journal, 127
  body mystery questions, 124
  Cheery Cathy, 126
  focusing contest, 126
  materials for, 123, 127
  outline, 123
  overview, 123
  questions and answers for, 127
  reflection for, 127
  Slow-Thinking Stewart, 126
  Soothies, the, 124
  therapist reminders for, 127
  thirst quenching contest, 126
  workbook, 124
sexual dysfunction, 28
Shakies, the, 7, 28, 80–81, 116, 117, 121
  body investigations, 117
  body lessons from, 84
Shelby, Rebecca, 28
short stature, 39

Simon says, 120
singing, 120
sleep, 106
  background information for session 7 and, 106
  before bed exercise routine investigation, 110–111
  promote restorative, 112
  scenario number one, 107
  scenario number two, 107–108
Sleep Match Ups, 108
Sleepy Steven, 107, 108, 110, 111, 112
Slow-Thinking Stewart, 123, 125, 126, 127
slurp, and burp, *72*
smiles, 126
snuggle propensity, 27
Solomon Satisfied, 59
Soothies, the, 7, 124
  Body investigations, 126
  body lessons from, 127
Sore Muscle Stan, 33, 98, *101*, 103, 104, 106, 117
  exercise routine, 111
  sleep and, 107
  vs Gassy Gus stretching routine, 108
sore muscles, power of, 101
sore throat, 38
stature, short, 39
stool, 38, 39
  blood in, 38
  gross blood in, 39
  occult blood in, 39
stool, for giardia antigen, 40
Strange Situation Test, 22
strep test, 40
streptococcal pharyngitis, 37, 39
stress, definition of, 18
Stressed-Out Stella, 81, 84, 87
Stuck Stephanie, 108, 110
  getting unstuck from, 112
superpowers, 48
  detecting threats and sensory, 69
  eating and sensory, 66
  emotional pain and sensory, 100
  intuitive decisions and, 17–19
  joyous emotions and, 116
  parenting a child with sensory, 26, 29, 89, 106
  power of sensory, 101–103
  recurrent pain and sensory, 106
  remembering beautiful moments with sensory, 124
  sensory, 6, 11–14, 16, 22, 30, 32–33, 35, *45*, 60, 126
  staying calm with sensory, 27
  trusting sensory, *46*
  visceral hypersensitivity as, 11
  visceral sensitivity as, 9–10

Tearful Tasha, 116, 117, 119, 121, 130
tenderness, 38
therapists
  dialogue about letting go, 119
  reminders for session 10, 131
  reminders for session 2, 64
  reminders for session 3, 77
  reminders for session 4, 87

reminders for session 5, 96
reminders for session 6, 104
reminders for session 7, 114
reminders for session 8, 122
reminders for session 9, 127
session 1 and, 43–44
thinking. *See also* Mind Racing Mikella
thirst, 61
  Thirsty Theo, 61
thirst quenching contest, 126
Thirsty Theo, investigations for, *61*
thoughts, slowing down, 126
threat hypervigilance, 123
threat perception, 32
Tina Tired. *See* Tired Tina
Tired Tina, 108, 109, 114
Tissue Transglutaminase IgA Antibodies (tTG IgA), 40
Tommy Thunderbolt, 81, 82, 87
Top-of-the-Wave, 85
trauma, 31

Umm-Ma Una, 61, *61*, 65, 124
  eating and, 65
  kiss, 64
unexpected
  creating, 121
  embracing the, *72*
unstuck, how to get, 112
urinalysis, 40
urinary frequency, 38
urinary tract infection (UTI), 39

validation, 25–26
  unintentional validation traps, *25*
Victor Vomit, 69–70, *69*, 71, 82, 132
viral exanthems, 39
visceral hypersensitivity, 6
  a sensory superpower, 16
  reframing of, 19
  sensory superpowers and, 11
visceral sensitivity
  as a sensory superpower, 9–10
  overview of, 9
vomit/vomiting, 38, 39, 40, 66, 67, 77, 82, 93, *See also* gag reflex, Victor Vomit
  appendicitis and, 38
  episodic, 39
  food poisoning and, 39

warmth
  and firmness, 29, *30*, 90, 94, 95
  feeling of, 95
weekly session, elements of, 6
weight gain, 37, 38
weight loss, 38, 39, 40
wondrous moments, strategies to remember, 121
workbook
  reading the, 57
  routines, 57

Zoomies, the, 7, 28, 80–81, 116, 117, *See also* Shakies, the
  body investigations, 117
  body lessons from, 84
  lessons from, 121